THE COMPLETE & UP-TO-DATE

FAT

BOOK

The information in this book is based on the research of the author, and does not substitute for personalized consultation with your physician. No endorsement is being made of any individual, institution, or product. The author and publisher do not claim to be licensed to give medical advice. Calories, fat content, and fat percentages for processed foods are subject to change and might in the future vary from listings within, which are based on research conducted in 1991. The authors and publisher disclaim any liability arising directly or indirectly from the use of this book.

THE COMPLETE & UP-TO-DATE

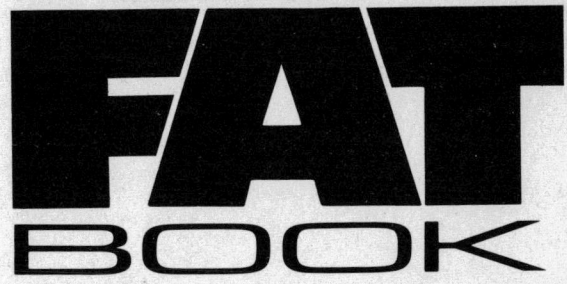

A GUIDE TO THE FAT, CALORIES, AND FAT PERCENTAGES IN YOUR FOOD

KAREN J. BELLERSON

AVERY PUBLISHING GROUP

Garden City Park, New York

SOURCES

Food manufacturers and processors direct, as well as their product labels.

United States Department of Agriculture Handbook No. 8, revised, "Composition of Foods, Raw, Processed, Prepared," sections 8-1 through 8-12; Agriculture Handbook No. 456, "Nutritive Value of American Foods In Common Units"; Home And Garden Bulletin No. 232, "Nutrition and Your Health: Dietary Guidelines for Americans."

Individual fast food chains.

Bowes and Church's *Food Values of Portions Commonly Used*, 15th Edition (1989), revised by Jean A. T. Pennington.

Cover designers: Rudy Shur and Evan Schwartz
In-house editor: Bonnie Freid
Typesetters: Evan Schwartz, Bonnie Freid, and Kerri Matheson

Library of Congress Cataloging-in-Publication Data

Bellerson, Karen J.
     The complete & up-to-date fat book / Karen J. Bellerson.
          p.   cm.
     ISBN 0-89529-483-4
     1. Food—Fat content—Tables. I. Title. II. Title: Complete and
up-to-date fat book.
TX551.B39 1991
641.1'4—dc20   91-24323
                                                                      CIP

Copyright © 1991 by Karen J. Bellerson

All rights reserved. No part of this publication may be reproduced, stored in a retrieval system, or transmitted, in any form or by any means, electronic, mechanical, photocopying, recording or otherwise, without the prior written permission of the copyright owner.

Printed in the United States of America

10   9   8   7   6   5

Contents

I wish to extend loving appreciation to my family for their continuous support. I also wish to give applause to those in the food industry who care enough to make the valuable nutritional information of their products available to the consumer, especially through the labeling of their products without mandatory governmental regulations.

Introduction

Lower your risk of:

Heart disease	High cholesterol	Strokes
High Blood Pressure	Diabetes	Obesity
Gallbladder ailments	Atherosclerosis	Osteoarthritis
Gout	Some forms of cancer (Breast, Colon, & Prostrate)	

simply by adopting a low-fat, nutritional lifestyle!

"The single most influential dietary change one can make to lower the risk of these diseases is to *reduce intake of foods high in fats* and to increase the intake of foods high in complex carbohydrates and fiber."
   –*The Surgeon General's Report On Nutrition and Health* (1988)

"It is calculated that, if intake of dietary fat were reduced from the present 40 percent of total calorie intake to 25 percent, about 9,000 lives would be saved annually."
   —National Cancer Institute, *Annual Review of Public Health*

"Reducing saturated fat is the single most important step Americans need to take in changing the way they eat."
   —Dr. Virgil Brown, professor of medicine at Mt. Sinai School of Medicine in New York (1989)

"Eating less fat can reduce the risk of colon, prostate, and breast cancer."
   —National Research Council, "Diet And Health" (1989)

Physicians, nutrition experts, and other health care professionals and organizations all promote the very real health benefits of a low-fat nutritional lifestyle.
   But, what is a "low-fat" nutritional lifestyle? How much fat is too much? How do you even begin to know what foods to eat and not to eat; and how do you go about changing eating habits of a lifetime?
   You have already begun! Just by being aware that there are necessary changes to be made in your eating habits and studying *The Fat Book* to educate yourself in

1

learning where the fat is in the foods you eat, you are on your way to a low-fat nutritional lifestyle!

Before we go into the simple guidelines, however, let's look at a few basic facts about fat.

FAT IS REQUIRED BY THE BODY

Our bodies use fat in numerous ways—ways in which most of us are not aware. We use fat in manufacturing antibodies to fight disease. Fats act as carriers for the fat-soluble vitamins A, D, E, and K. Fat deposits cushion, protect, and hold in place vital organs such as the kidneys, heart, and liver. Fat is the body's insulation against environmental temperature changes and is what gives the body its shape. While fat is one of the three nutrient energy sources, it also aids in digestion by slowing down the stomach's secretions of hydrochloric acid, which is what produces that satisfying feeling of "fullness" after a meal. So, as you can see, *fat should not be totally eliminated from our diets!*

There are two types of fat in the body. They are the nonessential fatty acids, which our body is able to manufacture, and the essential fatty acids, which we cannot make and have to get through our diets. These essential (unsaturated) fatty acids are necessary for normal growth, healthy skin, blood, arteries, and nerves, and for keeping our metabolism running smoothly.

Adults need a minimum daily intake of 15 to 25 grams of dietary fat to meet the body's needs.

Note: While a low-fat diet is recommended by health experts for almost everyone, the one exception is for children under the age of two years. Because of the possible interference with their growth development, *children under the age of two years should not have their dietary fat restricted.*

THERE ARE THREE TYPES OF DIETARY FAT

Foods containing fat contain mixtures of the following three types. No food is made up purely of saturated, monounsaturated, or polyunsaturated fat.

UNSATURATED FATS (divided into two categories)

POLYUNSATURATED: Found in most foods, including certain fish, but mainly in nuts, oils from plants, seeds, and soybeans. These fats are liquid at room temperature. Polyunsaturated fats reduce blood cholesterol, but an excess may lower the protective, "good," cholesterol.

MONOUNSATURATED: Found in most foods, but mainly in vegetable and nut oils such as olive, peanut, and canola. These fats are also liquid at room temperature. Monounsaturated fats reduce blood cholesterol while not having the side effect of lowering the protective cholesterol, as in the case of polyunsaturated fats.

Note: Both of these unsaturated fats can be hydrogenated. Hydrogenation is a process of adding hydrogen in order to make an oil more solid at room temperature and is done to make oil more usable in processing foods such as baked goods, non-dairy creamers, and whipped toppings. Hydrogenation of unsaturated fats makes them saturated. When reading your product labels, watch for the words "hydrogenated" or "partially hydrogenated."

SATURATED FATS (all foods from animal sources)

This includes all meats & dairy products, such as cheese, eggs, butter, cream, whole milk, and ice cream, which are all high in saturated fats. The "tropical oils"—coconut, palm, and palm kernel—are the oils highest in saturated fat and should be avoided. Cocoa butter, the oil used in making chocolate, is also a highly saturated fat source. Use powdered cocoa instead in all of your recipes calling for chocolate. Saturated fats are generally solid at room temperature. As mentioned before, some non-dairy products (i.e., non-dairy creamers and whipped toppings) are also high in saturated fat, through hydrogenation of the oils used in them. Check your labels carefully.

Note: You will find a chart of the most commonly used fats and oils, showing the percent of saturated fats and unsaturated fats contained by each on page 278.

SATURATED FATS CAUSE A RISE IN BLOOD CHOLESTEROL EVEN MORE THAN DOES DIETARY CHOLESTEROL

"Excessive saturated fat consumption is the major dietary contributor to total blood cholesterol levels. Dietary cholesterol raises blood cholesterol levels, but the effect is less pronounced than that of saturated fat."
   –The Surgeon General's Report on Nutrition and Health (1988)

"Don't make a fetish of removing all high cholesterol foods from your diet, because it is saturated fat, more than dietary cholesterol, that has the greatest effect in raising serum cholesterol."
   —James Cleeman, M.D., coordinator of the National Heart, Lung, and Blood Institute's National Cholesterol Education Program.

Dr. William P. Castelli, director of the illustrious Framingham (Massachusetts) Heart Study, fully agrees that it is the saturated fat in the food we eat, more than dietary cholesterol, that causes problems. "Most cholesterol in your body is produced by your cells. Saturated fat signals your cells to make more cholesterol and acts as the raw material for its manufacture. Trim the saturated fat in your diet and you automatically cut the cholesterol in your blood."

FAT SUBSTITUTES ("FAKE FATS")

In February of 1990, the Food and Drug Administration approved the first substitute fat for the United States market. This product, Simplesse, is manufactured by the NutraSweet Company, a subsidiary of Monsanto Company. Simplesse is made by cooking and blending egg-white and milk protein into a fluid that has the texture and taste of fat, but fewer calories and less cholesterol. Since the only fat content of Simplesse is the fat found naturally in skim milk, NutraSweet's ice cream has less than half of the calories of regular ice cream and a fat gram content of .6 for a 4 ounce serving size.

Because the heat used in baking or frying breaks down the droplets of Simplesse, however, it has been approved for use only in frozen desserts at this time.

Proctor & Gamble is presently working on the processing of Olestra, an ersatz fat, which has yet to be approved by the FDA. Although Olestra has the characteristics of fat, including taste and consistency, at present it cannot be digested or absorbed. If this problem is resolved, it is predicted that Olestra will be approved by the FDA within the next couple of years.

While some see this as an exciting new breakthrough, many of us in the field of nutrition are concerned over the prospect of additional approvals in the future for "fake fats" from Kraft, Inc., Proctor & Gamble Company, and others. There is a feeling that "fake fats" may cause a less than positive effect on efforts to improve the American diet.

New York University Professor Marion Nestle, managing editor of the Surgeon General's recent report on nutrition, expressed his concern that "what modern nutritionists are trying to do is change people's relationship with food and move them toward a diet that is more heavily based on fruits, vegetables, and grains. This is not going to do that. My prediction is that it is not going to reduce America's dietary intake of fat...This [fake fats] is about marketing. This is not about nutrition." The concern is that the reduction of fat in some foods will just encourage the consumer to eat more of other high-fat foods. This, of course, will not reduce total fat in the diet, but will continue the unhealthy balance of most American diets.

PROJECT LEAN

"Low-fat Eating for America Now" (LEAN) is a two-year program in several cities across the nation, funded by the Henry J. Kaiser Family Foundation. The program is a response to the Surgeon General's Report on Nutrition and Health, which advocated reduction of total dietary fat because of its relationship to life-threatening disease. The project's goal is to reduce the intake of dietary fat through education and the increased availability of low-fat foods in supermarkets, restaurants, and other away-from-home eating places such as employee cafeterias.

FOOD LABELING REFORMS

To further inform consumers about the nutritional contents of the foods they choose, the Federal Food and Drug Administration will be issuing new regulations for food manufacturers. These new regulations will include "mandatory and consistent" nutrition labels on nearly all packaged foods.

Products such as spices, teas, and other items of "limited nutritional value" would be exempt from the new rules. Products from the local retail bakeries and other small companies would also be exempt. The proposals offered will cover the following:

- Nutrition labels for most packaged foods. (Approximately 60 percent presently have labels.)
- New labeling to include amount of saturated fat, fiber, cholesterol, and the calories from fat.
- Definitions of food descriptions and claims such as "low fat," "high fiber," and "low cholesterol."
- Standardizing serving sizes to make food comparisons more exact.
- Test marketing different "easier-to-understand" label formats.

Since these proposals are very similar to those made by the FDA in 1979, consumer advocates are hoping that, this time, food-labeling legislation before Congress will result in more action being taken. It is predicted, however, that it will be at least two years before approval of federal regulations to set standards for nutritional data on food packaging.

Further, the United States Department of Agriculture (USDA) has proposed labeling requirements for processed meats and poultry products. These products include frozen dinners containing meat and/or poultry, luncheon meats, and canned soups containing meat and/or poultry.

Labeling for fresh meat and poultry will be on a voluntary basis. Brochures and shelf labels would be recommended to inform the consumer of the nutritional information for these products, but individual packages would not be required to carry nutritional information.

The USDA also wants clarification on the terms "light," "lean," and "low-calorie." Since these terms are not used to mean the same thing for all products, they add to consumer confusion over nutrition labels.

Again, don't expect these labeling reforms to take place before the latter part of 1993.

DIETARY FAT AND BODY METABOLISM

A recent study by Cornell University, to be published in the *American Journal of Clinical Nutrition*, claims that calorie-for-calorie, fat calories will make you fatter than the same number of calories of carbohydrates or protein, because of the way the body metabolizes fat.

Only about 3 percent of our body's energy is used to convert fat in foods to body fat; whereas 25 percent energy is needed to convert carbohydrate calories to body fat. What this means is that when you consume 100 fat calories (the amount in a tablespoon of butter, margarine, or oil) more than your body needs per day, 97 of them are stored as fat. But you can consume the extra 100 calories from a plain baked potato, essentially all carbohydrate calories, and only 75 calories will be stored as fat.

By following a low-fat diet, you can lose weight and eat even more—but more of the right foods!

WHAT IS A LOW-FAT LIFESTYLE?

As noted earlier, fat is a necessity for healthy body functions and should not be totally eliminated from our diets. *The Surgeon General's Report on Nutrition and Health* (1988) conveyed: "Adults need a minimum daily intake of 15 to 25 grams of fat to meet these necessities."

The American Heart Association, The American Health Foundation, The American Cancer Society, The National Heart, Lung, and Blood Institute, and the Surgeon General all recommend that:

No more than 30 percent of our daily calories should come from fat and no more than ⅓ of those fats (or 10 percent of our daily calories) should be saturated fats!

The following is a simple formula that lets you know exactly how many fat grams you should allow yourself on a daily basis, in order to follow these low-fat guidelines. In doing this, you are creating a "low-fat lifestyle" for yourself!

To find out your maximum daily allowance, multiply your daily calorie intake by .30, and divide that total by 9 (there are 9 calories in each gram of fat).

EXAMPLE: For a daily calorie intake of 1500, your equation would look like this:

1500 X .30 ÷ 9 = 50   *or*   1500 X .30 = 450.00 ÷ 9 = 50

Of course, to calculate your daily fat gram budget, you need to know your daily calorie intake. To determine this, multiply your present weight by your activity level factor.

Types of Activity	Activity Level Factor	Types of Activity	Activity Level Factor	Types of Activity	Activity Level Factor
Lightly Active =	13	*Moderately Active* =	15	*Very Active* =	20

Walking at a normal pace; typing; driving; light office or house work; bowling.	At least 20 minutes of walking briskly 3 times a week; heavier office, house, or lawn work; golf; doubles in tennis once a week.	Swimming; jogging; brisk walking of more than 30 minutes 4 times a week; singles in tennis 2 or more times a week; shoveling snow; heavy lawn work.

EXAMPLE: If your present weight is 175 pounds and you are moderately active (activity level factor of 15): 15 X 175 = 2625 calories are needed daily to maintain your present weight.

Further: 2625 X .30 ÷ 9 = 87.5 (rounded to 88) fat grams daily

If you want to lose weight and your "desired" weight is 120 pounds and you are moderately active (activity level factor of 15): 15 X 120 = 1800 calories are needed daily to achieve and maintain this desired weight.

Further: 1800 X .30 ÷ 9 = 60 fat grams daily

So you will have a means of comparison, I have taken the guess work out of it for you. On the next page is a chart of daily fat grams for a low-fat nutritional lifestyle.

MAXIMUM DAILY FAT GRAM BUDGET

DAILY CALORIE INTAKE	FAT GRAMS ALLOWED	CALORIES IN FAT*
1200	40	360
1300	43	387
1400	46	414
1500	50	450
1600	53	477
1700	56	504
1800	60	540
1900	63	567
2000	66	594
2100	70	630
2200	73	657
2300	76	684
2400	80	720
2500	83	747
2600	86	774
2700	90	810
2800	93	837
2900	96	864
3000	100	900

Note:
- This data has been rounded off by dropping all decimal places.
- This chart begins at 1200 calories, as it is not recommended for anyone to eat fewer than 1200 calories (women) or 1500 calories (men) in order to meet his or her daily nutritional needs.

To figure the number of fat calories in a food, multiply the number of fat grams by 9, since 1 fat gram = 9 calories.

How do these figures compare to your daily fat and calorie intake? First, using *The Fat Book*, figure out your daily calorie intake, and the number of grams of fat you consumed today. Then, figure out with the formula given before (or using this chart of daily fat grams) what your maximum daily allowance of fat should be. Do the actual fat grams in the food you ate during the day exceed your daily allowance of fat? Then you should revise your menu to include less fat, even if you do not decrease your total calorie intake.

As you begin to take stock of your eating habits, you will find that there are many low-fat foods you can substitute for high-fat foods. Here are just a few tips to practice, as you begin your quest for better nutrition:

- Eat more chicken, turkey, and fish in place of red meat. (Be sure to remove the skin on your chicken and turkey.) If you are having beef for dinner, make sure you have a leaner cut (check "BEEF") and prepare it without added fat.

  Please note that nutritionists recommend that you keep red meat consumption down to only once or twice a week. Since red meat is high in saturated fat, this will help you to control your saturated fat intake. Choose those leaner cuts and trim that fat. Be sure to watch for the "leaner" beef that is due to be on the market soon.

- Substitute plain low-fat yogurt, low-fat cottage cheese, or even skim milk for sour cream on a baked potato or in making tuna or potato salad. Don't forget the "fat-free" or reduced fat mayonnaise on the market today when throwing together a macaroni, potato, tuna, or turkey salad.

- Use a reduced-fat margarine or spread instead of butter or regular margarine. Try Kraft's Touch Of Butter or Land O Lakes' Spread with Sweet Cream for that "real butter" flavor. Try using smaller amounts and you will find yourself enjoying the taste of the food itself more. The reduced-fat margarines can be used in a lot of your cooking as well.

- There is a great selection of low-fat salad dressings available today; some are even "fat free"! They come in many flavors and styles; try them until you find one or more to your taste. Remember that you can save as many as 6 to 10 grams of fat *per tablespoon* by not using regular salad dressings!

- Instead of rich desserts like ice cream, try the wide range of frozen yogurts now available at your grocery store. There are also "lighter" ice creams now available. Food manufacturers are aware that the consumer is more health conscious today than ever before and are making a wide range of "fat-free" bakery goods available. *Read your labels!*

- Substitute low-fat, reduced fat, or no-fat cheese for those cheeses higher in fat. The fat saved here is between 6 and 10 grams per ounce!

- You will find most breads low in fat, but be careful when you reach for a croissant to make that sandwich. Croissants can have as many as 14 grams of fat. Do you really want it when you could replace it with two slices of almost any other kind of bread containing 1 gram of fat each?

- Dry cereals are great snack food at as little as 0 to 3 grams of fat per serving. Do monitor the granola-type cereals, as they are higher in fat. Reach for the pretzels and microwave "light" popcorn for other low-fat snacks. And don't forget the best low-fat snack as always is *fruit*!

- Go ahead and have your bacon for breakfast, but try Canadian bacon for a pleasant change in taste and fat gram count!

- Did you know you could have 10 french fries (8 fat grams) and eat less fat than if you ate 1.5 oz of potato chips (15 fat grams)!

These simple changes can easily be made. Learn the low-fat substitutes to use in your cooking at home and stay away from too many "bought" high-fat bakery products. *Read your labels!* It really can be done "without pain," and it gets easier once you have learned to recognize the fat content of the foods available to you by using *The Fat Book*. Making healthier eating choices will become a way of life!

As you select the foods you eat, keep in mind that while fat has a total of 9 calories per gram, complex carbohydrates and protein each have only 4 calories per gram. In choosing foods high in complex carbohydrates and protein, you will find yourself able to eat more without taking in more calories. In other words, you can actually eat more food by eating less fat!

HOW DO YOU CHANGE EATING HABITS OF A LIFETIME?

By following the suggestions in this book *a little at a time*. Now, don't think you have to throw the baby out with the bathwater by doing away with all of your favorite foods just because they might be high in fat. Acquaint yourself with *The Fat Book* by playing the "numbers" game. Check the fat content of the foods you usually eat against your daily fat gram budget and see what may need to be replaced by a lower-fat food. You will be surprised at exactly how much dietary fat you have been eating. You may have been aware of where the visible fat is—the butter, the mayonnaise, the cream cheese; but did you know how much fat is in processed and convenience foods, for example? Also, you will find that, if a favorite food takes a big enough bite out of your daily fat gram budget, you will want that favorite food less often and will automatically begin to make more nutritionally-sound food selections!

WRITE IT DOWN!

As you acquaint yourself with *The Fat Book*, you will find that keeping a daily account of your food intake is invaluable. Keep track of everything you eat as you count up the fat grams and calories for the day. This way, you are able to get a better idea of exactly what you are eating and where you need to adjust. Keeping close track of your eating habits, as you begin to form new ones, enables you to:

- Recognize your eating patterns.
- Gain control over what you eat.
- Budget your fat grams and calories more realistically.
- Think twice about deviating from a healthy low-fat lifestyle.
- Take pride in seeing your progress in writing.

In keeping a record of your daily fat grams and calories, you are making a further committment to changing to a healthier eating lifestyle. Research has shown over and over that keeping daily records is one of the most important components of changing our habits, especially those of long standing.

LET'S GET ACQUAINTED WITH *THE FAT BOOK*

Although extreme care has been taken in recording all data in *The Fat Book*, you may come across an occasional discrepancy between it and the nutritional data on product labels or other sources of nutritional information. There are a number of reasons why this might occur.

Manufacturers are given a slightly flexible range in which they are able to "round off" their data and still be in accordance with governmental regulations on product labeling. For example, if the fat gram data for a certain product is 2.3 grams, the manufacturer is able to list the fat content in this particular product as being 2 grams, dropping the .3. The same is done with data on calories. If a product serving has 134 calories, the manufacturer is able to list the calorie content of this product as being 130 or 135. Wherever possible, I have kept the whole nutritional data intact without "rounding off" for either fat or calorie content.

When I gathered data from product labeling and compared this with data I received directly from the manufacturer, there would occasionally be a difference between them. This difference was caused by the product label listing the nutritional data of the old formula, while the manufacturer was providing the most up-to-date data after the product formula had been changed. In these cases, the data directly from the manufacturer was always used.

Product serving sizes would also change and cause a change in nutritional data. So, be sure, when comparing products, that you are comparing the same serving size, i.e., ¼ cup against ¼ cup.

Other differences can be caused by analytical methods and sampling techniques used by the different nutritional sources.

The nutritional information in this book is offered as a ready reference and is not meant to be a substitute for seeking professional health care.

As you can see, data is listed in four columns. Amount means the serving size of food served or used in a recipe. Remember that any deviation of serving size will cause a change in the rest of the data given in all of the other columns. Fat content of each food is listed in fat grams (the measurement used for dietary fat); and the calorie column needs no explanation.

Further, I have listed the percentage of calories from fat under "% Fat Calories" for all listings. If you need to figure the percentage of fat in a food not listed, the formula is:

Fat Grams X 9 = Total Fat Calories (TFC);
Divide TFC by the total calorie content of your chosen food.

EXAMPLE: 1 oz Cheddar Cheese = 9 fat grams and 110 calories.
  9 X 9 = 81 TFC   81 divided by 110 = 73%

Since a high-fat food is any food containing 30 percent or more of its calories in fat, this cheddar cheese would be considered a high-fat food. Although, as I stated earlier, you need not deny yourself any food, high-fat foods should be monitored closely and included in your nutritional choices in small amounts. *Don't let high-fat foods keep you from eating an overall balanced diet by using up your fat gram budget!*

Remember that some of the data has been rounded off, as mentioned, and the percentage might be off slightly, but not to the point that it matters. For example, all oils and fats have 100 percent of their calories in fat. However, if you will look at a fat such as BUTTER, you will see that the "% Fat Calories" (100%) deviates slightly from the calculated amount—i.e., 11 fat grams X 9 = 99%. Because we know that all oils and fats contain 100 percent fat calories, I did not want to mislead you by using the rounded off data and listing 99% instead of the absolute 100%.

You will find both generic and brand name products in these tables. The listing of a product by brand name is not necessarily meant as an endorsement. Brand name products not listed had no nutritional data available to me at the time, and their omission is for that reason only.

HOW TO USE THIS BOOK

The *Complete and Up-to-Date Fat Book* is a comprehensive reference book for your nutritional needs. As you shop for and prepare low-fat foods, this book will be an invaluable source of information.

References for serving amount, fat grams, total calories, and % fat calories are under every entry. The foods are listed alphabetically for ready-reference convenience. You will also find a separate section of fast food franchises following the A to Z foods list.

Since cereals and soups are frequently prepared with milk, quick reference charts for adding milk can be found under these entries.

Since oils all have the same number of calories and the same number of fat grams, differing only in the saturated/unsaturated percentages, you will find oils broken down into % saturated and % unsaturated categories.

As far as style, the book is organized with main headings for foods capitalized and bold, and subheadings smaller and also capitalized and bold. Descriptions of foods are upper/lower case, with brand names in parentheses.

If you are unable to find a particular food, look for a listing of a similar food. The nutritional data should be close, if not exact, for any product not listed. When doing this, you want to make sure you are comparing the same serving sizes. Also, be sure you are comparing weight measure against weight measure and volume measure against volume measure. The Table Of Equivalent Measurements I have included should help you, not only in comparing serving sizes, but in making your exchanges easier as well. Note that all cooked vegetable amounts are drained of liquid, unless otherwise noted.

You will find *The Fat Book* a valuable companion as you begin to take control of your eating habits. And you will discover that adopting a low-fat nutritional lifestyle reaps you many other rewards while maximizing your good health! Rewards such as:

- Looking younger
- Having more energy
- Alleviating PMS symptoms
- Sleeping better
- Clearer skin
- Lower grocery bills
- Controlling weight
- Feeling sexier ... and much more!

"Dare to be wise; BEGIN! He who postpones the hour of living rightly is like the rustic who waits for the river to run dry before he crosses it!"
–Horace

EXPLANATION OF ABBREVIATIONS AND SYMBOLS USED

~	=	Approximate		Pkt	=	Packet
Dia	=	Diameter		Lb.	=	Pound
"	=	Inch		Tbs	=	Tablespoon
<	=	Less Than		Tsp	=	Teaspoon
Oz	=	Ounce		w/	=	With
Pkg	=	Package		w/o	=	Without

The term "Standard Home Recipe" (USDA) refers to bakery goods and other dishes that are made in the home. Since the homemade dishes listed in this guide are made with standard ingredients and not with low-fat substitutes, data will change when you replace certain ingredients with low-fat substitutes. The data listed is to be used as a viable guide for the same dish you might make in your home. You should also keep this in mind for the data on box mixes, as they are prepared according to package directions and, unless noted, low-fat ingredients are not used.

TABLE OF EQUIVALENT MEASURES

VOLUME

1 tablespoon	=	3 teaspoons
		½ fluid ounce
2 tablespoons	=	1 fluid ounce
4 tablespoons	=	¼ cup
		2 fluid ounces
16 tablespoons	=	1 cup
		½ pint
⅓ cup	=	5⅓ tablespoons
½ cup	=	8 tablespoons
		4 fluid ounces
⅔ cup	=	10⅔ tablespoons
¾ cup	=	12 tablespoons
1 cup	=	8 fluid ounces
2 cups	=	1 pint
2 pints	=	1 quart
4 quarts	=	1 gallon

WEIGHT

1 ounce	=	28.35 grams
3.5 ounces	=	100 grams
4 ounces	=	¼ pound
8 ounces	=	½ pound
12 ounces	=	¾ pound
16 ounces	=	1 pound
		454 grams

A

Food and Description	Amount	Fat Grams	Total Calories	% Fat Calories
ABALONE				
fried	3 oz	5.77	161	32%
raw	3 oz	1	90	10%
ACEROLA/raw	1	–	2	–
	1 cup	–	31	–
ACEROLA JUICE	8 oz	.7	51	12%
ACORN				
dried	1 oz	8.9	145	55%
raw	1 oz	6.8	105	58%
ACORN FLOUR				
full fat	1 oz	9	142	57%
ADZUKI BEANS				
boiled	½ cup	–	147	3%
canned-sweetened	½ cup	–	351	1%
(Arrowhead Mills)	2 oz	1	190	5%
raw	½ cup	–	325	1%
ALBACORE (See TUNA)				
ALE (See BEER, ALE, AND MALT LIQUOR)				
ALEWIFE(herring)/raw	4 oz	5.6	144	35%
ALFALFA SPROUTS/raw	1 cup	–	10	–
ALLIGATOR/raw	3 oz	3	200	14%
ALLSPICE	1 tsp	–	5	–
ALMOND				
blanched-slivered				
(Azar)	1 oz	15	170	79%
(Dole)	1 oz	14	170	74%
dried				
blanched	1 oz	14.9	166	81%
unblanched	1 oz	14.8	167	80%
dry roasted	1 oz	14.65	167	79%
(Blue Diamond)	1 oz	14	179	70%
hickory smoked	1 oz	15	166	81%
honey roasted (Eagle)	1 oz	12	150	72%
oil roasted-blanched	1 oz	16	174	83%

Food and Description	Amount	Fat Grams	Total Calories	% Fat Calories
(Planters)				
blanched				
sliced	1 oz	15	170	79%
slivered	1 oz	15	170	79%
whole	1 oz	15	170	79%
dry roasted	1 oz	15	170	79%
honey roasted	1 oz	13	170	69%
roasted-salted (Blue Diamond)	1 oz	15	150	90%
slices (Azar)	1 oz	15	170	79%
Smokehouse (Blue Diamond)	1 oz	14	150	84%
sour cream and onion (Blue Diamond)	1 oz	14	150	84%
toasted	1 oz	14	167	75%
ALMOND BUTTER				
honey & cinnamon	1 Tbs	8	96	75%
plain	1 Tbs	9.5	101	85%
raw (Hain)-natural	2 Tbs	18	190	85%
toasted blanched (Hain)	2 Tbs	19	210	81%
ALMOND MEAL/partially defatted	1 oz	5	116	39%
ALMOND PASTE	1 Tbs	7.7	127	55%
	1 cup	62	1010	55%
ALMOND POWDER				
full fat	1 oz	15	168	80%
	1 cup	34	385	80%
partially defatted	1 oz	5	112	40%
	1 cup	10	255	35%
ALOE VERA JUICE	2 oz	–	5	–
AMARANTH				
cooked	½ cup	–	14	–
raw	1 cup	–	7	–
ANCHOVY, EUROPEAN				
canned in oil	5 fish	1.9	42	41%
fresh-raw	3 oz	4	62	58%
pate	1 tsp	.8	14	51%
ANISE	1 tsp	–	7	–
APPLE				
canned-slices-sweetened	½ cup	.5	68	7%
cooked/without skin	1 cup	.6	91	6%
dried				
cooked	1 cup	–	144	–
cooked w/sugar	1 cup	–	232	–
uncooked	1 cup	–	209	–
uncooked	10 rings	–	155	–
(Del Monte)-sliced	2 oz	–	140	–
(Mariani)	¼ cup	–	150	–

Food and Description	Amount	Fat Grams	Total Calories	% Fat Calories
(Nature's Favorite) Apple Chips				
cinnamon	1 oz	5	120	38%
golden delicious	1 oz	5	120	38%
original	1 oz	5	120	38%
(Sun Maid)-chunks	2 oz	–	150	–
(Weight Watcher's)	.5 oz	< 1	50	9%
fried-canned (Luck's)	8 oz	–	190	–
raw with skin	1	.5	81	6%
slices	1 cup	–	64	–
raw without skin	1	–	72	–
slices	1 cup	–	62	–
APPLE-BERRY DRINK				
Appleberry (Juice Works)	6 oz	–	96	–
APPLE-BOYSENBERRY JUICE				
(Knudsen)	8 oz	–	110	–
APPLE BUTTER	1 Tbs	–	33	–
	1 cup	2	525	3%
(Smucker's)-Autumn Harvest Natural & Cider Apple Butter	1 tsp	–	12	–
(Smucker's)-Spiced	2 tsp	–	25	–
APPLE-CHERRY DRINK	8 oz	–	116	–
APPLE-CINNAMON JUICE				
Nectar/bottled	6 oz	–	110	–
APPLE-CRANBERRY DRINK				
(Mott's)	10 oz	–	176	–
	9.5 oz	–	167	–
(Tropicana)-single serve	10 oz	–	175	–
APPLE-CRANBERRY JUICE				
(Mott's)	6 oz	–	80	–
	8.45 oz	–	136	–
(Tree Top)	6 oz	–	100	–
APPLE DRINK				
Apple (Juice Works)	6 oz	–	97	–
(Alpine) Spiced Cider Mix	8 oz	–	80	–
low cal	8 oz	–	16	–
APPLE DUMPLINGS (Pepperidge Farm)				
frozen	3 oz	13	260	45%
Standard Home Recipe (USDA)	1 average	16	275	52%
APPLE-GRAPE JUICE				
Juicy Juice (Libby's)	6 oz	–	90	–
(Mott's)	6 oz	–	86	–
	8.45 oz	–	128	–
(Tree Top)	6 oz	–	100	–

Food and Description	Amount	Fat Grams	Total Calories	% Fat Calories
APPLE JUICE				
Apple Cider/sweet	8 oz	–	124	–
(Tree Top)	6 oz.	–	90	–
Apple Juice				
canned or bottled	6 oz	–	116	–
frozen				
(Birds Eye)	6 oz	–	80	–
(Seneca)	6 oz	–	90	–
(Tree Top)	6 oz	–	90	–
Juice Bowl-Apple (Campbell's)	6 oz	–	110	–
(Kraft) Pure 100%	6 oz	–	80	–
(Mott's)	8.45 oz	–	124	–
natural style	6 oz	–	88	–
(Ocean Spray)-unsweetened	6 oz	–	90	–
(S&W)	6 oz	–	85	–
(Seneca)	6 oz	–	90	–
Sparkling	6 oz	–	80	–
(Sippin' Pak) from concentrate	8.45 oz	–	110	–
(Sunglo)	8.45 oz	–	130	–
(Sunkist)				
from frozen concentrate	8 oz	–	79	–
(Tropicana)	8 oz	–	116	–
Apple Nectar (Kern's)	6 oz	–	110	–
APPLE-PEAR JUICE (Tree Top)	6 oz	–	90	–
APPLE-RASPBERRY DRINK (Mott's)	10 oz	–	158	–
	9.5 oz	–	150	–
APPLE-RASPBERRY JUICE				
(Mott's)	8.45 oz	–	120	–
(Tree Top)	6 oz	–	100	–
APPLESAUCE				
canned				
sweetened	1 cup	–	194	–
unsweetened	1 cup	–	106	–
(Del Monte)				
sweetened	½ cup	–	90	–
Lite	½ cup	–	50	–
(Hunt's) Snack Pack				
natural	4.25oz	–	50	–
regular	4.25 oz	–	80	–
raspberry	4.25 oz	–	80	–
strawberry	4.25 oz	–	80	–
(Mott's)				
chunky	4 oz	–	57	–
cinnimon	4 oz	–	72	–

Food and Description	Amount	Fat Grams	Total Calories	% Fat Calories
natural	4 oz	–	44	–
regular	4 oz	–	88	–
(Nutradiet)-unsweetened	½ cup	–	55	–
(S&W)				
sweetened	½ cup	–	90	–
unsweetened	½ cup	–	55	–
(Seneca)				
cinnamon	½ cup	–	90	–
100% natural	½ cup	–	50	–
McIntosh	½ cup	–	90	–
regular	½ cup	–	90	–
sweetened	½ cup	–	90	–
(Tree Top)				
cinnamon	½ cup	–	80	–
natural	½ cup	–	60	–
original	½ cup	–	80	–
(Wilderness)				
raspberry	½ cup	–	82	–
strawberry	½ cup	–	90	–
APRICOT				
candied	1oz	–	96	–
canned				
(Del Monte)				
halves unpeeled	½ cup	–	100	–
whole unpeeled	½ cup	–	100	–
(Del Monte)-Lite halves				
unpeeled	½ cup	–	60	–
(Nutradiet)				
halves	½ cup	–	35	–
whole peeled	½ cup	–	28	–
(S&W)				
halves unpeeled in heavy syrup	½ cup	–	110	–
whole peeled-in heavy syrup	½ cup	–	100	–
canned in water w/o skin	1 cup	–	51	–
canned in water w/skin	1 cup	–	65	–
in juice	1 cup	–	119	–
in light syrup	1 cup	–	160	–
in heavy syrup	1 cup	–	214	–
dried				
cooked	½ cup	–	106	–
uncooked	½ cup	.6	155	4%
(Del Monte)	2 oz	–	140	–
(Mariani)	¼ cup	–	140	–
(Sun Maid)	2 oz	–	140	–

Food and Description	Amount	Fat Grams	Total Calories	% Fat Calories
fresh	3 fruit	.5	51	9
	1 cup	–	74	–
frozen, sweetened	½ cup	–	119	–
APRICOT JUICE				
Apricot Juice/unsweetened	8 oz	–	123	–
APRICOT NECTAR	1 cup	–	141	–
(Del Monte)	6 oz	–	100	–
(Libby's)	8 oz	–	140	–
(S&W)	6 oz	–	100	–
APRICOT-ORANGE NECTAR (Kern's)	6 oz	–	112	–
APRICOT-PINEAPPLE NECTAR				
(Kern's)	6 oz	–	110	–
(Nutradiet)	½ cup	–	35	–
(S&W)	6 oz	–	120	–
ARMADILLO/raw	3 oz	4	150	24%
ARROWHEAD				
cooked	Medium Corm	.5	9	50%
raw	Medium Corm	.5	12	38%
ARTICHOKE				
canned-marinated crowns				
(Cara Mia)	1oz	–	12	–
fresh-cooked	Medium	–	53	–
frozen-cooked	½ cup	–	36	–
Jerusalem Artichoke raw/slices	½ cup	–	57	–
raw	Medium	–	65	–
ARTICHOKE HEARTS				
canned-marinated				
(Cara Mia)	1 oz	2	27	67%
(S & W)	3.5 oz	25	225	100%
fresh-cooked	½ cup	–	37	–
frozen (Birds Eye)	3 oz	–	30	–
ASPARAGUS				
canned	½ cup	.78	24	29%
All Green (Nutradiet)	½ cup	–	17	–
All Green Fancy (S & W)	½ cup	–	18	–
All Green cut spears (Del Monte)	½ cup	–	20	–
spears & tips (Del Monte)	½ cup	–	20	–
Colossal Spears (S&W)	½ cup	–	20	–
Green Tipped (Del Monte)	½ cup	–	20	–
50% Less Salt (Green Giant)	½ cup	–	20	–
spears (Green Giant)	½ cup	–	20	–
whole spears (Thank You)	½ cup	–	25	–

Food and Description	Amount	Fat Grams	Total Calories	% Fat Calories
fresh-cooked/cuts & tips	½ cup	–	22	–
	4 spears	–	15	–
frozen cuts (Birds Eye)	½ cup	–	25	–
frozen spears				
(Birds Eye)	3.3 oz	–	25	–
(Pictsweet)	3.3 oz	–	25	–
raw	½ cup	–	15	–
	4 spears	–	13	–

ASPARAGUS SOUP, CREAM OF (*See* SOUP)
AVOCADO
California

mashed	1 cup	36	407	80%
raw	1	30.79	324	86%
Florida	1	27	340	72%

B

Food and Description	Amount	Fat Grams	Total Calories	% Fat Calories
BABY FOOD				

(NOTE: A low-fat nutrition program is not recommended for any child under two years of age.)

BAKED GOODS
(Gerber)

Animal Crackers	.4 oz	2	50	36%
Animal Shaped Cookies	.4 oz	2	60	30%
Arrowrood Cookies	.4 oz	2	50	36%
Pretzels	.4 oz	–	50	–
Toddler Biter Biscuits	.4 oz	1	50	18%
Zwieback Toast	.5 oz	2	70	26%
(Nabisco)				
Zwieback Teething Toast	2 pieces	1	60	15%

CEREALS
(Beech-Nut Stages)
Dry-Ready-To-Serve

Barley-dry	½ oz	–	50	–
w/whole milk	2.4 oz	3	100	27%
High Protein-dry	½ oz	1	50	18%
w/whole milk	2.4 oz	4	100	36%
Mixed-dry	½ oz	1	50	18%

Food and Description	Amount	Fat Grams	Total Calories	% Fat Calories
w/whole milk	2.4 oz	4	100	36%
Oatmeal-dry	½ oz	1	50	18%
w/whole milk	2.4 oz	4	100	36%
Oatmeal w/Bananas-dry	½ oz	1	60	15%
w/whole milk	2.4 oz	4	100	36%
Rice-dry	½ oz	1	60	15%
w/whole milk	2.4 oz	4	100	36%
Rice w/Bananas-dry	½ oz	–	60	15%
w/whole milk	2.4 oz	4	100	36%
Stage 2				
Mixed w/Applesauce & Bananas	4.5 oz	–	80	–
Oatmeal w/Applesauce & Bananas	4.5 oz	1	90	10%
Rice w/Applesauce & Bananas	4.5 oz	–	100	–
(Gerber)				
Dry-Ready-To-Serve (½ oz = 4 Tablespoons)				
Barley-dry	½ oz	1	60	15%
w/whole milk	2.4 oz	4	100	36%
High Protein-dry	½ oz	1	50	18%
w/whole milk	2.4 oz	4	100	36%
High Protein w/Apple & Orange-dry	½ oz	1	60	15%
w/whole milk	2.4 oz	4	100	36%
Mixed-dry	½ oz	1	60	15%
w/whole milk	2.4 oz	4	100	36%
Oatmeal-dry	½ oz	1	60	15%
w/whole milk	2.4 oz	4	100	36%
Oatmeal w/Banana-dry	½ oz	1	60	15%
w/whole milk	2.4 oz	4	100	36%
Rice-dry	½ oz	1	60	15%
w/whole milk	2.4 oz	4	100	36%
Rice w/Banana-dry	½ oz	1	60	15%
w/whole milk	2.4 oz	4	100	36%
Junior With Fruit				
Mixed w/Applesauce & Bananas	6 oz	2	140	13%
Oatmeal w/Applesauce & Bananas	6 oz	2	130	14%
Rice w/Mixed Fruit	6 oz	1	140	6%
Strained With Fruit				
Mixed w/Applesauce & Bananas	1 jar/4.5 oz	1	100	9%
Oatmeal w/Applesauce & Bananas	1 jar/4.5 oz	1	100	9%
Rice w/Applesauce & Bananas	1 jar/4.5 oz	1	100	9%
(Heinz)				
Instant				
Barley-dry	½ oz	1	60	15%
w/whole milk	2.4 oz	4	100	36%
Mixed-dry	⅓ oz	1	50	18%

Food and Description	Amount	Fat Grams	Total Calories	% Fat Calories
w/whole milk	2.4 oz	4	90	40%
Oatmeal-dry	½ oz	2	60	30%
w/whole milk	2.4 oz	5	100	45%
Rice-dry	½ oz	1	60	15%
w/whole milk	2.4 oz	4	100	36%
Instant With Fruit				
Mixed w/Bananas & Apple Juice	½ oz	1	50	18%
Rice w/Bananas & Apple Juice	½ oz	1	60	15%
Oatmeal w/Bananas & Apple Juice	½ oz	1	60	15%
Rice w/Bananas & Apple Juice	½ oz	1	60	15%
Rice w/Pears & Apple Juice	½ oz	1	50	18%
DESSERTS				
Apple Betty				
junior	~ 7.8 oz	–	153	–
strained	~ 4.8 oz	–	97	–
(Beech-Nut Stages)				
Caramel Pudding				
junior	~ 7.5 oz	1.9	167	10%
strained	~ 4.8 oz	.9	104	8%
Cherry Vanilla Pudding				
junior	~ 7.8 oz	< 1	152	3%
strained	~ 4.8 oz	< 1	91	5%
Chocolate Custard				
junior	~ 7.8 oz	3.5	195	16%
strained	~ 4.5 oz	2	107	17%
Stage 2				
Banana Custard Pudding	4.5 oz	1	120	8%
Banana Pineapple	4.5 oz	–	100	–
Dutch Apple	4.5 oz	–	80	–
Guava Tropical Fruit	4.5 oz	–	100	–
Mango Tropical Fruit	4.5 oz	–	90	–
Mixed Fruit & Yogurt	6 oz	1	140	6%
	4.5 oz	1	110	8%
Papaya Tropical Fruit	4.5 oz	–	80	–
Peaches & Yogurt	4.5 oz	1	110	8%
Vanilla Custard Pudding	4.5 oz	3	130	21%
Stage 3				
Banana Custard	7.5 oz	2	200	9%
Mixed Fruit & Yogurt	7.5 oz	1	170	5%
Peaches & Yogurt	7.5 oz	2	190	10%
Vanilla Custard	7.5 oz	5	210	21%
(Heinz)				
Instant (Dry Serving Size)				
Banana Pudding	4 Tbs	1	60	15%
Dutch Apple Pie	4 Tbs	–	50	–

Food and Description	Amount	Fat Grams	Total Calories	% Fat Calories
Peach Cobbler	4 Tbs	1	60	15%
Vanilla Custard	4 Tbs	2	60	30%
(Gerber)				
Junior				
Dutch Apple	6 oz	2	130	14%
Fruit	6 oz	1	130	7%
Hawaiian Delight	6 oz	1	150	6%
Peach Cobbler	6 oz	1	130	7%
Vanilla Custard Pudding	6 oz	2	150	7%
Strained				
Banana Apple	4.5 oz	1	90	10%
Cherry Vanilla Pudding	4.5 oz	1	90	10%
Chocolate Custard Pudding	4.5 oz	2	110	16%
Dutch Apple	4.5 oz	2	100	18%
Fruit	4.5 oz	1	100	9%
Hawaiian Delight	4.5 oz	1	120	8%
Orange Pudding	4.5 oz	1	110	8%
Peach Cobbler	4.5 oz	1	100	9%
Vanilla Custard Pudding	4.5 oz	1	100	9%
Peach Melba				
junior	~ 7.8 oz	–	132	–
strained	~ 4.8 oz	–	81	–
Pineapple Pudding				
junior	~ 7.8 oz	.9	192	4%
strained	~ 4.5 oz	< 1	104	4%
DINNERS				
(Beech-Nut Stages)				
Stage 2				
Beef & Egg Noodles w/Vegetables	4.5 oz	4	90	40%
Beef Dinner Supreme	4.5 oz	7	120	53%
Chicken & Rice w/Vegetables	4.5 oz	3	80	34%
Chicken Noodle w/Vegetables	4.5 oz	3	90	30%
Macaroni, Tomato, & Beef	4.5 oz	3	90	30%
Turkey Dinner Supreme	4.5 oz	5	110	41%
Turkey Rice w/Vegetables	4.5 oz	2	70	26%
Vegetable Beef	4.5 oz	3	90	30%
Vegetble Chicken	4.5 oz	3	90	30%
Vegetable Ham	4.5 oz	3	90	30%
Vegetable Lamb	4.5 oz	3	90	30%
Stage 3				
Beef & Egg Noodles w/Vegetables	6 oz	8	150	48%
	7.5 oz	5	150	30%
Beef Dinner Supreme	7.5 oz	9	180	45%
Chicken Noodles w/Vegetables	6 oz	2	100	18%
	7.5 oz	4	140	26%

Food and Description	Amount	Fat Grams	Total Calories	% Fat Calories
Macaroni, Tomato, & Beef	6 oz	8	160	45%
	7.5 oz	5	150	30%
Spaghetti, Tomato, & Beef	7.5 oz	5	170	27%
Turkey Dinner Supreme	7.5 oz	8	190	38%
Turkey Rice w/Vegetables	7.5 oz	4	130	28%
Vegetable Bacon	7.5 oz	9	180	45%
Vegetable Beef	6 oz	7	160	39%
	7.5 oz	5	150	30%
Vegetable Chicken	6 oz	2	90	20%
	7.5 oz	5	140	32%
Vegetable Lamb	7.5 oz	5	140	32%
Table Time				
Beef Stew	6 oz	4	140	26%
Pasta Squares in Meat Sauce	6 oz	4	140	26%
Soups				
Hearty Chicken w/stars	6 oz	9	180	45%
Hearty Vegetable	6 oz	–	70	–
Spaghetti Rings in Meat Sauce	6 oz	4	160	23%
Vegetable Stew w/Chicken	6 oz	8	190	38%
(Gerber)				
Chunky Products				
Homestyle Noodles & Beef	6 oz	6	150	36%
Macaroni Alphabets w/beef & tomato sauce	6.25 oz	4	140	26%
Noodles & Chicken w/Carrots & Peas	6 oz	3	110	25%
Rice w/Beef & Tomato Sauce	6.25 oz	4	140	26%
Saucy Rice w/Chicken	6 oz	3	120	23%
Spaghetti-Tomato Sauce & Beef	6.25 oz	5	160	28%
Vegetables & Beef	6.25 oz	5	130	35%
Vegetables & Chicken	6.25 oz	5	140	32%
Vegetables & Ham	6.25 oz	5	130	35%
Vegetables & Turkey	6.25 oz	4	120	30%
Junior				
Beef Egg Noodle	6 oz	4	120	30%
Chicken Noodle	6 oz	3	100	27%
Macaroni Tomato Beef	6 oz	2	110	16%
Spaghetti Tomato Sauce Beef	6 oz	3	120	23%
Split Peas Ham	6 oz	3	130	21%
Turkey Rice	6 oz	4	110	33%
Vegetable Bacon	6 oz	6	140	39%
Vegetable Beef	6 oz	3	110	25%
Vegetable Chicken	6 oz	3	100	27%
Vegetable Ham	6 oz	4	120	30%

Food and Description	Amount	Fat Grams	Total Calories	% Fat Calories
Vegetable Lamb	6 oz	5	120	38%
Vegetable Turkey	6 oz	3	100	27%
Junior Lean Meat Dinners				
Beef w/Vegetables	4.5 oz	3	100	27%
Chicken w/Vegetables	4.5 oz	3	90	30%
Ham w/Vegetables	4.5 oz	4	110	33%
Turkey w/Vegetables	4.5 oz	4	100	36%
Strained				
Beef Egg Noodle	4.5 oz	3	90	30%
Chicken Noodle	4.5 oz	3	90	30%
Macaroni Cheese	4.5 oz	3	90	30%
Macaroni Tomato Beef	4.5 oz	2	80	23%
Turkey Rice	4.5 oz	3	80	34%
Vegetable Bacon	4.5 oz	5	100	45%
Vegetable Beef	4.5 oz	4	90	40%
Vegetable Chicken	4.5 oz	2	80	23%
Vegetable Ham	4.5 oz	3	80	34%
Vegetable Lamb	4.5 oz	4	90	40%
Vegetable Liver	4.5 oz	1	60	15%
Vegetable Turkey	4.5 oz	2	70	26%
Strained Lean Meat Dinners				
Beef w/Vegetables	4.5 oz	3	90	30%
Chicken w/Vegetables	4.5 oz	3	90	30%
Ham w/Vegetables	4.5 oz	4	100	36%
Turkey w/Vegetables	4.5 oz	4	100	36%
(Heinz)				
Instant (Dry Serving Size)				
Beef Noodle	5 Tbs	3	70	39%
Chicken Noodle	5 Tbs	2	70	26%
Chicken Rice	6 Tbs	2	60	30%
Tuna Noodle	6 Tbs	1	60	15%
Turkey Rice	5 Tbs	2	70	26%
Vegetables & Beef	5 Tbs	3	70	39%
Vegetables & Chicken	5 Tbs	2	70	26%
Vegetables & Ham	5 Tbs	2	70	26%
Vegetables & Turkey	5 Tbs	2	60	30%
FINGER FOODS				
(Gerber)				
Toddler				
Chicken Sticks	2.5 oz	8	120	60%
Meat Sticks	2.5 oz	7	110	57%
Turkey Sticks	2.5 oz	9	120	68%
FRUIT JUICES				
(Beech-Nut Stages)				
Stage 1				

Food and Description	Amount	Fat Grams	Total Calories	% Fat Calories
Apple	4.2 oz	–	60	–
Pear	4.2 oz	–	60	–
White Grape	4.2 oz	–	60	–
Stage 2				
Juice Plus	4 oz	–	80	–
Unstaged				
Apple	4 oz	–	60	–
Apple Banana	4.2 oz	–	60	–
Apple Cherry	4.2 oz	–	50	–
Apple Cranberry	4.2 oz	–	60	–
Apple Grape	4.2 oz	–	60	–
Apple Pear	4.2 oz	–	60	–
Mixed Fruit	4.2 oz	–	60	–
Orange	4.2 oz	–	60	–
Pear	4 oz	–	60	–
Tropical Blend	4 oz	–	70	–
(Gerber)				
Strained				
Apple	4.2 oz	–	60	–
Apple-Apricot	4.2 oz	–	60	–
Apple-Banana	4.2 oz	–	70	–
Apple-Cherry	4.2 oz	–	60	–
Apple-Grape	4.2 oz	–	60	–
Apple-Peach	4.2 oz	–	60	–
Apple-Pineapple	4.2 oz	–	60	–
Apple-Plum	4.2 oz	–	60	–
Apple-Prune	4.2 oz	–	70	–
Mixed Fruit	4.2 oz	–	70	–
Orange	4.2 oz	–	70	–
Pear	4.2 oz	–	60	–
Toddler				
Apple	4 oz	–	60	–
Apple-Cherry	4 oz	–	60	–
Apple-Grape	4 oz	–	60	–
Apple'N Berry	4 oz	–	60	–
Fruits-A-Plenty	4 oz	–	60	–
Fruits Of The Sun	4 oz	1	60	15%
Mixed Fruit	4 oz	1	60	15%
Pear	4 oz	–	60	–
FRUITS				
(Beech-Nut Stages)				
Stage 1				
Barlett Pears	2.8 oz	–	50	–
	4.5 oz	–	60	–
Chiquita Bananas	2.8 oz	–	70	–

Food and Description	Amount	Fat Grams	Total Calories	% Fat Calories
	4.5 oz	–	100	–
Golden Delicious Applesauce	2.8 oz	–	45	–
	4.5 oz	–	60	–
Yellow Cling Peaches	2.8 oz	–	40	–
	4.5 oz	–	60	–
Stage 2				
Apples & Grapes	4.5 oz	–	90	–
Apples & Strawberries	4.5 oz	–	90	–
Applesauce & Apricots	4.5 oz	–	60	–
Applesauce & Bananas	4.5 oz	–	60	–
Applesauce & Cherries	4.5 oz	–	70	–
Apples, Mandarin Oranges, & Bananas	4.5 oz	–	90	–
Apples, Peaches, & Strawberries	4.5 oz	–	100	–
Apples, Pears, & Bananas	4.5 oz	–	90	–
Apricots, w/Pears & Applesauce	4.5 oz	–	70	–
Bananas w/Pears & Applesauce	4.5 oz	–	90	–
Bartlett Pears & Pineapple	4.5 oz	–	70	–
Cottage Cheese w/Pineapple	4.5 oz	1	110	8%
Fruit Dessert	4.5 oz	–	80	–
Island Fruits	4.5 oz	–	90	–
Pears & Applesauce	4.5 oz	–	70	–
Plums w/rice	4.5 oz	–	110	–
Prunes w/Pears	4.5 oz	–	120	–
Stage 3				
Apples & Grapes	7.5 oz	–	190	–
Apples & Strawberries	7.5 oz	–	160	–
Applesauce	6 oz	–	80	–
	7.5 oz	–	100	–
Applesauce & Bananas	7.5 oz	–	110	–
Applesauce & Cherries	7.5 oz	–	110	–
Apples, Mandarin Oranges, & Bananas	7.5 oz	–	150	–
Apples, Peaches, & Strawberries	7.5 oz	–	160	–
Apples, Pears, & Bananas	7.5 oz	–	160	–
Apricots w/Pears & Apples	6 oz	–	110	–
	7.5 oz	–	120	–
Bananas w/Pears & Apples	6 oz	–	120	–
	7.5 oz	–	160	–
Bartlett Pears	6 oz	–	90	–
	7.5 oz	–	110	–
Bartlett Pears & Pineapple	7.5 oz	–	120	–
Cottage Cheese w/Pineapple	6 oz	2	160	11%
	7.5 oz	2	190	10%

Food and Description	Amount	Fat Grams	Total Calories	% Fat Calories
Fruit Dessert	7.5 oz	–	130	–
Island Fruits	7.5 oz	–	150	–
Peaches	6 oz	–	100	–
	7.5 oz	–	150	–
(Gerber)				
First Foods				
Applesauce	2.5 oz	–	40	–
Bananas	2.5 oz	–	60	–
Peaches	2.5 oz	–	30	–
Pears	2.5 oz	–	40	–
Prunes	2.5 oz	–	70	–
Junior				
Apple Blueberry	6 oz	1	80	11%
Applesauce	6 oz	1	90	10%
Apricots w/Tapioca	6 oz	1	130	7%
Bananas w/Tapioca	6 oz	1	140	6%
Bananas w/Pineapple & Tapioca	6 oz	1	90	10%
Peaches	6 oz	1	110	8%
Pear Pineapple	6 oz	1	100	9%
Pears	6 oz	1	100	9%
Plums w/Tapioca	6 oz	1	130	7%
Strained				
Apple Blueberry	4.5 oz	1	60	15%
Applesauce	4.5 oz	1	60	15%
Applesauce & Apricot	4.5 oz	1	70	13%
Apricots w/Tapioca	4.5 oz	1	90	10%
Bananas w/Tapioca	4.5 oz	1	110	8%
Bananas w/Pineapple & Tapioca	4.5 oz	–	60	–
Peaches	4.5 oz	1	90	10%
Pear Pineapple	4.5 oz	1	80	11%
Pears	4.5 oz	1	80	11%
Plums w/Tapioca	4.5 oz	–	90	–
Prunes w/Tapioca	4.5 oz	1	100	9%
Strained Tropical Fruits				
Guava w/Tapioca	4.5 oz	1	90	10%
Mango Bananas & Passion Fruit w/Tapioca	4.5 oz	–	100	–
Mango w/Tapioca	4.5 oz	1	90	10%
Papaya w/Tapioca	4.5 oz	1	80	11%
Peaches Mango w/Tapioca	4.5 oz	1	100	9%
Tropical Fruits w/Tapioca	4.5 oz	1	80	11%
(Heinz)				
Instant				
Apples	1 serving	–	50	–

Food and Description	Amount	Fat Grams	Total Calories	% Fat Calories
Bananas	1 serving	–	50	–
Peaches	1 serving	–	50	–
Pears	1 serving	–	50	–
Instant Fruit Combinations				
Apples & Apricots	1 serving	–	50	–
Apples & Bananas	1 serving	–	50	–
Apples & Peaches	1 serving	–	50	–
Apples & Pears	1 serving	–	50	–
Apricots w/Pears & Bananas	1 serving	–	50	–
Mixed Fruit	1 serving	–	50	–
Peaches & Pears	1 serving	1	50	18%
Pears & Pineapple	1 serving	–	50	–
MEATS				
(Beech-Nut Stages)				
Stage 1				
Beef	2.8 oz	7	100	63%
	3.5 oz	8	120	60%
Chicken	2.8 oz	6	90	60%
	3.5 oz	6	110	49%
Lamb	2.8 oz	6	90	60%
	3.5 oz	8	130	55%
Turkey	2.8 oz	6	100	54%
	3.5 oz	7	120	53%
Veal	2.8 oz	7	100	63%
	3.5 oz	7	120	53%
(Gerber)				
Junior Meats				
Beef	2.5 oz	4	80	45%
Chicken	2.5 oz	7	110	57%
Ham	2.5 oz	5	90	50%
Turkey	2.5 oz	6	100	54%
Veal	2.5 oz	4	80	45%
Strained Meats & Egg Yolks				
Beef	2.5 oz	4	80	45%
Chicken	2.5 oz	7	110	57%
Egg Yolks	2.25 oz	11	130	76%
Ham	2.5 oz	5	90	50%
Lamb	2.5 oz	3	70	39%
Pork	2.5 oz	5	90	50%
Turkey	2.5 oz	6	100	54%
Veal	2.5 oz	4	80	45%
Ham				
junior	~ 3.5 oz	6.6	123	48%
strained	~ 3.5 oz	5.7	110	48%

Food and Description	Amount	Fat Grams	Total Calories	% Fat Calories
Liver				
strained	~ 3.5 oz	3.7	100	33%
VEGETABLES				
(Beech-Nut Stages)				
Stage 1				
Butternut Squash	2.8 oz	–	20	–
	4.5 oz	–	40	–
Green Beans	4.5 oz	–	40	–
Regal Imperial Carrots	4.5 oz	–	40	–
Sweet Potatoes	2.8 oz	–	40	–
	4.5 oz	–	70	–
Tender Sweet Peas	4.5 oz	–	70	–
Stage 2				
Creamed Corn	4.5 oz	–	90	–
Garden Vegetables	4.5 oz	–	60	–
Mixed Vegetables	4.5 oz	–	50	–
Peas & Carrots	4.5 oz	–	60	–
Stage 3				
Carrots	7.5 oz	–	60	–
Green Beans	7.5 oz	–	60	–
Mixed Vegetables	7.5 oz	–	90	–
Sweet Potatoes	7.5 oz	–	120	–
(Gerber)				
First Foods				
Carrots	2.5 oz	1	40	23%
Green Beans	2.5 oz	–	20	–
Peas	2.5 oz	1	40	23%
Squash	2.5 oz	–	20	–
Sweet Potatoes	2.5 oz	–	50	–
Junior				
Carrots	6 oz	1	50	18%
Creamed Green Beans	6 oz	1	80	11%
Mixed Vegetables	6 oz	1	70	13%
Peas	6 oz	1	90	10%
Squash	6 oz	1	60	15%
Sweet Potatoes	6 oz	1	110	8%
Strained				
Beets	4.5 oz	1	60	15%
Carrots	4.5 oz	1	40	23%
Creamed Corn	4.5 oz	1	80	11%
Creamed Spinach	4.5 oz	1	60	15%
Garden Vegetables	4.5 oz	1	50	18%
Green Beans	4.5 oz	1	50	18%
Mixed Vegetables	4.5 oz	1	60	15%
Peas	4.5 oz	1	60	15%

Food and Description	Amount	Fat Grams	Total Calories	% Fat Calories
Squash	4.5 oz	1	40	23%
Sweet Potatoes	4.5 oz	1	80	11%
(Heinz)				
Instant (Dry Serving Size)				
Beets	3 Tbs	–	50	–
Carrots	5 Tbs	2	70	26%
Creamed Corn	6 Tbs	1	60	15%
Creamed Peas	5 Tbs	1	60	15%
Creamed Spinach	6 Tbs	2	60	30%
Garden Vegetables	5 Tbs	1	60	15%
Green Beans	4 Tbs	1	60	15%
Mixed Vegetables	5 Tbs	2	70	26%
Peas & Carrots	5 Tbs	1	60	15%
Squash	5 Tbs	1	50	18%
Sweet Potatoes	4 Tbs	1	60	15%
Spinach				
junior	~ 7.5 oz	3	90	30%
strained	~ 4.5 oz	1.7	48	32%
BACON (See also LUNCHEON MEAT)				
Breakfast Strips				
cooked	3 slices	12.5	156	72%
(Ekcrich) Sizzlean-cooked	2 slices	8	90	80%
(Oscar Meyer)-Lean & Tasty				
heated	1 slice	4	50	72%
(Swift)-Premium-brown				
sugar cured	2 slices	9	110	74%
Canadian Bacon				
cold	2 slices/ 2 oz	3.95	89	40%
grilled	2 slices/ 2 oz	3.9	86	41%
(Hormel)	1 oz	2	45	40%
(Oscar Meyer) 93% fat-free	1 oz	1	35	26%
Cured Breakfast Strips				
pan-fried or roasted	3 Medium Slices	9	109	74%
Black Label (Hormel)-cooked	2 slices	5	60	75%
Range Brand (Hormel)-cooked	2 slices	9	110	74%
Red Label (Hormel)-cooked	3 slices	10	110	82%
Thick-sliced	1 slice	19	190	90%
BACON BITS				
Homestyle	1 Tbs	2	30	60%
(Hormel)	1 Tbs	2	30	60%
(Oscar Meyer)	¼ oz	1	21	43%

Food and Description	Amount	Fat Grams	Total Calories	% Fat Calories
BACON-LIKE BITS	1 Serving	.5	10	45%
BACON SUBSTITUTES				
Bacon Bits				
(Betty Crocker)	2 tsp	1	25	36%
Bacon Flavor Sprinkles				
(Molly McButter)	½ tsp	–	4	–
BacOs				
(Betty Crocker)	2 tsp	1	25	36%
(Durkee) Imitation Bacon Bits	1 tsp	.5	8	56%
(Durkee) Bacon Chips	1 Tbs	2	44	41%
BAGEL				
Chips/(New York Style)				
Garlic	¾ oz	3	90	30%
Hot'N Spicy	¾ oz	2	90	20%
Plain	¾ oz	3	90	30%
Plain - 3" dia.	1	.8	64	11%
Pumpernickel - 3" dia.	1	.5	152	3%
Sea Salt	¾ oz	3	90	30%
Whole Wheat - 3" dia.	1	.6	152	–
Frozen (Lenders)-Bagelettes	1	.5	70	6%
Big 'N Crusty	1	1	230	3%
Blueberry	1	1	190	4%
Cinnamon Raisin	1	1	200	4%
Egg	1	1	150	6%
Garlic, Onion	1	1	160	5%
Oat Bran	1	2	170	10%
Plain	1	1	150	6%
Poppy	1	1	160	5%
Pumpernickel	1	1	160	5%
Raisin & Honey	1	1	190	4%
Rye	1	1	150	6%
Sesame	1	1	160	5%
Soft	1	3	210	13%
Wheat & Honey	1	1	190	4%
(Sara Lee)				
Cinnamon & Raisin	1	2	240	7%
Egg	1	2	250	7%
Oat Bran	1	1	220	4%
Onion	1	1	230	4%
Plain	1	1	230	4%
Poppy Seed	1	1	230	4%
Sesame Seed	1	3	260	10%
BAKE & FRY MIX (Krusteaz)	2 Tbs	–	48	–

Food and Description	Amount	Fat Grams	Total Calories	% Fat Calories
BAKING MIX/dry				
Arrowhead-Biscuit Mix	2 oz	1	100	9%
Bisquick	2 oz	8	240	30%
Feam				
Brown rice	½ cup	3	215	13%
Rice	½ cup	1	260	4%
Whole wheat	½ cup	2	210	9%
Hain-whole wheat	1.5 oz	1	150	6%
Jiffy	1 oz	3	115	24%
BAKING POWDER	1 tsp	–	5	–
Calumet	1 tsp	–	4	–
Davis	1 Tbs	–	15	–
BAKING SODA	1 tsp	–	5	–
BALSAMPEAR/raw	1 cup	–	15	–
leaf tips				
cooked	½ cup	–	10	–
raw	½ cup	–	7	–
pods				
cooked	½ cup	–	12	–
raw	½ cup	–	8	–
BAMBOO SHOOT				
canned	1 cup	< 1	25	18%
canned (La Choy)	¾ cup	–	6	–
cooked	1 cup	–	14	–
raw	½ cup	–	21	–
BANANA				
(Del Monte)				
fresh	1 medium	< 1	101	5%
chips-freeze dried	¼ cup	4	124	29%
flakes	⅓ cup	1	22	75%
fresh	1	.55	105	5%
mashed	1 cup	1	207	4%
powder	2 oz	–	194	–
sliced	1 cup	–	130	–
Plantain Banana	1	1	220	4%
cooked-sliced	1 cup	< 1	180	3%
BANANA-ORANGE DRINK	8 oz	–	126	–
BANANA-PINEAPPLE JUICE				
Nectar (Kern's)	6 oz	–	120	–
BARBECUE LOAF (See LUNCHEON MEATS)				
BARBECUE SAUCE (See SAUCE)				
BARLEY (pearled)	1 serving	1	170	5%
	2 oz	1	200	5%
Quaker/Scotch-medium pearled	¼ cup	1	170	5%

Food and Description	Amount	Fat Grams	Total Calories	% Fat Calories
BARRACUDA				
baked or broiled	3 oz	5	135	33%
breaded & fried	3 oz	7.5	169	40%
BASIL				
ground	1 tsp	–	3	–
leaves	1 tsp	–	3	–
BASS				
Black				
cooked-dry heat	3 oz	14.5	215	61%
raw	3 oz	1	80	11%
Freshwater				
raw	3 oz	3	97	28%
Mixed				
raw	3 oz	3	97	28%
Striped				
cooked-dry heat	3 oz	1.98	82	22%
BAY LEAF / crumbled	1 tsp	–	2	–
BEAN (*See* individual names)				
BEAN, BAKED & VARIETY				
canned				
baked				
(B&M) baked				
BBQ	~ 1 cup	6	310	17%
Honey	~ 1 cup	2	280	6%
Red Kidney	~ 1 cup	7	290	22%
Small Pea	~ 1 cup	8	330	22%
Tomato	~ 1 cup	3	230	12%
Vegetarian	~ 1 cup	2	280	6%
Yellow Eye	~ 1 cup	7	362	17%
(Green Giant)				
w/bacon & brown sugar	1/2 cup	1	130	7%
(S&W) Brick Oven	½ cup	2	160	11%
(Stagg)	½ cup	2.5	145	16%
(Van Camp's)	1 cup	2	260	7%
Deluxe	1 cup	4	320	11%
Garden Style Special Recipe	½ cup	.8	110	7%
baked w/brown sugar	½ cup	2.5	142	16%
baked w/crumbled bacon	½ cup	4	160	23%
baked w/molasses & brown sugar	½ cup	1.5	133	10%
barbecue (Campbell's)	7⅞ oz	4	210	17%
Boston Baked	½ cup	6.7	193	31%
(Health Valley)	½ cup	1	110	8%
Boston Baked-No Salt				
(Health Valley)	½ cup	1	110	8%

Food and Description	Amount	Fat Grams	Total Calories	% Fat Calories
Cajun Beans and Sauce (Lipton)	½ cup	.6	130	4%
homestyle (Campbell's)	½ cup	2	115	16%
	8 oz	4	230	16%
Maple Sugar (S&W)	½ cup	1	150	6%
New England Style				
(Special Recipe)	½ cup	2.5	148	15%
Old Fashioned (Campbell's)	½ cup	1.5	115	12%
Old Fashioned (Campbell's)	8 oz	3	230	12%
Pork & Beans				
(Campbell's)	8 oz	3	190	14%
(Heinz)	8 oz	4	250	14%
(Hunt's)	4 oz	1	140	6%
(Van Camp's)	1 cup	2	220	8%
Pork & Molasses (Libby)	½ cup	2	140	13%
Pork & Tomato Sauce (Libby)	½ cup	2	140	13%
Pork'N Beans (S&W)	½ cup	2	130	14%
Ranchero (Campbell's)	7¾ oz	4	190	19%
Smokey Ranch (S&W)	½ cup	2	130	14%
Texas Style Barbecue (S&W)	½ cup	1	135	7%
vegetarian				
(Heinz)	8 oz	1	230	4%
(Libby)	½ cup	1	130	7%
vegetarian seasoned in tomato sauce				
(Campbell's)	½ cup	1	210	4%
Vegetarian Style Beans				
(Van Camp's)	1 cup	1	210	4%
Vegetarian w/miso				
(Health Valley)	½ cup	1	90	10%
canned				
w/beef	½ cup	4.59	161	26%
w/franks	½ cup	8	182	40%
w/pork	½ cup	1.96	133	13%
w/pork & sweet sauce	½ cup	1.85	140	12%
w/pork and tomato sauce	½ cup	1	123	7%
homemade (includes white beans, molasses, brown				
sugar, salt pork, & spices)	½ cup	6.5	190	31%
BEAN MEALS, BAKED				
Beanee Weenee /canned (Van Camp's)	1 cup	15	330	41%
Beans'N Franks (Heinz)	7¾ oz	15	330	41%
BEAN SALAD, MIXED				
Four Bean Salad				
canned				
(Hanover)	½ cup	–	80	–
(Joan of Arc)	½ cup	–	100	–

Food and Description	Amount	Fat Grams	Total Calories	% Fat Calories
Garden Salad-marinated				
jar (S&W)	½ cup	1	90	10%
Mixed Bean Salad-marinated				
canned (S&W)	½ cup	1	90	10%
Mixed Beans (Pinto & Great Northern) seasoned w/pork				
canned (Luck's)	7.25 oz	5	200	23%
	7.5 oz	7	220	29%
Three Bean Salad				
canned				
(Green Giant)	½ cup	–	70	–
(Joan Of Arc)	½ cup	–	80	–
homemade	1 cup	15	300	45%
BEAN SOUP (See SOUP)				
BEAN SPROUT				
Kidney/boiled	4 oz	< 1	37	–
raw	1 cup	< 1	53	–
Mung/boiled	1/2 cup	–	13	–
canned (Arrowhead Mills)	1/2 cup	–	25	–
raw	4 oz	–	40	–
stir fried	1/2 cup	–	31	–
Navy/boiled	1 cup	< 1	88	5%
raw	4 oz	< 1	70	6%
Pinto/boiled	4 oz	–	25	–
raw	4 oz	1	70	13%
Soy/boiled	1/2 cup	2	38	47%
raw	10 sprouts	.6	12	45%
stir fried	4 oz	8	143	50%
BEAVER/roasted	3 oz	11.6	211	50%
BEECHNUT				
dried	1 oz	14	164	77%
BEEF				

(Note: Serving sizes are for cooked beef, unless otherwise stated. "Lean only" means beef trimmed of all separable fat before cooking. "Lean and fat" means untrimmed and cooked or eaten as purchased. Prime cuts have the most fat, Choice cuts less, and Select/Good cuts the least amount of all cuts.)

BEEF CUTS				
Brisket				
Whole/lean and fat-braised	3 oz	27.6	332	75%
Whole/lean only-braised	3 oz	10.9	205	48%
Chuck				
Arm pot roast/lean and fat				
Choice	3 oz	22.5	301	67%
Good	3 oz	20.8	287	65%
Arm pot roast/lean only				
Choice-braised	3 oz	8.8	199	40%

Food and Description	Amount	Fat Grams	Total Calories	% Fat Calories
Good-braised	3 oz	7.6	189	36%
Blade/lean and fat				
All grades-braised	3 oz	25.9	325	72%
Blade/lean only				
All grades-braised	3 oz	13	230	51%
Rib roast or steaks/lean and fat				
Choice-braised	3 oz	31	364	77%
Good-braised	3 oz	25.8	321	72%
Rib roast or steaks/lean only				
Choice-braised	3 oz	15.6	218	64%
Good-braised	3 oz	8.7	187	42%
Stew meat-boneless/Lean and fat				
Braised or stewed	3 oz	20	279	65%
Lean only				
Braised or stewed	3 oz	8	183	39%
Club Steak/lean and fat				
Choice-broiled	3 oz	34.5	386	30%
Corned Beef				
Boneless/roasted	3 oz	25.8	316	74%
Flank/lean and fat				
Lean and fat/Choice				
Braised	3 oz	13	218	54%
Broiled	3 oz	13.9	216	58%
Lean only				
Choice-braised	3 oz	11.8	208	51%
Choice-broiled	3 oz	12.7	207	55%
Ground (Note: 4 oz raw ground meat is equal to 3 oz cooked ground meat.)				
Extra lean 15% fat				
Broiled medium	3 oz	13.9	215	58%
Broiled well-done	3 oz	13	225	52%
Fried medium	3 oz	14	216	58%
Fried well done	3 oz	13.6	224	55%
Raw	4 oz	19	265	65%
Extra Lean 10% Fat				
Raw	4 oz	11	202	49%
Broiled well-done	3 oz	9.6	186	46%
Lean 21% Fat				
Raw	4 oz	24	303	71%
Broiled medium	3 oz	15.7	231	61%
Broiled well-done	3 oz	15	238	57%
Fried medium	3 oz	16	234	62%
Fried well-done	3 oz	15	235	57%
Regular				
Raw	4 oz	30	351	77%

Food and Description	Amount	Fat Grams	Total Calories	% Fat Calories
Broiled medium	3 oz	17.6	246	64%
Broiled well-done	3 oz	16.5	248	60%
Fried medium	3 oz	19	260	66%
Fried well-done	3 oz	16	243	59%
Lite Beef (Golden Trim)-Raw				
Bottom Round Roast	3 oz	4	110	33%
Bottom Round Rump Roast	3 oz	4	110	33%
Bottom Round Steak	3 oz	4	110	33%
Chopped Sirloin Steak	3 oz	5	110	41%
Chuck Eye Steak	3 oz	7	120	53%
Chuck Shoulder Steak or Roast	3 oz	4	110	33%
Chuck Top Blade Steak or Roast	3 oz	7	120	53%
Eye of Round Roast	3 oz	4	110	33%
Eye of Round Steak	3 oz	4	110	33%
Filet Mignon	3 oz	3	100	27%
Hamburger	3 oz	5	110	41%
Kabob Beef	3 oz	3	100	27%
Loin Porterhouse Steak	3 oz	6	120	45%
Loin T-Bone Steak	3 oz	6	120	45%
Rib Eye Roast	3 oz	8	140	51%
Rib Eye Steak	3 oz	8	140	51%
Round Tip Roast	3 oz	2	90	20%
Round Tip Steak	3 oz	2	90	20%
Stew Meat	3 oz	5	120	38%
Striploin Steak	3 oz	5	120	38%
Top Loin Steak	3 oz	5	120	38%
Top Round/London Broil	3 oz	2	100	18%
Top Round Roast	3 oz	2	100	18%
Top Round Steak	3 oz	2	100	18%
Top Sirloin Steak	3 oz	4	100	36%
London Broil, 100%lean				
Choice-braised	3 oz	6	167	32%
Rib				
Whole/lean and fat				
Choice-broiled	3 oz	26	313	75%
Choice-roasted	3 oz	27.6	328	76%
Good-broiled	3 oz	26	313	75%
Good-roasted	3 oz	24.9	306	73%
Whole/lean only				
Choice-broiled	3 oz	11.5	198	52%
Choice-roasted	3 oz	12.6	209	54%
Rib Eye				
Lean and fat				
Choice-broiled	3 oz	17.5	250	63%

Food and Description	Amount	Fat Grams	Total Calories	% Fat Calories
Lean only				
Choice-broiled	3 oz	9.9	191	47%
Ribs, Short				
Lean and fat				
Choice-braised	3 oz	35.7	400	80%
Lean only				
Choice-braised	3 oz	15	251	54%
Round				
Bottom/lean and fat				
Choice-braised	3 oz	13	224	52%
Good-braised	3 oz	12	215	50%
Prime	3 oz	16	253	57%
Bottom/lean only				
Choice-braised	3 oz	8	191	38%
Good-braised	3 oz	7	182	35%
Prime-braised	3 oz	11	212	47%
Eye Of/lean and fat				
Choice-roasted	3 oz	12	207	52%
Good-roasted	3 oz	12	201	54%
Prime-roasted	3 oz	13	213	55%
Eye of/lean only				
Choice-roasted	3 oz	6	156	35%
Good-roasted	3 oz	5	150	30%
Prime-roasted	3 oz	7	168	38%
Full Cut/lean and fat				
Choice-broiled	3 oz	15.5	233	60%
Good-broiled	3 oz	14	222	57%
Full Cut/lean				
Choice-broiled	3 oz	6.8	165	37%
Good-broiled	3 oz	5.9	157	34%
Tip/lean and fat				
Choice-broiled	3 oz	8	181	40%
Good-broiled	3 oz	7	156	40%
Prime-broiled	3 oz	10	201	45%
Tip/lean only				
Choice-broiled	3 oz	5	165	27%
Good-broiled	3 oz	5	156	29%
Prime-broiled	3 oz	8	183	39%
Top/lean and fat				
Choice-roasted	3 oz	13	216	54%
Good-roasted	3 oz	12	205	53%
Prime-roasted	3 oz	16	242	60%
Top/lean only				
Choice-roasted	3oz	7	164	38%

Food and Description	Amount	Fat Grams	Total Calories	% Fat Calories
Good-roasted	3 oz	6	156	35%
Prime-roasted	3 oz	9	181	45%
Rump Roast				
Lean and fat				
Choice-roasted	3 oz	23	295	70%
Good-roasted	3 oz	19.9	269	67%
Lean only				
Choice-roasted	3 oz	7.9	177	40%
Good-roasted	3 oz	6	162	33%
Shank Crosscuts				
Lean and fat				
Choice-simmered	3 oz	10	208	43%
Lean only				
Choice-simmered	3 oz	5	171	26%
Sirloin				
Lean and fat				
All grades-broiled	3 oz	15	238	57%
Lean only				
All grades-broiled	3 oz	7	177	36%
Steak				
Porterhouse/lean and fat				
Choice-broiled	3 oz	18	254	64%
Porterhouse /lean only				
Choice-broiled	3 oz	9	185	44%
T-bone/lean and fat				
Choice-broiled	3 oz	20.9	276	68%
T-bone/lean only				
Choice-broiled	3 oz	8.8	182	44%
Tenderloin				
Lean and fat				
Choice-broiled	3 oz	15	230	59%
Choice-roasted	3 oz	19	262	65%
Good-broiled	3 oz	13	216	54%
Good-roasted	3 oz	17	245	62%
Prime-broiled	3 oz	19.9	270	66%
Lean only				
Choice-broiled	3 oz	8	176	41%
Choice-roasted	3 oz	9.9	189	47%
Good-broiled	3 oz	7	167	38%
Good-roasted	3 oz	8.6	177	44%
Prime-broiled	3 oz	10.5	197	48%
Top Loin				
Lean and fat				
Choice-broiled	3 oz	16.6	243	62%

Food and Description	Amount	Fat Grams	Total Calories	% Fat Calories
Good-broiled	3 oz	14	223	57%
Prime-broiled	3 oz	22	288	69%
Lean only				
Choice-broiled	3 oz	8	176	41%
Good-broiled	3 oz	6	162	33%
Prime-broiled	3 oz	11.6	208	50%
Wedge-Bone Sirloin				
Lean and fat				
Choice-broiled	3 oz	16	240	56%
Good-broiled	3 oz	15	232	58%
Prime-broiled	3 oz	19	271	63%
Lean only				
Choice-broiled	3 oz	6	178	30%
Good-broiled	3 oz	7	170	37%
Prime-broiled	3 oz	10	201	45%
BEEF CUTS, OTHER				
Brains				
Fried	3 oz	13.5	167	73%
Simmered	3 oz	10.6	136	70%
Heart/braised	3 oz	4.8	148	29%
Kidneys/simmered	3 oz	2.9	122	21%
Liver				
Braised	3 oz	4	137	26%
Fried	3 oz	6.8	184	33%
Lungs/braised	3 oz	3	102	27%
Pancreas/braised	3 oz	14.7	232	57%
Spleen/braised	3 oz	4	123	29%
Sweetbreads/braised	3 oz	19.7	272	65%
Thymus/braised	3 oz	21	273	69%
Tongue				
Braised-medium fat	3 oz	22	208	95%
Simmered	3 oz	17.6	241	66%
Tripe/raw	4 oz	4	111	32%
BEEF BROTH (*See* SOUP)				
BEEF DISHES				
Beef Bourguignoine				
Standard Home Recipe (USDA)	¾ cup	8	194	37%
Beef Pot Pie				
Frozen (Swanson)	7 oz	20	380	47%
	16 oz	36	700	46%
Standard Home Recipe (USDA)				
(⅓ of 9" dia pie)	~7 oz	30	515	52%
Beef Stew-Vegetable				
Canned				
(Bounty)	7.6 oz	3	144	19%

Food and Description	Amount	Fat Grams	Total Calories	% Fat Calories
(Estee)	7.5 oz	11	210	47%
(Libby's)	7.5 oz	5	160	28%
(Heinz)	7.5 oz	9	210	34%
Beef Stew				
Canned				
(Chef Boyardee)-Meat Ball	8 oz	24	350	62%
(Dinty Moore)-24 oz can	8 oz	12	220	49%
(Dinty Moore)-40 oz can	8 oz	11	210	47%
	8 oz	6	170	32%
Frozen				
(Banquet)	7 oz	5	140	32%
Standard Home Recipe (USDA)	1 cup	11	220	45%
Beef Stroganoff				
Frozen (Weight Watchers)	9 oz	13	320	37%
Standard Home Recipe (USDA)				
w/noodles	1 cup	20	342	53%
Beef Wellington				
Standard Home Recipe (USDA)	4 oz	18	325	50%
Beefaroni				
Canned (Chef Boyardee)	7 oz	6	200	27%
Beef-o-getti				
Canned (Chef Boyardee)	7 oz	9	210	39%
Breaded Beef Steaks				
Frozen (Hormel)	4 oz	30	370	73%
Chipped & Creamed Beef				
Frozen (Banquet) Cookin' Bag	4 oz	4	100	36%
Creamed Dried Beef				
Standard Home Recipe (USDA)	¾ cup	18	275	59%
Dinty Moore				
Beef Stew				
24 oz can	8 oz	12	220	49%
40 oz can	8 oz	11	210	47%
Meatball Stew				
24 oz can	8 oz	15	240	56%
Goulash				
Canned				
(Heinz)	7.5 oz	11	240	41%
(Hormel)-Short Order	7.5 oz	12	230	47%
Great Beginnings (Hormel) Box prepared				
w/Chunky Beef	5 oz	7	136	46%
International Lites - Microwavable Box				
Beef Stroganoff	10 oz	8	260	28%
Enchilada Acapulco	10 oz	8	250	29%
Milano Lasagna	10 oz	7	280	23%

Food and Description	Amount	Fat Grams	Total Calories	% Fat Calories
Kid's Kitchen (Hormel) - Microwavable Box				
Beef Ravioli	7.5 oz	2	160	11%
Chunky Vegetables & Beef	7.5 oz	1	120	8%
Spaghetti w/meatballs	7.5 oz	8	200	36%
Lemon Ginger Beef				
Frozen (Kibun)	8 oz	4	230	16%
Light Balance, Microwaveable lunch buckets				
Beef Americana	8.25 oz	3	190	14%
Beef & Pasta Bordeaux	8.25 oz	1	180	5%
Chicken Caciatore	8.25 oz	1	210	4%
Chicken Fiesta	8.25 oz	4	210	18%
Pasta & Garden Vegetables	8.25 oz	1	170	5%
BEEF, FROZEN ENTREE (*See* FROZEN ENTREE/DINNER, BEEF)				
BEEF PRODUCTS (*See also* LUNCHEON MEATS)				
Beef Spread				
Underwood				
Corned beef	2.25 oz	10	120	75%
Roast beef	2.4 oz	10	140	64%
Beef Tallow	1 cup	205	1849	100%
	1 Tbs	12.8	115	100%
Breakfast Strips				
(Oscar Meyer)-Lean'N Tasty	1 slice	4	45	80%
Dried or Chipped Beef	2.5 oz	4	145	25%
Dried Sliced				
(Armour Star)	8 slices	2	60	30%
(Hormel)	1 oz	1	45	20%
Smoked Chopped Beef	1 oz	1	38	24%
Smoked Sliced Beef (Hormel)	1 oz	3	50	54%
Steak-Umm (Gagliardi)				
Frozen-sandwich steaks	2 oz	16	180	80%
Summer Sausage	1 oz	7.6	86	80%
BEEF SOUP (*See* SOUP)				
BEER, ALE, AND MALT LIQUOR				
Ale-generic	12 fl oz	–	155	–
Amstel Light	12 fl oz	–	95	–
Anheuser-Busch	12 fl oz	–	153	–
Anheuser-Busch Natural Light	12 fl oz	–	110	–
Beck's	12 fl oz	–	143	–
Beer-generic				
Light	12 fl oz	–	100	–
Regular	12 fl oz	–	146	–
Black Horse	12 fl oz	–	158	–
Black Label	12 fl oz	–	136	–
Blatz	12 fl oz	–	142	–

Food and Description	Amount	Fat Grams	Total Calories	% Fat Calories
Blatz Light	12 fl oz	–	96	–
Bud Light	12 fl oz	–	108	–
Budweiser	12 fl oz	–	144	–
Busch	12 fl oz	–	144	–
Busch Light	12 fl oz	–	110	–
Champale-Extra dry	12 fl oz	–	169	–
Cheers (non-alcoholic)	12 fl oz	–	55	–
Classic	12 fl oz	–	144	–
Colt 45	12 fl oz	–	156	–
Coors Light	12 fl oz	–	105	–
Coors Premium	12 fl oz	–	141	–
Coqui	12 fl oz	–	208	–
Corona Light	12 fl oz	–	105	–
Hamm's Light	12 fl oz	–	96	–
Heidelberg Light	12 fl oz	–	115	–
Heileman's				
Old Style	12 fl oz	–	146	–
Light	12 fl oz	–	99	–
Special Export	12 fl oz	–	155	–
Light	12 fl oz	–	115	–
Special Export-Dark	12 fl oz	–	155	–
Herman Joseph's	12 fl oz	–	157	–
King Cobra	12 fl oz	–	160	–
Kingsbury (non-alcoholic malt)	12 fl oz	–	60	–
Knickerbocker	12 fl oz	–	140	–
LA	12 fl oz	–	112	–
Lite Genuine Draft	12 fl oz	–	98	–
Michelob	12 fl oz	–	160	–
Michelob Classic Dark	12 fl oz	–	164	–
Michelob Light	12 fl oz	–	134	–
Mickeys Malt Liquor	12 fl oz	–	156	–
Miller Lite	12 fl oz	–	96	–
Milwaukee's Best-Light	12 fl oz	–	98	–
Molson Light	12 fl oz	–	109	–
Moussy (non-alcoholic)	11.1 fl oz	–	50	–
Natural Light (Anheuser-Busch)	12 fl oz	–	110	–
Near Beer	12 fl oz	–	32	–
Nordik Wolf Light	12 fl oz	–	110	–
Old Milwaukee-Light	12 fl oz	–	120	–
Old Style Light	12 fl oz	–	115	–
Olympia Gold Light	12 fl oz	–	70	–
Ortieb's	12 fl oz	–	140	–
Pabst Blue Ribbon	12 fl oz	–	144	–
Pabst Blue Ribbon Extra Light	12 fl oz	–	70	–

Food and Description	Amount	Fat Grams	Total Calories	% Fat Calories
Pabst NA (non-alcoholic)	12 fl oz	–	55	–
Piels Light	12 fl oz	–	136	–
Prior Double Dark	12 fl oz	–	171	–
Rainier	12 fl oz	–	142	–
Red White & Blue Light	12 fl oz	–	115	–
Rheingold	12 fl oz	–	148	–
Rheingold Light	12 fl oz	–	96	–
Schaefer Light	12 fl oz	–	112	–
Schmidt	12 fl oz	–	142	–
Schmidt Light	12 fl oz	–	96	–
Schmidt Select (non-alcoholic malt)	12 fl oz	–	80	–
Sharp's (Miller) (non-alcoholic)	12 fl oz	–	74	–
Stroh's American Lager	12 fl oz	–	145	–
Tiger Head Ale	12 fl oz	–	166	–
BEERWURST (*See* LUNCHEON MEAT)				
BEET				
canned	½ cup	–	36	–
canned-crinkle sliced				
pickled (Del Monte)	½ cup	–	80	–
canned-Harvard-slices	½ cup	–	89	–
canned-Julienne French Style (S&W)	½ cup	–	40	–
canned-Party sliced pickled w/red				
wine vinegar (S&W)	½ cup	–	70	–
canned				
pickled	½ cup	–	75	–
(Libby & Seneca)	½ cup	–	35	–
pickled-sliced (Libby)	½ cup	–	80	–
pickled-sliced				
w/red wine vinegar (S&W)	½ cup	–	70	–
pickled-Whole-Extra Small (S&W)	½ cup	–	70	–
canned sliced				
(Del Monte)	½ cup	–	35	–
(Libby)	½ cup	–	35	–
(Nutradiet)	½ cup	–	35	–
canned				
small sliced (Freshlike)	½ cup	–	40	–
small Tender sliced (S&W)	½ cup	–	40	–
small whole				
(Freshlike)	½ cup	–	40	–
(S&W)	½ cup	–	40	–
canned-Tender diced (S&W)	½ cup	–	40	–
canned-whole or tiny whole				
(Del Monte)	½ cup	–	35	–
fresh /cooked	½ cup	–	26	–

Food and Description	Amount	Fat Grams	Total Calories	% Fat Calories
BEET DISHES				
Beets in Orange Sauce/frozen				
(Birds Eye) Specialty Classics	5 oz	3	110	25%
BEET GREENS				
fresh				
cooked	½ cup	–	20	–
raw	½ cup	–	4	–
BERRY DRINK				
Berries & Berries (Tropicana)-				
single serve	10 oz	–	156	–
Berry Blend-(Crystal Light)				
–mix-diet	8 oz	–	3	–
BERRY JUICE				
Juicy Juice (Libby's)	6 oz	–	90	–
BISCUITS				
Baking mix (Krusteaz) 2" dia	1	4	110	33%
BixMix (Martha White)	1	3	100	27%
Frozen-(Bridgeford)				
–heat & serve-microwave	1	6	190	28%
Homemade 2" dia	1	5	100	45%
Mix	1	3	95	28%
refrigerated-Plain	1	2	65	29%
Baking Powder (1869 Brand)	2	10	210	43%
Big Country Butter Tastin' (Pillsbury)	2	8	190	38%
Big Country Southern Style				
(1869 Brand)	2	8	200	36%
Big Premium Heat'n Eat (Pillsbury)	2	15	280	48%
Butter (Pillsbury)	1	1	50	18%
Butter Tastin' (1869 Brand)	2	10	210	43%
Butter Tastin' Flaky (Hungry Jack)	1	4	90	40%
Buttermilk (1869 Brand)	2	10	210	43%
Buttermilk (Pillsbury)	1	1	50	18%
Buttermilk, Extra Rich (Hungry Jack)	1	1	50	18%
Buttermilk, Flaky (Hungry Jack)	1	4	90	40%
Buttermilk, Fluffy (Hungry Jack)	1	4	80	45%
Buttermilk, Big Country (Hungry Jack)	2	8	200	36%
Buttermilk, Deluxe Heat 'n Eat				
(Pillsbury)	2	14.8	281	47%
Buttermilk, Heat'nEat (Pillsbury)	1	2.5	85	27%
Buttermilk, Flaky Extra Lights				
(Pillsbury)	2	4	110	33%
Buttermilk, Tenderflake (Pillsbury)	2	5	110	41%
Country (Pillsbury)	1	1	50	18%
Flaky (Hungry Jack)	1	4	80	45%

Food and Description	Amount	Fat Grams	Total Calories	% Fat Calories
Good'N Buttery	2	10	180	50%
OvenReady (Ballard)	1	1	50	18%
OvenReady, Buttermilk (Ballard)	1	1	50	18%
Tender Layer Buttermilk (Pillsbury)	1	2	60	30%
Tenderflake Baking Powder (Pillsbury)	2	5	110	41%
BLACK BEAN / boiled	½ cup	< 1	113	4%
BLACK BEAN SOUP (*See* SOUP)				
BLACK CHERRY JUICE				
(Smucker's)	8 oz	–	130	–
BLACK TURTLE SOUP				
boiled	½ cup	< 1	121	4%
canned	½ cup	–	109	–
(Arrowhead Mills)	2 oz	1	190	8%
(Progresso)	8 oz	1	205	4%
BLACKBERRY				
fresh	1 cup	1	75	12%
canned in water	1 cup	1.5	60	23%
canned in juice	½ cup	< 1	41	11%
canned in heavy syrup	½ cup	< 1	94	5%
frozen/no sugar	½ cup	< 1	97	5%
BLACKBERRY JUICE				
canned	½ cup	1	46	20%
canned (Smucker's)	8 oz	1.5	91	15%
BLACK-EYED PEA				
canned				
(Progresso)	8 oz	1	165	6%
Seasoned w/Pork (Luck's)	7.5 oz	6	200	27%
dried-boiled	½ cup	.6	100	5%
dried-raw	½ cup	1	131	7%
dry (Joan of Arc/Green Giant)	½ cup	1	90	10%
frozen-cooked	½ cup	1	115	8%
frozen (Freshlike)	3.3 oz	1	95	10%
young pods with seeds				
boiled	1 cup	–	32	–
raw	1 cup	–	42	–
BLACK-EYED PEA DISHES				
Black-eyed Peas & Corn seasoned with w/pork				
canned (Luck's)	7.5 oz	7	220	29%
BLUEBERRY				
canned				
in heavy syrup	1 cup	< 1	225	2%
(S&W)	½ cup	< 1	111	4%

Food and Description	Amount	Fat Grams	Total Calories	% Fat Calories
in water	1 cup	< 1	94	5%
fresh	1 cup	< 1	82	6%
frozen				
no sugar	1 cup	< 1	88	5%
	3.5 oz	< 1	50	9%
sweetened	1 cup	< 1	190	2%
BLUEFISH//raw	3 oz	3.6	105	31%
BOCKWURST (See LUNCHEON MEATS)				
BOLOGNA (See also LUNCHEON MEAT)				
4" dia	1 slice	8	89	81%
4½" dia	1 slice	6.5	72	81%
BORAGE				
cooked	½ cup	1	25	36%
raw	½ cup	< 1	9	50%
BORSCHT (See SOUP)				
BOYSENBERRY				
canned				
in water	1 cup	–	90	–
in heavy syrup	1 cup	–	226	–
fresh	½ lb	–	125	–
frozen				
no sugar	1 cup	–	66	–
sweetened	1 cup	–	144	–
BOYSENBERRY DRINK				
Boysenberry Plus-Nice & Natural	6 oz	–	60	–
BOYSENBERRY JUICE				
Boysenberry (Smucker's)	8 oz	–	120	–
Boysenberry Delight	6 oz	–	80	–
BRAN				
(Miller's) unprocessed/dry	1 oz=6 Tbs	1	70	13%
Oat				
Golden Harvest	1 oz	2	90	20%
Quaker	½ cup	3.8	165	21%
Roman Meal	¼ cup	3	115	24%
Rice	3 oz	19	375	46%
Golden Harvest	½ cup	8	120	60%
Rite Bran				
Uncle Ben's	½ cup	9	100	81%
Toasted Wheat (Kretchmer)	⅓ cup	2	60	30%
Unprocessed				
Miller's	1 oz/ 6 Tbs	1	70	13%
Quaker	2 Tbs	–	8	–
BRANDY (See DISTILLED LIQUOR)				

Food and Description	Amount	Fat Grams	Total Calories	% Fat Calories
BRATWURST (See LUNCHEON MEAT)				
BRAZIL NUT				
dried	1 oz	18.8	186	91%
BREAD				
Date Nut/homemade	1 slice	3	100	27%
Date Walnut (Pepperidge Farm)	2 slices	7	180	35%
Dijon Party Slices (Pepperidge Farm)	4 slices	1	70	13%
(Earth Grains)-Barley Bran	1 slice	1	70	13%
–Canadian Oat	1 slice	1	70	13%
Cracked Wheat	1 slice	1	70	13%
Deli Rye	1 slice	1	70	13%
Gold'N Bran	1 slice	1	70	13%
Honey N'Bran	1 slice	1	70	13%
Honey Multi-Grain	1 slice	1	70	13%
Honey Oat & Nut	1 slice	2	80	23%
Honey Oatberry	1 slice	1	70	13%
Oat & Nut	1 slice	2	80	23%
Oat Bran	1 slice	2	80	23%
Raisin Cinnamon Swirl	1 slice	2	80	23%
Wheat Berry	1 slice	1	70	13%
Yogurt Bran	1 slice	1	70	13%
Egg	1 slice	2.6	75	31%
Five Star Fibre-(Pepperidge Farm)-				
Apple Spice Swirl	1 slice	2	70	26%
Harvest Wheat	1 slice	2	70	26%
Orchard Fruit & Nut	1 slice	2	70	26%
White	1 slice	2	60	30%
French (5x2 ½x1")	1 slice	.8	100	7%
(International Hearth)	1 slice	1	70	13%
(Le Francais)-Francisco Square	2 oz	1	150	6%
refrigerated Crusty (Pillsbury)	1 slice	.5	60	7%
Frozen bread doughs - baked				
French (Bridgeford)	2 slices	1	150	6%
Honey Wheat (Bridgeford)	1 slice	1	75	12%
(Rhodes)	1 slice	.5	75	6%
White (Bridgeford)	1 slice	1	75	12%
(Rhodes)	1 slice	.5	80	6%
(Rich's)	1 slice	.5	58	8%
Garlic	1 slice	3.8	100	34%
(Cole's)/frozen-butter				
flavored mini loaf	1 oz	3	90	10%
(Oh Boy!)/frozen w/cheese	2 oz	11	202	49%
Gluten	1 slice	1	69	13%
Granola (Country Hearth)	1 slice	1	70	13%

Food and Description	Amount	Fat Grams	Total Calories	% Fat Calories
(Pepperidge Farm)				
Oat & Honey	1 slice	2	65	28%
Wheat & Honey	1 slice	2	60	30%
(Grant's Farm)-Buttermilk	1 slice	1	80	11%
Honey Cracked	1 slice	1	70	13%
Oat Bran	1 slice	1	70	13%
Oatmeal & Toasted Almonds	1 slice	2	80	23%
Stoneground Wht & 7 Grain	1 slice	1	70	13%
Health Nut (Brownberry)	1 slice	2	70	26%
Hearth Breads-(Pepperidge Farm) -				
Baked-French Style Enriched	1 slice	1	75	12%
Sourdough French Style	1 slice	.5	75	6%
Twin French Style Enr	1 slice	1	75	12%
Vienna	1 slice	1	70	13%
Brown & Serve-French Enr	1 slice	1	90	10%
Italian Enr	1 slice	1	75	12%
Hi-Fibre (Monk's Bread)	1 slice	1	50	18%
Hillbilly (Holsum)	1 slice	1	70	13%
Homestyle Buttermilk	1 slice	1	75	12%
Honey Apple (Brownberry)	1 slice	1	60	15%
Honey Bran (Pepperidge Farm)				
1-1/2 lb loaf	1 slice	1	90	10%
Honey Oat Bran (Roman Meal)	1 slice	1	71	13%
Honey, Nut & Oat (Roman Meal)	1 slice	1.5	72	19%
Honey Wheat Berry	1 slice	1	70	13%
(Pepperidge Farm)	1 slice	1	65	14%
(Roman Meal)	1 slice	1	66	14%
Honey-Buttered Split Top White				
(Family Recipe)	1 slice	1	80	11%
Wheat	1 slice	1	70	13%
Honeybran-Light (Roman Meal)	1 slice	–	40	–
Hush Puppies	1 slice	7	145	34%
Italian (4 1/2x3 1/4x3/4")	1 slice	–	85	–
King's Hawaiian	1/2 oz	1	43	21%
Low Sodium	1 slice	.8	70	10%
Mixed Grain	1 slice	1	65	14%
(Mrs. Wright's)-Crushed Wheat	1 slice	1	80	11%
Crushed Wheat Sandwich	1 slice	1	70	13%
French Enriched	1 slice	1	70	13%
Homestyle Butter Top Wheat	1 slice	1	70	13%
Homestyle Butter Top White	1 slice	1	80	11%
Honey Bran	1 slice	1	90	10%
Honey Wheat Berry	1 slice	1	70	13%
Jewish Rye w/Seeds	1 slice	1	60	15%

Food and Description	Amount	Fat Grams	Total Calories	% Fat Calories
Lite	1 slice	–	40	–
Multi Meal Sandwich	1 slice	1	70	13%
Old Fashioned Italian	1 slice	1	100	9%
Old World Style Black	1 slice	1	60	15%
Raisin	1 slice	1	70	13%
Roundtop Wheat	1 slice	1	80	11%
Sandwich Wheat	1 slice	1	80	11%
Supersoft Sandwich	1 slice	1	60	15%
Supersoft White	1 slice	1	80	11%
Unsalted Grain	1 slice	1	70	13%
Unslated White	1 slice	1	80	11%
Multi-Bran (Roman Meal)	1 slice	1	64	14%
Multi-Grain (Pepperidge Farm)				
Very Thin	1 slice	.5	40	11%
Oat (Roman Meal)	1 slice	1	70	13%
Oat Bran-Light (Rainbo/Colonial)	1 slice	.5	40	11%
Oat Bran & Honey				
(Roman Meal-Light)	1 slice	.5	40	11%
Oatmeal (Brownberry)	1 slice	1	60	15%
(Pepperidge Farm)	1 slice	1	65	14%
1-1/2 lb loaf	1 slice	1.5	85	17%
Oatmeal and Oat Bran	1 slice	1	65	14%
(Oatmeal Goodness)				
Cinnamon Oatmeal	1 slice	2	90	20%
Oatmeal Bran	1 slice	2	90	20%
Oatmeal & Sunflower Seeds	1 slice	2	90	20%
Thinner Sliced White Oatmeal	1 slice	1	80	11%
Wheat Oatmeal	1 slice	2	90	20%
Oatnut Bread (Oroweat)	1 slice	2	100	28%
(Oroweat)-Light				
Country Oat	1 slice	–	40	–
Hearty Rye	1 slice	–	40	–
9 Grain	1 slice	–	40	–
100% Whole Wheat	1 slice	–	40	–
Sour Dough	1 slice	–	40	–
Pita-6 1/2"dia	1 slice	.5	165	3%
8 1/2" dia	1 slice	1	232	4%
Pita, Sesame-6 1/2" dia	1 slice	1	140	6%
Pita, whole wheat-8 1/2" dia	1 slice	2	200	9%
Potato	1 slice	.8	70	10%
Pumpernickel	1 slice	1	80	11%
(Pepperidge Farm)				
Classic Dark	1 slice	1	75	12%
party slices	4 slices	1	70	13%

Food and Description	Amount	Fat Grams	Total Calories	% Fat Calories
Pumpernickel-Rye (Earth Grains)	1 slice	1	70	13%
Pumpkin-homemade	1 slice	5	130	35%
Quick Breads-box mix-(Pillsbury) -				
Applesauce Spice	1 slice	3	150	18%
Apricot Nut	1 slice	4	160	23%
Banana	1 slice	5	160	28%
Blueberry Nut	1 slice	4	150	24%
Carrot Nut	1 slice	4	150	24%
Cherry Nut	1 slice	5	180	25%
Cranberry	1 slice	3	160	17%
Date	1 slice	3	160	17%
Honey Granola	1 slice	4	170	21%
Nut	1 slice	6	170	32%
(Rainbo)				
IronKids	1 slice	1	60	15%
Light Sourdough	1 slice	< 1	40	11%
Raisin	1 slice	1	65	14%
homemade	1 slice	2	135	13%
(Monks' Bread)	1 slice	2	70	26%
Raisin Cinnamon (Brownberry)	1 slice	1	70	13%
(Pepperidge Farm)	1 slice	1.5	70	19%
Raisin Walnut (Brownberry)	1 slice	3	80	21%
(Pepperidge Farm)				
Bountiful Breads	1 slice	2.5	80	28%
Round Top (Roman Meal)	1 slice	1	68	13%
(Rubschlager)				
Cocktail Pumpernickel	2 slices	1	60	15%
Cocktail Rye	1 slice	1	50	18%
Danish Pumpernickel	1 slice	1	70	13%
European Style Whole Grain	1 slice	2	80	23%
German Style Komissbrot	1 slice	1	70	13%
Jewish Deli Rye	1 slice	1	70	13%
Sandwich Malt	1 slice	2	90	20%
Sandwich Rye	1 slice	2	90	20%
Sandwich Wheat	1 slice	2	90	20%
Sweedish Limpa Rye	1 slice	1	60	15%
Westphalian Pumpernickel	1 slice	1	70	13%
Rye	1 slice	–	63	14%
Family w/Seeds				
(Pepperidge Farm)	1 slice	1	8	11%
Family Seedless				
(Pepperidge Farm)	1 slice	1	75	12%
Natural UnSeeded				
(Brownberry)	1 slice	1	70	13%

Food and Description	Amount	Fat Grams	Total Calories	% Fat Calories
Natural UnSeeded Thin				
(Brownberry)	1 slice	1	50	18%
(Pepperidge Farm)				
party slices	4 slices	1	60	18%
Rye, Caraway-Natural				
(Brownberry)	1 slice	1	70	13%
Rye, Dijon-(Pepperidge Farm)	1 slice	1	50	18%
Hearty-(Pepperidge Farm)	1 slice	1	70	13%
Seven Grain (Roman Meal)	1 slice	1	68	13%
Light	1 slice	.5	40	11%
Sour Dough	1 slice	.8	72	10%
French (Colombo)				
brown n'serve	2 oz	–	150	–
(Earth Grains)	1 slice	1	70	13%
mini loaf (Earth Grains)	1 oz	1	80	11%
Spoonbread-homemade				
w/whole-ground cornmeal	2 oz	7	117	54%
Sprouted Wheat (Pepperidge Farm)	1 slice	1.5	60	23%
Sun Grain (Roman Meal)	1 slice	1	68	13%
Sunflower & Bran (Monks' Bread)	1 slice	1	70	13%
Triticale	1 slice	.5	61	7%
12 Grain (Aunt Hattie's)	1 slice	< 1	100	4%
Vienna (4¾x4x½")	1 slice	1	70	13%
(Weight Watchers)				
Cinnamon Raisin	1 slice	1	60	15%
Light Cinnamon Raisin	1 slice	< 1	40	11%
Multi-grain	1 slice	< 1	40	11%
thin slice	2 slices	< 1	80	6%
Rye	1 slice	< 1	40	11%
thin slice	2 slices	< 1	40	6%
Wheat	1 slice	< 1	40	11%
thin slice	2 slices	< 1	80	6%
White	1 slice	< 1	40	11%
thin slice	2 slices	< 1	80	6%
Wheat (Pepperidge Farm)				
1-½ lb loaf	1 slice	1.5	90	15%
Family-2 lb loaf	1 slice	1	65	14%
Wheat berry	1 slice	1	70	13%
light (Rainbo/Colonial)	1 slice	.5	40	11%
(Roman Meal)	1 slice	–	39	–
Wheat Breads				
Beefsteak Hearty Wheat	1 slice	1	70	13%
Beefsteak Multigrain	1 slice	1	70	13%
Beefsteak Soft	1 slice	1	70	13%

Food and Description	Amount	Fat Grams	Total Calories	% Fat Calories
Country Grain,	1 slice	1	70	13%
Cracked Wheat	1 slice	1	70	13%
Family Wheat	1 slice	1	70	13%
Fresh & Natural	1 slice	1	70	13%
High Fiber Wheat	1 slice	–	40	–
Home Pride	1 slice	1	70	13%
Home Pride Butter Top	1 slice	1	70	13%
Home Pride 7 Grain	1 slice	1	70	13%
Stoneground	1 slice	1	70	13%
100% Whole Wheat	1 slice	1	70	13%
100% Whole Wheat-soft	1 slice	1	70	13%
Wheat Light	1 slice	–	40	–
Wheat Germ-(Pepperidge Farm)	1 slice	.5	60	7%
Wheat Oatmeal (Oatmeal Goodness)	1 slice	2	90	20%
White	1 slice	1	65	14%
(Fresh Horizons)	1 slice	1	50	18%
light (Rainbo/Colonial)	1 slice	.5	40	11%
(Roman Meal)	1 slice	–	40	–
(Pepperidge Farm)	1 slice	1.5	75	18%
Large Family-2 lb loaf	1 slice	1.5	75	18%
Very Thin	1 slice	.5	30	15%
refrigerated Pipin' Hot (Pillsbury)	1 slice	2	80	23%
Sandwich (Pepperidge Farm)	1 slice	1	65	14%
Sandwich (Roman Meal)	1 slice	1	55	16%
Toasting (Pepperidge Farm)	1 slice	1	85	11%
very thin (Earth Grains)	1 oz	1	80	11%
White Breads				
Beefsteak Robust	1 slice	1	70	13%
Home Pride Butter Top	1 slice	1	70	13%
Wonder High Fiber	1 slice	–	40	–
Wonder Thin Sliced	1 slice	1	50	18%
Wonder White	1 slice	1	70	13%
Wonder White Light	1 slice	–	40	–
Wonder White W/Butermilk	1 slice	1	70	13%
Whole Bran-Natural (Brownberry)	1 slice	1	60	15%
Whole Grain (Roman Meal)	1 slice	1	66	14%
Whole Wheat	1 slice	1	65	14%
homemade	1 slice	1.6	67	22%
pound loaf	1 slice	1	70	13%
(Fresh Horizons)	1 slice	1	50	18%
(Pepperidge Farm)	1 slice	1	60	15%
Very Thin	1 slice	.5	30	15%
refrigerated Pipin' Hot (Pillsbury)	1 slice	2	80	23%
(Rainbo/Colonial-Light)	1 slice	.5	40	11%

Food and Description	Amount	Fat Grams	Total Calories	% Fat Calories
(Roman Meal)	1 slice	1	66	14%
(Roman Meal)-Light	1 slice	–	40	–
(Sunbeam-Reduced Calorie)	1 slice	.5	40	11%
Very Thin (Earth Grains)	1 oz	1	70	13%
(Wonder)				
Rye Breads-Wonder Rye, Beefsteak Onion Rye, Beefsteak Soft Rye, Beefsteak Hearty Rye, Beefsteak Mild Rye, Beefsteak Wheatberry Rye, & Braun's Old Allegheny	1 slice	1	70	13%
SPECIALTY BREADS				
Apple Walnut Cinnamon Swirl (Pepperidge Farm)				
Bountiful Breads	2 slices	6	160	34%
Banana Nut /homemade	1 slice	2	180	9%
Black	1 slice	–	64	–
Box mix-Quick (Pillsbury)				
Banana	½ loaf	6	170	32%
Blueberry Nut	½ loaf	4	150	24%
Cherry Nut	½ loaf	5	180	25%
Cranberry	½ loaf	4	160	23%
Date	½ loaf	3	160	17%
Nut	½ loaf	6	170	32%
Bran	1 slice	2.9	110	24%
Bran & Honey (Roman Meal)	1 slice	1	66	14%
Bran'ola-Original (Brownberry)	1 slice	1	90	10%
Country Oat (Brownberry)	1 slice	2	90	20%
Hearty Wheat (Brownberry)	1 slice	1.5	90	15%
Cinnamon Raisin	1 slice	1	80	11%
DiCarlo Parisian French	1 slice	1	70	13%
DiCarlo Sour Dough	1 slice	1	70	13%
Hollywood Dark	1 slice	1	70	13%
Hollywood Light	1 slice	1	70	13%
Oatmeal Goodness	1 slice	2	90	20%
Wonder Family Italian	1 slice	1	70	13%
Wonder French	1 slice	1	70	13%

BREAD COATINGS (*See* individual seasoning listings, i.e. chicken, fish, meat)

BREADCRUMBS

Food and Description	Amount	Fat Grams	Total Calories	% Fat Calories
(Contadina)-seasoned	1 cup	3.6	426	6%
	1 Tbs	–	35	–
dry	1 cup	5	390	12%
(Friday's)-Seasoned	1 oz	–	56	–
(Kellog's) corn flake crumbs	1 oz	–	111	–
(Old London)	1 oz	2	210	9%
soft-cubes	1 cup	1	81	9%
soft-crumbs	1 cup	1	122	7%
BREAD CUBES (Brownberry)	1 oz	1	110	8%

Food and Description	Amount	Fat Grams	Total Calories	% Fat Calories
BREADFRUIT/raw	¼ small	–	99	–
	1 cup	.5	227	2%
BREAD PUDDING (*See* PUDDING)				
BREADSTICKS				
Brown/canned				
(S&W) New England Recipe	2 slices	–	76	–
(B&M)-plain	½" slice	–	80	–
w/raisins	½" slice	–	80	–
Boston (3 ¼x½")	1 slice	1	95	10%
Brown 'N Serve - unsliced loaves 8 oz -				
(Wonder)-du Jour Austrian	1 slice	1	70	13%
–du Jour French	1 slice	1	70	13%
Cheese	1 slice	1	72	13%
(Lance)	1	1	10	90%
(Oroweat)	1 oz	2	110	16%
Cinnamon	1 slice	.8	75	18%
Swirl-(Pepperidge Farm)	1 slice	2.5	80	28%
Cinnamon-raisin	1 slice	1	80	11%
(Fattorie & Pandea)-				
traditiional	3	1	60	15%
whole wheat	3	1	57	16%
garlic (Lance)	1	1	15	60%
(Oroweat)	1 oz	2	113	16%
hard-large	1	1	43	21%
onion (Stella D'Oro)	1	1	40	23%
pizza (Stella D'Oro)	1	1	43	21%
plain (Lance)	1	1	15	60%
(Oroweat)	1 oz	2	110	16%
(Stella D'Oro)	1	1	41	22%
refrigerated soft (Pillsbury)	1	2	100	18%
sesame (Lance)	2	1	15	60%
(Oroweat)	1 oz	2	120	15%
(Stella D'Oro)	3	7	170	29%
	1	2	51	35%
soft oat bran	1	1	59	15%
wheat (Stella D'Oro)	1	1	42	21%
BREAD STUFFING (*See also* STUFFING)				
dry	1 cup	31	500	56%
moist	1 cup	26	420	56%
BREAKFAST BAR				
Carnation Breakfast Bars				
Chocolate chip	1 bar	11	200	50%
Chocolate crunch	1 bar	10	190	47%
Peanut butter crunch	1 bar	11	190	52%

Food and Description	Amount	Fat Grams	Total Calories	% Fat Calories
Peanut butter w/chocolate chips	1 bar	11	200	50%
Carnation Slender				
Chocolate, Chocolate chip	1 bar	7	135	47%
Chocolate peanut butter, Vanilla	1 bar	7.5	135	50%
Fi-Bar Morning Granola Snack Bar				
Apple Oatmeal & Spice	1 bar	3	150	18%
Raisin Nut	1 bar	4	150	24%
Strawberry Oatmeal Almond	1 bar	4	150	24%
Figurines				
Chocolate	1 bar	5	100	45%
Chocolate caramel	1 bar	6	100	54%
Chocolate peanut butter	1 bar	6	100	54%
S'Mores	1 bar	5	100	45%
Vanilla	1 bar	5	100	45%
Granola Bar, Chewy (Quaker)				
Maple Oatmeal	1 bar	4	130	28%
Health Valley				
Fat-Free Fruit	1 bar	< 1	95	5%
Fruit & Fitness Energy	2 bars	5	200	23%
Oat Bran Fruit				
Apples/dates	1 bar	4	150	24%
Fruit and nuts	1 bar	4	150	24%
Raisin/cinnamon	1 bar	4	140	26%
Jack La Lane-High Energy Bar				
Original	1 bar	6	165	33%
(Kelloggs) Nutri-grain				
Apple	1 bar	5	150	30%
Blueberry	1 bar	5	150	30%
Raspberry	1 bar	5	150	30%
Strawberry	1 bar	5	150	30%
Natural Nectar Fi-Bar				
Apple	1 bar	3.5	99	32%
Apple w/oat bran	1 bar	3.5	99	32%
Cocoa almond crunch	1 bar	4.9	130	34%
Cocoa peanut butter	1 bar	5.88	130	41%
Mandarin orange	1 bar	3.5	99	32%
Raspberry	1 bar	3.5	99	32%
Raspberry w/oat bran	1 bar	3.5	99	32%
Strawberry	1 bar	3.5	99	32%
Vanilla almond crunch	1 bar	4.9	130	41%
Vanilla peanut butter	1 bar	5.88	130	41%
Vanilla peanut crunch	1 bar	5.88	130	41%
Oat Bran Bar (Grist Mill)				
Cinnamon	1 bar	4	110	33%

Food and Description	Amount	Fat Grams	Total Calories	% Fat Calories
Honey	1 bar	4	110	33%
Peanut	1 bar	5	115	39%
Smart Start Cereal Bars				
Corn Flakes	1 bar	7	180	35%
Nutri Grain-blueberry	1 bar	7	170	37%
Nutri Grain-strawberry	1 bar	7	170	37%
Oat bran	1 bar	6	170	32%
Raisin Bran	1 bar	6	170	32%
Rice Krispies	1 bar	6	130	42%
Strawberry	1 bar	7	180	35%
Sunbelt				
Baked apple bar	1.31 oz bar	2	130	14%
Macaroon	2 oz bar	16	288	50%
Peanut butter naturals	1.25 oz bar	10	170	53%
Tiger's Milk				
Peanut butter	1 bar	7	160	39%
Peanut butter & honey	1 bar	5	160	28%
Protein rich	1 bar	6	160	34%
Raisin nut crunch	1 bar	9	170	48%
Worthington-Natural Touch				
Caroby Milk Bar	1 bar	9	150	54%

BREAKFAST DRINK(See also BREAKFAST BAR, NUTRITIONAL SUPPLEMENT)
NOTE:Drinks and mixes prepared according to package directions.

Food and Description	Amount	Fat Grams	Total Calories	% Fat Calories
Alba				
Chocolate, Marshmallow, Milk				
Chocolate, Rich chocolate	1	1	110	8%
Alba 77 Fit n Frosty				
Chococolate	1	1	70	13%
Chocolate marshmallow	1	1	70	13%
Double fudge	1	1	70	13%
Strawberry & vanilla	1	–	70	–
Carnation Instant Breakfast				
All flavors				
Dry	1 envl.	1	130	7%
w/whole milk	8 oz	9	280	29%
No sugar				
Chocolate, Chocolate malted	1 envl	1	70	13%
Strawberry, Vanilla	1 envl	–	70	–
Carnation Slender				
Can				
Banana, Chocolate, Chocolate malt,				
Chocolate fudge, Milk chocolate,				
Strawberry, Peach, Vanilla	10 oz	4	220	16%

Food and Description	Amount	Fat Grams	Total Calories	% Fat Calories
Dry				
Chocolate	1 envl	1	110	8%
Dutch chocolate	1 envl	1	110	8%
French vanilla	1 envl	.5	110	4%
Milk & Egg				
Dry	2 Tbs	–	100	–
w/8 oz non-fat milk	1 serving	–	190	–
Lucerne Instant Breakfast				
Chocolate	1 serving	1	130	7%
Coffee	1 serving	–	130	–
Vanilla	1 serving	–	130	–
Mus-L-On-Vanilla				
Dry	5 Tbs	4	330	11%
w/16 oz whole milk	1 serving	22	650	31%
Nutrament Energy Food				
Chocolate	12 oz	10	360	25%
Vanilla	12 oz	10	360	25%
Meritene				
Milk chocolate	4 Tbs	1	120	8%
Vanilla	4 Tbs	1	120	8%
Pillsbury Instant Breakfast				
Chocolate, Chocolate malt				
Dry	1 package	–	130	–
w/8 oz whole milk	1 serving	9	290	28%
Strawberry				
Dry	1 package	–	130	–
w/ 8 oz whole milk	1 serving	9	290	28%
Vanilla				
Dry	1 package	–	140	–
w/ 8 oz whole milk	1 serving	9	300	27%
Resource				
Chocolate	1 packet	8.8	250	32%
Vanilla	1 packet	8.8	250	32%
Super High-Instant				
Dry	3 Tbs	–	90	–
w/8 oz non-fat milk	1 serving	–	180	–
Sustacal				
Chocolate	32 oz	22	960	21%
BREAKFAST SANDWICH (*See also* EGGS, FAST FOOD)				
Biscuits				
(Jimmy Dean)-microwaveable				
Chicken	1	8	170	42%
Sausage	1	14	210	60%
Steak	1	11	190	52%

Food and Description	Amount	Fat Grams	Total Calories	% Fat Calories
Great Starts-Sausage	1	22	410	48%
(Hormel) New Traditions				
Canadian bacon/egg/cheese	1	16	350	41%
Sausage & Egg	1	19	350	49%
(Owens)-microwaveable				
Ham 'N Cheese	1	6	150	36%
Sausage'N Biscuit	1	14	210	60%
Smoked Sausage	1	12	200	54%
(Schwan's)				
Country Steak	1	24	430	50%
Haugin's Farm Sausage	1	11	180	55%
Weight Watchers Sausage	1	11	220	45%
Muffins				
(Jimmy Dean)-microwaveable				
Ham & cheese	1	4	130	28%
Sausage	1	11	190	52%
(Weight Watchers) English				
Muffin Sandwich	1	8	230	31%
Tacos				
(Owens) Border Breakfasts				
Ham	1	6	90	60%
Sausage	1	12	190	57%
BROADBEAN				
boiled	½ cup	< 1	93	5%
canned	½ cup	< 1	91	5%
raw				
immature	8 oz	1	238	4%
mature	8 oz	3.8	766	5%
BROCCOLI				
cooked/chopped	½ cup	–	23	–
frozen				
(Pictsweet)				
Express microwave	2.5 oz	–	20	–
frozen/baby spears				
(Birds Eye)	3.3 oz	–	30	–
frozen/chopped	3.3 oz	–	25	–
(Pictsweet)	3.3 oz	–	25	–
frozen/cut				
(Harvest Fresh)	½ cup	–	18	–
frozen/cuts				
(Green Giant)	½ cup	–	12	–
(Pictsweet)	3.3 oz	–	25	–
frozen/Florentine				
(Pictsweet)	3.2 oz	–	30	–

Food and Description	Amount	Fat Grams	Total Calories	% Fat Calories
frozen/florets (Birds Eye)	3.3 oz	–	25	–
frozen/spears				
(Birds Eye)	3.3 oz	–	25	–
(Harvest Fresh)	½ cup	–	20	–
(Pictsweet)	3.3 oz	–	25	–
frozen individually/spears (Green Giant)	½ cup	–	12	–
frozen w/butter sauce	½ cup	–	58	–
raw/chopped	½ cup	–	12	–
BROCCOLI DISHES				
Broccoli Crisp				
frozen				
(Ore Ida)	3 oz	11	190	52%
Broccoli Cuts in Cheese Sauce				
One serving				
vegetables/frozen				
(Green Giant)	5 oz	3	70	39%
Broccoli in butter sauce, one serving				
vegetables/frozen				
(Green Giant)	4.5 oz	2	45	40%
Broccoli in cheese sauce, frozen				
(Birds Eye)	5 oz	6	120	45%
Broccoli in cheese sauce, frozen				
Micro Quick (Freshlike)	4.5 oz	3	70	39%
Broccoli in cheese flavored sauce, frozen				
(Green Giant)	½ cup	2	60	30%
Broccoli in creamy Italian sauce, frozen				
(Birds Eye)	4.5 oz	6	90	60%
Broccoli in White Cheddar Cheese Flavored Sauce, frozen				
(Green Giant)	½ cup	3	50	54%
Broccoli Stuffed Shells, frozen				
(Celentano)	6.75 oz	15	280	48%
BROCCOLI SOUP (*See* SOUP)				
BROTWURST (*See* LUNCHEON MEATS)				
BROWNIE(*See also* COOKIE)				
Box Mix				
(Betty Crocker)				
Chocolate Chip	¹⁄₂₄ pkg	6	140	39%
Frosted (Stir'n Frost)	⅙ pkg	9	250	22%
Frosted	¹⁄₂₄ pkg	6	160	34%
Fudge (regular size)	¹⁄₁₆ pkg	6	150	36%
Fudge (family size)	¹⁄₂₄ pkg	5	130	35%
German Chocolate	¹⁄₂₄ pkg	7	160	39%
Supreme Fudge	¹⁄₂₄ pkg	3	120	23%
Walnut	¹⁄₂₄ pkg	7	140	45%

Food and Description	Amount	Fat Grams	Total Calories	% Fat Calories
(Betty Crocker)-Bake Shop Brownie Mix				
Caramel Pecan	1/16 pkg	8	220	33%
Chunky Chocolate Walnut	1/16 pkg	10	230	39%
(Betty Crocker)-Microwave				
Frosted	1/8 pkg	7	180	35%
Fudge	1/8 pkg	5	140	32%
Walnut	1/8 pkg	7	160	39%
(Betty Crocker)-Microrave Singles				
w/hot fudge topping	1	12	350	31%
(Duncan Hines)				
Chewy Recipe Fudge	1	5	130	35%
Gourmet Truffle	1	13	280	42%
Gourmet Turtle	1	9	200	41%
Gourmet Vienna White	1	12	240	45%
Milk Chocolate	1	7	160	39%
Original Double Fudge	1	6	150	36%
Peanut Butter Fudge	1	8	150	48%
(Estee)-2"x2"	1	2	45	40%
(Pillsbury)				
Deluxe Family-Sized Fudge	2" square	7	150	42%
Deluxe Fudge Brownie	2" square	6	150	36%
Deluxe Fudge Brownie w/walnuts	2" square	8	150	48%
Lovin' Lites-Fudge	1	2	100	18%
Ultimate Caramel Fudge Chunk	2" square	7	170	37%
Ultimate Chunky Triple Fudge	2" square	7	170	37%
Ultimate Double Fudge	2" square	6	160	34%
Ultimate Rocky Road Fudge	2" square	8	170	42%
commercial-w/frosting	~ 3/4 oz	4	100	36%
fudge (Little Debbie)	2 oz	8	260	28%
	3 oz	12	350	31%
frozen (Weight Watchers)				
chocolate	1.25 oz	3	100	27%
cheesecake	3.5 oz	6	200	27%
homemade-w/frosting (1-3/4x1-3/4x7/8")	1	6	95	57%
butterscotch (1-3/4x1-3/4x7/8")	1	5	115	39%
microwave (Pillsbury)				
Fudge brownie	1	9	190	43%
Fudge brownie w/chocolate				
fudge frosting	1	11	240	41%
Walnut brownie	1	12	210	51%
microwave ready fudge brownie				
w/choc flavored chips (Pillsbury)	1	9	180	45%
pouch mix (Robin Hood/Gold Medal) prepared				
Fudge Brownie	1	4	100	36%

Food and Description	Amount	Fat Grams	Total Calories	% Fat Calories
ready-to-eat				
Brownie Nut Bar (Bakery Wagon)	1 cookie	4	97	37%
Fudge Brownie (Break Cake)	1-2.8 oz	18	370	44%
BRUSSELS SPROUTS				
fresh-cooked	½ cup	–	30	–
frozen				
(Green Giant)	½ cup	–	25	–
(Freshlike)	3.3 oz	–	35	–
(Pictsweet)	3.3 oz	–	35	–
(Pictsweet)				
Express Microwave	2.5 oz	–	30	–
frozen-cooked	½ cup	–	33	–
BRUSSELS SPROUTS DISHES				
Baby Brussels Sprouts in cheese sauce, frozen				
(Birds Eye)	4.5 oz	6	110	49%
Brussels Sprouts in butter sauce, frozen				
(Green Giant)	½ cup	1	40	23%
Brussels Sprouts in cheese flavored sauce, frozen				
(Green Giant)	½ cup	2	70	26%
BUCKWHEAT KERNELS				
Kasha roasted (Wolff's)	¼ cup	–	145	–
BUFFALO (BISON)/raw	3 oz	1.8	93	17%
BULGAR/canned	1 serving	0.9	227	4%
BURBOT/raw	3 oz	.68	76	8%
BURDOCK-root				
cooked	1 cup	< 1	110	4%
raw	1 cup	< 1	85	5%
BURGER-LIKE MEAL ENHANCER	~ 4 oz	< 1	90	5%
BURGER MIX	1 oz	.7	90	7%
BUTTER (*See also* BUTTER BLENDS, BUTTER SUBSTITUTE, MARGARINE)				
sweet/salted and unsalted	1 pat	4	36	100%
	1 Tbs	11	100	100%
	1 stick/			
	4 oz	92	810	100%
	1 Tbs	11	100	100%
(Hotel Bar/Keller's)	1 tsp	4	35	100%
(Land O'Lakes)	1 Tbs	11	100	100%
	1 tsp	4	35	100%
whipped	1 pat	3	27	100%
	1 stick/			
	4 oz	61	542	100%
	1 Tbs	9	81	100%
(Land O'Lakes)	1 Tbs	7	60	100%
	1 tsp	3	25	100%

Food and Description	Amount	Fat Grams	Total Calories	% Fat Calories
BUTTER BEAN				
canned				
(Joan of Arc/Green Giant)	½ cup	–	80	–
(S&W)				
tender cooked-dry	½ cup	–	100	–
(Van Camp's)	1 cup	1	160	6%
Speckled/canned Seasoned				
–w/Pork (Luck's)	7.5 oz	8	230	31%
BUTTER BLENDS				
(Blue Bonnet)				
Stick and Tub	1 Tbs	11	90	100%
	4 oz	44	360	100%
(Buttery Blend), liquid	1 Tbs	14	120	100%
honey butter (Downey's)				
cinnamon	1 Tbs	1	50	18%
original	1 Tbs	1	50	18%
(Kraft) Touch of Butter Spread				
bowl	1 Tbs	6		50%
stick-50% fat	1 Tbs	7	60	100%
(Land O'Lakes) Country Morning Blend				
stick				
light	1 tsp	2	20	100%
salted	1 Tbs	11	100	100%
unsalted	1 Tbs	11	100	100%
	1 tsp	4	35	100%
tub				
light	1 tsp	2	20	100%
salted	1 Tbs	10	90	100%
unsalted	1 Tbs	10	90	100%
	1 tsp	3	30	100%
(Land O'Lakes) Spread				
w/sweet cream	1 tsp	3	25	100%
BUTTER SUBSTITUTE				
Best of Butter/plain	½ tsp	< 1	4	100%
cheddar cheese flavor	½ tsp	< 1	6	75%
sour cream flavor	½ tsp	< 1	4	100%
Butter Buds Butter Flavored Mix	1 Tbs=			
	½ oz	–	6	–
Butter Buds Sprinkles	½ tsp	–	4	–
Butter Flavored Salt	no set			
	amount	–	–	–
Buttery Spray				
(Weight Watchers)	1 second			
	spray	.5	2	100%

Food and Description	Amount	Fat Grams	Total Calories	% Fat Calories
Imitation Butter Flavor Salt	no set amount	–	–	–
Molly McButter/butter	½ tsp	–	4	–
Cheese flavor	½ tsp	–	4	–
sour cream flavor	½ tsp	–	4	–
BUTTERBUR				
cooked	½ cup	< 1	8	56%
raw	1 cup	< 1	13	35%
BUTTERFISH				
raw	3 oz	6.8	124	49%
BUTTERNUTS				
dried	1 oz	16	174	83%

C

Food and Description	Amount	Fat Grams	Total Calories	% Fat Calories
CABBAGE				
Chinese				
raw/shredded	1/12 cup	–	5	–
fresh-cooked	½ cup	–	10	–
Red, raw/shredded	½ cup	–	10	–
Savoy, raw	1 cup	–	12	–
Spoon, raw	1 cup	–	37	–
Swamp, fresh-cooked	1 cup	–	21	–
White				
raw/shredded	½ cup	–	12	–
fresh-cooked	½ cup	–	16	–
CABBAGE DISHES, Stuffed, homemade	~ 5 oz	18	310	52%
CAKE AND CAKE PASTRY (*See also* PASTRY SHEET; PASTRY SHELL; PASTRY,TOASTER)				
CAKE				
(NOTE: Cakes, both homemade and from mix, were made with vegetable shortening. The frostings were made with margarine. Homemade cookies were made with margarine. All pie crusts were made with enriched flour & vegetable shortening.)				
Angelfood (Break Cake)	1 oz	–	70	–
Angelfood-box mix (Betty Crocker)-				
Chocolate	1/12 cake	–	150	–
Confetti	1/12 cake	–	160	–
Lemon Custard	1/12 cake	–	150	–

Food and Description	Amount	Fat Grams	Total Calories	% Fat Calories
Strawberry	1/12 cake	–	150	–
Traditional	1/12 cake	–	130	–
White	1/12 cake	–	150	–
(Duncan Hines)	1/12 cake	–	140	–
Apple Cinnamon Coffee cake-box mix-				
(Pillsbury)	1/8 cake	7	240	20%
Applesauce	3 oz	12	400	27%
Baklava/homemade	2 oz	18	250	65%
Banana-frozen-(Sara Lee)	1 slice	6	170	32%
Black Forest-frozen-(Sara Lee)	1 slice	8	190	38%
frozen (Weight Watchers)	3 oz	5	180	25%
Boston Cream Pie (See PIE)				
frozen-(Pepperidge Farm)	2 7/8 oz	14	290	43%
(Weight Watchers)	3 oz	4	190	19%
Box mixes				
(Betty Crocker)-Classics Dessert Mixes				
Boston Cream Pie	1/8 pkg	6	270	20%
Golden Pound Cake	1/12 cake	9	200	41%
Lemon Chiffon Cake	1/12 cake	4	200	18%
Pineapple Upside-Down Cake	1/9 cake	10	250	36%
(Betty Crocker)-Microrave Singles				
Chocolate w/chocolate frosting	1 cake	18	440	37%
Yellow w/ chocolate frosting	1 cake	19	440	39%
(Betty Crocker)-Pudding Cake Mixes				
Chocolate and lemon	1/6 cake	5	230	20%
(Betty Crocker)-Snackin' Cake				
Applesauce Raisin	1/9 cake	6	190	28%
Banana Walnut	1/9 cake	7	200	25%
Golden Chocolate Chip	1/9 cake	5	190	24%
(Betty Crocker)-Stir 'N Frost (with frosting)				
Chocolate Devil's Food				
w/choc frosting	1/6 cake	5	210	21%
Spice Cake w/vanilla frosting	1/16 cake	9	280	28%
Yellow Cake w/chocolate frosting	1/16 cake	8	220	33%
(Betty Crocker)-Supermoist				
Apple Cinnamon	1/12 cake	10	250	36%
Butter Brickle	1/12 cake	10	250	36%
Butter Pecan	1/12 cake	11	250	40%
Butter Recipe/chocolate	1/12 cake	13	270	43%
Butter Recipe/yellow	1/12 cake	11	260	38%
Carrot	1/12 cake	11	250	40%
Cherry Chip	1/12 cake	3	190	14%
Chocolate Chip	1/12 cake	14	280	45%
Chocolate Choc Chip	1/12 cake	12	260	42%

Food and Description	Amount	Fat Grams	Total Calories	% Fat Calories
Chocolate Fudge	1/12 cake	12	260	42%
Devil's Food	1/12 cake	12	260	42%
German Chocolate	1/12 cake	12	260	42%
Golden Vanilla	1/12 cake	14	280	45%
Lemon	1/12 cake	11	260	38%
Marble	1/12 cake	11	250	40%
Milk Chocolate	1/12 cake	12	260	42%
Rainbow Chip	1/12 cake	11	250	40%
Sour Cream Choc	1/12 cake	12	260	42%
Sour Cream White	1/12 cake	3	180	15%
Spice	1/12 cake	11	260	38%
White	1/12 cake	9	240	34%
Yellow	1/12 cake	11	260	38%
(Betty Crocker)-Supermoist Light Mixes				
Devils Food				
No Cholesterol	1/12 cake	3	180	15%
Standard Recipe	1/12 cake	4	190	19%
White	1/12 cake	3	180	15%
Yellow				
No Cholesterol	1/12 cake	3	180	15%
Standard Recipe	1/12 cake	4	190	19%
(Dromedary) - Carrot Cake	1 piece	15	232	58%
(Duncan Hines)-Delights				
Devil's Food	1/12 cake	5	180	25%
Fudge Marble	1/12 cake	4	180	20%
Lemon	1/12 cake	4	180	20%
Yellow	1/12 cake	4	180	20%
(Duncan Hines) - (Original Directions)				
Angel Food	1/12 cake	–	140	–
Butter Recipe				
Fudge	1/12 cake	13	270	43%
Golden	1/12 cake	13	270	43%
Dark Dutch Fudge	1/12 cake	15	280	48%
Devil's Food	1/12 cake	15	280	48%
Fudge Marble	1/12 cake	11	260	38%
French Vanilla	1/12 cake	11	260	38%
Lemon Supreme	1/12 cake	11	260	38%
Pineapple Supreme	1/12 cake	11	260	38%
Spice	1/12 cake	11	260	38%
Strawberry Supreme	1/12 cake	11	260	38%
Swiss Chocolate	1/12 cake	15	280	48%
White	1/12 cake	10	250	36%
Yellow	1/12 cake	11	260	38%

Food and Description	Amount	Fat Grams	Total Calories	% Fat Calories
(Duncan Hines)-Tiarra Dessert Mixes				
Black Forest Mousse	1/12 cake	13	260	45%
Cherries & Cream	1/12 cake	11	250	40%
Chocolate Mousse	1/12 cake	16	270	53%
Chocolate Amaretto Mousse	1/12 cake	16	270	53%
(Entenmann's)-Fat Free				
Apple Cinnamon Twist	1.1 oz	–	90	–
Apple Spice	1 oz	–	80	–
Blueberry Crunch Coffee Cake	1 oz	–	90	–
Cheese Filled Crumb Coffee Cake	1.3 oz	–	90	–
Cherry Cheese Coffee Cake	1.3 oz	–	90	–
Cinnamon Apple Coffee Cake	1.3 oz	–	90	–
Chocolate Loaf	1 oz	–	70	–
Fudge Iced Gold Cake	1.4 oz	–	90	–
Golden Loaf	1 oz	–	80	–
Lemon Twist Coffee Cake	1.1 oz	–	90	–
Louisiana Crunch	1 oz	–	80	–
Marble Loaf	1 oz	–	70	–
Orange Cake	1 oz	–	70	–
Pineapple Cheese Coffee Cake	1.3 oz	–	90	–
Pineapple Crunch Cake	1 oz	–	70	–
Raspberry Twist	1.1 oz	–	90	–
(Estee)-Chocolate-box mix	1/10 cake	2	100	18%
all other flavors	1/10 cake	2	100	18%
(Hostess) 97% fat free				
Cinnamon Crumb Coffee Cake	1 cake	1	80	11%
(Pillsbury)-Mix				
Bundt				
Chocolate Caramel	1/16 cake	16	310	46%
Chocolate Eclair	1/16 cake	10	270	33%
Lovin' Lites				
Chocolate				
Egg White Recipe	1/12 cake	2	160	11%
Egg Recipe	1/12 cake	3	170	16%
Yellow				
Egg White Recipe	1/12 cake	2	170	11%
Egg Recipe	1/12 cake	3	180	15%
Lovin' Loaf-Angel Food	1/8 cake	–	90	–
Microwave Snack Cakes				
Banana Walnut	1/9 cake	12	210	51%
Carrot	1/9 cake	11	200	44%
Streusel Coffee Cake (Refrigerated)				
Cinnamon Swirl	1 slice	9	180	45%
Pecan Crumb	1 slice	9	180	45%

Food and Description	Amount	Fat Grams	Total Calories	% Fat Calories
(Pillsbury Plus)				
Applesauce	1/12 cake	11	250	40%
Applesauce Spice	1/12 cake	11	250	40%
Banana	1/12 cake	11	250	40%
Butter Recipe	1/12 cake	12	260	42%
Carrot & Spice	1/12 cake	11	260	38%
Chocolate Chip	1/12 cake	14	270	47%
Confetti	1/12 cake	9	240	34%
Dark Chocolate	1/12 cake	12	250	43%
Devil's Food	1/12 cake	14	270	47%
Fudge Marble	1/12 cake	12	270	40%
German Choc	1/12 cake	11	250	40%
Lemon	1/12 cake	11	250	40%
Strawberry	1/12 cake	11	260	42%
White				
Basic Recipe	1/12 cake	10	230	39%
No Cholesterol Recipe	1/12 cake	4	190	19%
Yellow	1/12 cake	12	260	42%
Brownie Cheese Cake/frozen				
(Weight Watchers)	3.5 oz	6	220	25%
(Bundt) Ring				
Black Forest Cherry	1/16 cake	8	240	30%
Boston Cream	1/16 cake	10	270	33%
Chocolate Macaroon	1/16 cake	10	240	38%
Pineapple	1/16 cake	9	260	31%
Pound	1/16 cake	9	230	35%
(Royal)-No Bake				
Cheese Cake-Lite	1 piece	10	210	43%
Real	1 piece	9	280	29%
(Streusel Swirl)				
Cinnamon	1/16 cake	11	260	38%
Lemon	1/16 cake	11	270	37%
Tunnel of Fudge	1/16 cake	12	260	42%
Tunnel of Lemon	1/16 cake	9	270	30%
Butterscotch Pecan-frozen				
(Pepperidge Farm)	1 5/8 oz	7	160	40%
Caramel Cake-homemade				
no icing 8" dia	1/12 cake	10	218	42%
w/caramel icing	1/12 cake	12	315	34%
Carrot w/cream cheese frosting				
frozen-(Pepperidge Farm)	1 3/8 oz	8	140	51%
homemade (10"dia)	1/10 cake	21	385	49%
Carrot Cakes (Break Cake)	2 cakes	12	370	29%
frozen-(Sara Lee)	1 slice	13	260	45%

Food and Description	Amount	Fat Grams	Total Calories	% Fat Calories
(Weight Watchers)	3 oz	5	170	27%
Cheesecake, (9" dia)	1/12 cake	18	280	58%
box mix (Jell-O) 8" w/whole milk	1/8 cake	13	280	42%
(Jell-O) real fruit topping				
Cherry/dry	1/8 pkg	4	220	16%
-prepared w/ whole milk	1/8 pkg	13	330	35%
Strawberry/dry	1/8 pkg	4	220	16%
-prepared w/ whole milk	1/8 pkg	13	330	35%
(Formagg) Le Creame				
Amaretto/almond	2 oz	6	130	42%
Pineapple	2 oz	6	130	42%
Plain	2 oz	6	130	42%
Strawberry	2 oz	6	130	42%
frozen (Weight Watchers)	3.9 oz	7	220	29%
French-frozen (Sara Lee)	1 slice	13	200	59%
New York-box mix				
(Jell-O)- No Bake	1/8 cake	14	290	43%
Cheesecake-Strawberry-frozen				
(Weight Watchers)	3.9 oz	5	180	25%
Cherries & Cream Cake/frozen				
(Weight Watchers)	3.5 oz	5	190	24%
Chocolate				
frozen				
(Pepperidge Farm)	2 7/8 oz	17	310	49%
(Sara Lee) Free & Light	1 slice/1 oz	–	110	–
(Weight Watchers)	2.5 oz	5	190	24%
homemade-no icing (9"dia)	1/12 cake	13	272	43%
w/chocolate icing	1/12 cake	16	365	40%
Chocolate Fudge-frozen				
(Pepperidge Farm)	1 5/8 oz	10	180	50%
Chocolate Fudge Stripe-frozen				
(Pepperidge Farm)	1 5/8 oz	9	170	48%
Chocolate Mint-frozen				
(Pepperidge Farm)	1 5/8 oz	9	170	48%
Chocolate Mousse-frozen (Sara Lee)	1 slice	14	200	63%
Coconut-frozen-(Pepperidge Farm)	1 5/8 oz	8	180	40%
Coffeecake-box mix				
(Pillsbury)-Apple Cinn.	1/8 cake	7	240	26%
Coffeecake-crumb	~ 2.5 oz	7	230	27%
frozen-(Sara Lee)				
Apple Cinnamon	1 cake	13	290	40%
Butter Streusel	1 cake	12	230	47%
Pecan	1 cake	16	280	51%

Food and Description	Amount	Fat Grams	Total Calories	% Fat Calories
(Weight Watcher)-w/cinnamon streusel	2.25 oz	7	190	33%
Cottage Pudding/homemade				
no sauce	3 oz	8	251	29%
w/chocolate sauce	3 oz	8.7	315	25%
Cupcakes (See SNACK CAKES)				
Devil's Food				
frozen-(Pepperidge Farm)	1⅝ oz	9	180	45%
homemade w/choc icing (9" dia)	1/16 cake	8	235	31%
Pound Cake/frozen (Sara Lee)				
Free & Light	1 slice/1 oz	–	70	–
Fruitcake				
homemade-dark (7.5" dia)	1/32 cake	7	165	38%
(Manor)				
plain	2 oz	11	240	41%
Cherry Rapture	2 oz	15	260	52%
deluxe	2 oz	6	210	26%
French Apple Walnut	2 oz	16	260	55%
Macadamia Surprise	2 oz	14	240	53%
German Chocolate				
(Pepperidge Farm)	1⅝ oz	10	180	50%
frozen (Weight Watchers)	2.5 oz	7	200	32%
Gingerbread-/homemade 8"square	⅑ cake	4	175	21%
box mix (Betty Crocker)	⅑ pkg	7	220	29%
box mix (Pillsbury)	3" square	4	190	19%
Golden-frozen-(Pepperidge Farm)	1⅝ oz	9	180	45%
Lemon Coconut-frozen				
(Pepperidge Farm)	3 oz	13	280	42%
Microwave box mixes (Pillsbury)				
Chocolate Cake	⅛ cake	13	210	56%
Double Chocolate Supreme	⅛ cake	19	330	52%
Double Lemon Supreme	⅛ cake	15	300	45%
Lemon	⅛ cake	13	220	53%
Streusel Swirl-Cinnamon	⅛ cake	11	240	41%
Tunnel of Fudge Bundt	⅛ cake	17	290	53%
Yellow	⅛ cake	13	220	53%
Microwave box mixes w/frosting				
(Betty Crocker)-Microrave				
Chocolate Fudge w/vanilla frst	⅙ cake	16	310	47%
Lemon w/lemon frosting	⅙ cake	16	300	48%
German Choc w/coconut pecan frst	⅙ cake	17	310	49%
Devil's Food w/choc frosting	⅙ cake	16	300	48%
Golden Vanilla w/rainbow chip frst	⅙ cake	16	310	47%
Yellow w/chocolate fosting	⅙ cake	16	300	48%

Food and Description	Amount	Fat Grams	Total Calories	% Fat Calories
(Pillsbury) -				
Chocolate cake w/choc frosting	1/8 cake	17	300	51%
Chocolate cake				
w/choc fudge frosting	1/8 cake	17	300	51%
Chocolate cake w/vanilla frosting	1/8 cake	17	300	51%
Lemon cake w/lemon frosting	1/8 cake	17	300	51%
Yellow cake w/choc frosting	1/8 cake	17	300	51%
Peach Melba-frozen (Pepperidge Farm)	3½ oz	7	270	23%
(Pepperidge Farm)-Dessert Light-individual servings-frozen				
Apple'n Spice	1 pkg	2	170	11%
Cherry Cake Supreme	1 pkg	2	170	11%
Lemon Cake Supreme	1 pkg	5	170	27%
Peach Parfait	1 pkg	5	150	30%
Raspberry Vanilla Swirl	1 pkg	5	160	28%
Strawberry ShortCake	1 pkg	5	170	27%
Pineapple Cream-frozen (Pepperidge)	2 oz	7	190	33%
Pound-8½x3½x3¼"	1/17 cake	5	120	38%
Butter-frozen (Pepperidge Farm)	1	7	130	49%
Butter-frozen (Sara Lee)	1 slice	7	130	49%
Cholesterol Free				
frozen-(Pepperidge Farm)	1	6	110	49%
Mix (Martha White)	1/10 cake	4	120	30%
w/blueberry topping/frozen				
(Weight Watchers)	2.5 oz	6	180	30%
Prune Whip (baked)/homemade				
hot	1 cup	–	140	–
cold	1 cup	–	203	–
Raspberry Mocha-frozen				
(Pepperidge Farm)	3⅛ oz	14	310	41%
(Sara Lee) Lights-frozen				
Chocolate Mousse	1 pkg	9	180	45%
Double Chocolate	1 pkg	5	160	28%
French Cheese Cake	1 pkg	6	180	30%
Lemon Cream Cake	1 pkg	7	190	–
Strawberry	1 pkg	4	160	23%
Sheet				
w/no-cook white frosting 9"sq.	1/9 cake	14	445	28%
w/o frosting	1/9 cake	12	315	34%
CAKE PASTRY				
Cinnamon bun	1/~ 2 oz	5	174	26%
frosted	1/~ 2 oz	5	185	24%
refrig w/icing (Hungry Jack)	2	14	290	43%
refrigerated w/icing (Pillsbury)	1	4.5	115	35%
Coffee Cakes (See CAKE)				

Food and Description	Amount	Fat Grams	Total Calories	% Fat Calories
Cream Puff w/custard filling				
(3⅓" dia 2" high)	1	18	303	54%
shell only	2 oz	10	136	66%
frozen (Rich's)	1	8	146	49%
Danish (4½"dia)	1/~2 oz	12	220	49%
frozen (Sara Lee)				
Apple	1	6	120	45%
Apple (Free & Light)	1	–	130	–
Cheese	1	8	130	31%
Cinnamon Raisin	1	8	150	27%
refrigerated-(Pillsbury)				
Best Apple	1	11	240	41%
Best Quick Cinnamon	1	9	210	39%
Caramel w/nuts	2	16	310	47%
Cinnamon Raisin w/icing	2	14	290	43%
Orange	2	14	290	43%
Danish				
(Earth Grains)				
Apple	2 oz	8	210	34%
Bear Claw	2.25 oz	11	260	38%
Cheese	1.92 oz	10	220	41%
Cherry	1.92 oz	8	210	34%
Cinnamon	1.67 oz	9	200	41%
Raisin Nut	1.67 oz	10	210	43%
(Hostess)				
Apple	1 Danish	20	360	50%
Butterhorn	1 Danish	18	330	49%
Raspberry	1 Danish	7	270	23%
Raisin Rounds	1	2	140	13%
Danish with fruit (4 ½"dia)	1/~2oz	13	235	50%
Eclair-chocolate icing/custard filling	1	13.6	239	51%
chocolate/frozen (Rich's)	1	10	210	43%
Honey Buns (Break Cake)	1-3 oz	28	410	62%
Hot Cross Bun	2 oz	8	190	38%
Napoleon	1 medium	15	285	47%
Sweet Rolls				
Apple Sweet Roll				
frozen-(Weight Watchers)	4.5 oz	4	160	23%
Cheese Sweet Roll (Weight Watchers)				
frozen	5 oz	5	180	25%
Cinnamon Nut Rolls (Break Cake)	2-3 oz	11	330	33%
Cinnamon Roll-frozen-(Sara Lee)				
All Butter	1	10	230	39%
w/icing	1	10	290	31%

Food and Description	Amount	Fat Grams	Total Calories	% Fat Calories
Turnovers				
frozen-(Pepperidge Farm)				
Apple	1	17	300	51%
Blueberry	1	19	320	53%
Cherry	1	19	310	55%
Peach	1	19	320	53%
Raspberry	1	18	320	51%
refrigerated-(Pillsbury)-All flavors	1	8	170	42%
CAKE ICING				
DECORATORS-CAKE & COOKIE (Pillsbury)				
Chocolate	1 Tbs	2	60	30%
Other flavors	1 Tbs	2	70	26%
FROSTING-BOX MIX				
(Betty Crocker)				
Chocolate fudge	1/12 cake	6	180	30%
Chocolate fudge creamy	1/12 cake	6	170	32%
Chocolate sour cream	1/12 cake	8	160	45%
Coconut pecan	1/12 cake	8	150	48%
Creamy cherry	1/12 cake	6	180	30%
Creamy vanilla	1/12 cake	5	170	27%
Creamy white creamy	1/12 cake	6	190	28%
Fluffy	1/12 cake	–	70	–
Lemon	1/12 cake	6	10	54%
Milk chocolate	1/12 cake	5	170	27%
Rainbow chip	1/12 cake	6	180	30%
Sour cream chocolate fudge	1/12 cake	6	180	30%
Sour cream white	1/12 cake	5	170	27%
(Estee)- all flavors	1½ Tbs	1-2	50-60	18%-30%
(Pillsbury)				
Chocolate/Frost It Hot	1/8 cake	–	50	–
Coconut almond	1/12 cake	10	160	56%
Coconut pecan	1/12 cake	7	150	42%
Fluffy white	1/12 cake	–	60	–
Fluffy white/Frost It Hot	1/8 cake	–	50	–
Standard Home Recipe (USDA)				
Boiled	1/4 cup	–	74	–
Caramel	1/4 cup	6	306	18%
Chocolate	1/4 cup	9.5	259	33%
Coconut	1/4 cup	3	151	18%
White	1/4 cup	5	300	15%
FROSTING-READY-TO-SPREAD				
(Betty Crocker)				
Amaretto almond	1/12 cake	6	160	34%
Butter pecan	1/12 cake	7	170	37%
Caramel nut	1/12 cake	8	160	45%

Food and Description	Amount	Fat Grams	Total Calories	% Fat Calories
Cherry	1/12 cake	6	160	34%
Chocolate	1/12 cake	7	160	39%
Chocolate coconut almond	1/12 cake	8	160	45%
Coconut pecan	1/12 cake	9	160	51%
Chocolate sour cream fudge	1/12 cake	8	160	45%
Cream cheese	1/12 cake	6	160	34%
Creamy white	1/12 cake	6	190	28%
Dark dutch fudge	1/12 cake	7	160	39%
Double chocolate chip	1/12 cake	8	170	42%
Lemon	1/12 cake	6	160	34%
Milk chocolate	1/12 cake	6	160	34%
Rainbow chip	1/12 cake	7	170	37%
w/mini morsels	1/2 cake	7	170	37%
Rocky road	1/12 cake	7	150	42%
w/mini morsels	1/12 cake	8	160	45%
Sour cream chocolate	1/2 cake	7	160	39%
Sour cream white	1/12 cake	6	160	34%
Vanilla	1/12 cake	6	160	34%
(Betty Crocker) Creamy Deluxe				
Light Chocolate	1/12 cake	2	130	14%
Light Vanilla	1/12 cake	2	140	13%
Party Frosting				
Chocolate w/Dinosaurs	1/12 cake	7	160	39%
Vanilla w/Teddy Bears	1/12 cake	6	160	34%
(Duncan Hines)				
Chocolate	1/12 cake	7	160	39%
Cream cheese	1/12 cake	8	160	45%
Dark Dutch fudge	1/12 cake	7	160	39%
Milk chocolate	1/12 cake	7	160	39%
Polka dot pink & vanilla	1/12 cake	7	160	39%
Vanilla	1/12 cake	7	160	39%
(Pillsbury)				
Chocolate fudge	1/8 cake	5	110	41%
Chocolate fudge funfetti	1/12 cake	6	140	39%
Frosting supreme				
Caramel pecan	1/12 cake	8	160	45%
Chocolate chip	1/12 cake	5	150	30%
Chocolate fudge	1/12 cake	6	150	36%
Chocolate mint	1/12 cake	7	150	42%
Chocolate mocha	1/12 cake	6	150	36%
Coconut almond	1/12 cake	9	150	54%
Coconut pecan	1/12 cake	10	160	56%
Cream cheese	1/12 cake	6	160	34%
Double Dutch	1/12 cake	6	140	39%

Food and Description	Amount	Fat Grams	Total Calories	% Fat Calories
Lemon	1/12 cake	6	160	34%
Milk chocolate	1/12 cake	6	150	36%
Sour cream vanilla	1/2 cake	6	160	34%
Strawberry	1/12 cake	6	160	34%
Vanilla	1/12 cake	6	160	34%
Vanilla	1/8 cake	5	120	38%
Vanilla funfetti	1/12 cake	6	150	36%
(Lovin Lites)				
Chocolate	1/12 cake	2	120	15%
Vanilla	1/12 cake	2	130	14%
Swirl				
Milk Chocolate w/Fudge	1/12 cake	6	150	36%
Vanilla w/Fudge	1/12 cake	6	150	36%
CALIFORNIA RED BEAN, boiled	1/2 cup	–	109	–
CANDY				
Almond Joy (Peter Paul)	1 oz	7	132	48%
(Andes) Creme De Menthe	1 oz	9	150	54%
Baby Ruth	1 oz	6	130	42%
Baby Ruth	2.2 oz	13	300	39%
nuggets	1 oz	6	130	42%
Bar None	1.5 oz	14	240	53%
Bit-O-Honey Bar (Nestle)	1.7 oz	4	200	18%
Black Cow-sucker	1 oz	3	127	21%
Bonkers!/all flavors	1	–	20	–
(Bounty)-dark chocolate & coconut bar	2.1 oz	8	150	48%
milk chocolate & coconut bar	2.1 oz	8	150	48%
(Brach's) candies-Bridge Mix	1 oz	6	130	42%
Broxie-Big	1 oz	8	150	48%
Little	1 oz	8	150	48%
Butterscotch Disks	1 oz	–	110	–
Candy corn	1 oz	–	100	–
Choc Cov'd Buttercream Egg	1 oz	3	120	23%
Choc Cov'd Chelsea Chips	1 oz	6	140	39%
Chocolate Covered Cherries	1 oz	2	110	16%
Choc Cov'd Cherry Cream Egg	1 oz	2	110	16%
Choc Cov'd Coconut Cream Egg	1 oz	3	110	16%
Choc Cov'd Fruit & Nut Cream Egg	1 oz	2	110	16%
Choc Cov'd Maple Cream Eggs	1 oz	2	110	16%
Choc Cov'd Mint Patties	1 oz	2	110	16%
Choc Cov'd Vanilla Cream	1 oz	2	110	16%
Chocolate Cov'd Mint Cremes	1 oz	2	110	16%
Chocolate Cov'd Mints	1 oz	2	110	16%
Choc Cov'd Orange Sticks	1 oz	2	110	16%
Choc Cov'd Thin Mints	1 oz	2	110	16%

Food and Description	Amount	Fat Grams	Total Calories	% Fat Calories
Chocolate Creme Cherries	1 oz	2	110	16%
Chocolate Jots	1 oz	5	130	35%
Chocolate Malted Milk Eggs	1 oz	5	130	35%
Christmas Jots	1 oz	5	130	35%
Christmas Mint Pearls	1 oz	1	110	8%
Christmas Nougats	1 oz	2	110	16%
Christmas Ornaments	1 oz	8	150	48%
Cinnamon Disks	1 oz	–	110	–
Cinnamon Imperials	1 oz	–	110	–
Coffee	1 oz	2	120	15%
Crazy Pumpkin Heads	1 oz	1	100	9%
Creme De Menthe Mint	1 oz	9	150	54%
Dark Choc Covered Cherries	1 oz	2	110	16%
Dark Choc Cov'd Hulachews	1 oz	8	140	51%
Dark Chocolate Nonpariels	1 oz	6	140	39%
Dark Choc X-Mas Nonpariels	1 oz	6	140	39%
Dessert mints	1 oz	–	110	–
Easter Nougats	1 oz	1	100	9%
Filled Peanuts	1 oz	1	110	8%
French Burnt Peanuts	1 oz	5	130	35%
Fruit Bunch	1 oz	–	100	–
Gumdinger Gum Balls	1 oz	2	110	16%
Gummy Worms	1 oz	–	100	–
Heart Box Candies	1 oz	2	110	16%
Holiday Mints	1 oz	1	110	8%
Jelly Beans	1 oz	–	100	–
Jelly Nougats	1 oz	1	100	–
Jordan Apples	1 oz	2	120	15%
Jube Jels	1 oz	–	100	–
Lemon Drops	1 oz	–	110	–
Lollydrops	1 oz	–	110	–
Love	1 oz	8	150	48%
Kentucky Mints	1 oz	–	110	–
Licorice Twists	1 oz	1	100	9%
Marshmallow Eggs	1 oz	3	120	23%
Marshmallow Rabbits	1 oz	3	120	23%
Marshmallow Santas	1 oz	3	120	23%
Milk Choc Cashew Clusters	1 oz	5	130	35%
Milk Choc Covered Cherries	1 oz	2	110	16%
Milk Choc Covered Malt Balls	1 oz	5	130	35%
Milk Choc Covered Peanuts	1 oz	9	150	54%
Milk Choc Covered Putters	1 oz	9	150	54%
Milk Choc Peanut Clusters	1 oz	9	150	54%
Milk Chocolate Stars	1 oz	8	150	48%

Food and Description	Amount	Fat Grams	Total Calories	% Fat Calories
Milk Maid Caramels	1 oz	2	110	16%
chocolate	1 oz	3	110	25%
Mint Filled Straws	1 oz	1	110	8%
Mint Jots	1 oz	2	120	15%
Mint Parfait	1 oz	9	150	54%
Mint Pearls	1 oz	2	120	15%
Neapolitan Coconuts	1 oz	2	120	15%
Nut Goodies	1 oz	4	130	28%
Orangettes	1 oz	–	100	–
PBM Easter Eggs	1 oz	10	160	56%
PBM Heart	1 oz	9	150	54%
PBM Santas	1 oz	10	160	56%
PBM Squares	1 oz	9	150	54%
Panned Peanuts	1 oz	7	140	45%
Pastel Fiesta Eggs	1 oz	3	120	23%
Peanut Caramel Clusters	1 oz	8	150	48%
Peanut Clusters	1 oz	9	150	54%
Peanut Butter Kisses	1 oz	2	110	16%
Peanut Jots	1 oz	6	140	39%
Peanut Parfait	1 oz	10	160	56%
Peanuts-chocolate covered	1 oz	10	160	56%
small	1 oz	7	140	45%
Peppermint Kisses	1 oz	1	100	9%
Petite	1 oz	9	150	54%
Raisins-chocolate covered	1 oz	5	130	35%
Red Laces	1 oz	–	100	–
Red Twists	1 oz	–	100	–
Robin's Eggs	1 oz	6	140	39%
Royals	1 oz	2	110	16%
Salt Water Taffy	1 oz	1	100	9%
Santa's Assortment	1 oz	2	110	16%
Santas-foiled-tray of 8	1 oz	7	140	45%
Snappy Tarts	1 oz	–	100	–
Solid Chocolate Eggs	1 oz	8	150	48%
Solid Chocolate Bells-foiled	1 oz	8	150	48%
Spearmint Leaves	1 oz	–	100	–
Spicettes	1 oz	–	100	–
Starlight Mints	1 oz	–	110	–
Targets	1 oz	3	120	23%
Ting-A-Ling	1 oz	8	150	48%
Toffee	1 oz	2	110	16%
Valentine Hearts	1 oz	2	110	16%
Valentine Nougat Kisses	1 oz	2	110	16%

Food and Description	Amount	Fat Grams	Total Calories	% Fat Calories
Breath Savers Mints-sugar-free				
all flavors	1	–	8	–
Butterfinger	1 oz	5	134	34%
	2 oz	11	270	37%
Butternut	2 oz	13	270	43%
Butterscotch	1 oz	1	113	8%
(Cadbury)-Dairy Milk	1 oz	8	150	48%
Roast Almond	1 oz	9	150	48%
Candy Corn	¼ cup	1	180	5%
Carmello (Cadbury's)	1 oz	7	140	45%
Caramels-(Kraft)	1	1	35	26%
Chocolate Fudgies	1	1	35	26%
Caravelle	1 oz	5	127	35%
Charleston Chew/all flavors	2 oz	6	240	23%
Cherries-chocolate covered	1	3	90	30%
	1 oz	4	126	29%
Cherry Bites (Y&S)	1 oz	–	100	5%
Chocolate-dark sweet	1 oz	10	150	60%
milk-dairy (Cadbury)	1 oz	8	150	48%
milk-plain	1 oz	9	145	50%
milk w/almonds	1 oz	10	150	60%
milk w/peanuts	1 oz	11	155	64%
milk w/rice cereal	1 oz	7	140	45%
Roast Almonds (Cadbury)	1 oz	9	150	54%
Special Dark-(Hershey)	1 Bar	12	220	49%
Chocolate-Covered-almonds	1 oz	12	161	67%
Peanuts-(Nestle)-Goobers	1⅜ oz	13	220	53%
Chocolate-Discs-sugar coated	1 oz	5.6	132	38%
Chocolate Mint Patty	1	1	50	18%
Chuckles-jellied candied				
fruit flavors	1 oz	–	100	–
jellied eggs	1 oz	–	110	–
Jujubes	1 oz	–	110	–
Juju Softees	1 oz	–	100	–
Licorice	1 oz	–	100	–
Chunky-milk chocolate	1 oz	4	120	30%
original	1 oz	7	143	44%
peanut	1 oz	9	151	54%
pecan	1 oz	8	148	49%
Clark Bar	1 oz	5	134	34%
(Estee)-Chocolate Bars	2 squares	4-6	60	60%-90%
Chocolate Covered Raisins	6 pieces	2	30	60%
Crunch Chocolate Bar	2 squares	3	45	60%
Estee-ets	5 pieces	2	35	51%

Food and Description	Amount	Fat Grams	Total Calories	% Fat Calories
Gummy Bears	4 pieces	–	20	–
(Featherweight)-Sweet Pretenders -				
Chewy Caramels	1 piece	1	30	30%
Chocolate-flavored Almond Bar	¼ bar	7	90	70%
	2 oz	28	360	70%
Chocolate-flavored Crunch Bar	¼ bar	6	80	68%
	2 oz	24	320	68%
Milk Chocolate-flavored Bar	¼ bar	6	80	68%
	2 oz	24	320	68%
Peppermint Swirls	1 piece	–	20	–
5th Avenue	1.93 oz	9	270	30%
	1.16 oz/2 bars	7	160	39%
Fruit & Nut Bar (Cadbury)	1 oz	8	150	48%
Fudge-caramel & peanuts	1 oz	5	123	37%
chocolate	1 oz	4.5	122	33%
chocolate w/nuts	1 oz	5.9	128	42%
vanilla	1 oz	3	113	24%
vanilla w/nuts	1 oz	5	120	38%
Good & Plenty	1 oz	< 1	106	4%
Gum Drops/all flavors	1 oz	–	100	–
(Estee)	4 pieces	–	25	–
Hard candy	1 oz	–	110	–
(Estee)	2 pieces	–	25	–
Hot Tamales	1 oz	–	109	–
Jaw Breaker	1	–	20	–
Jelly Beans/all flavors	1 oz	–	100	–
	1 cup	1	807	1%
Junior Mints	1 oz	3	120	23%
Kisses (Hershey's)-plain	1 kiss	1	25	36%
	9 pieces	13	220	53%
	1 oz/			
	~6 pieces	9	150	54%
w/almonds	1 oz	10	160	56%
Kit-Kat	2/snack size	9	170	48%
	1.62 oz	13	250	47%
Krackel Chocolate Bar	1 oz	8	150	48%
	1.65 oz	14	250	50%
Kudos, Nutty Fudge	1 oz	12	200	54%
Licorice-black	1 oz	< 1	100	5%
Life Savers/all flavors	1 piece	–	9	–
Lollipops-(Estee)	1	–	25	–
M & M's (Hershey)				
Almond	1 oz	8	150	48%
Creamy Peanut	1 oz	7	140	45%

Food and Description	Amount	Fat Grams	Total Calories	% Fat Calories
Mint	1 oz	6	140	39%
Peanut	1.6 oz	12	240	45%
Plain	1 oz	6	140	39%
Malt Balls-chocolate covered	2 pieces	4	50	72%
Marathon	1.38 oz	7	179	35%
Mars Bar	1.76 oz	11	240	41%
Mike & Ike	1 oz	–	109	–
Milk Chocolate Bar				
(Cadbury)	1 oz	8	150	48%
	1 oz	9	150	54%
(Hershey)	1.65 oz	14	250	50%
with almonds	1.55 oz	15	250	54%
(Nestle)	1.45 oz	13	220	53%
with almonds	1.45 oz	14	230	55%
Milk Chocolate Stars	1 oz	8	160	45%
Milk Duds	1 oz	4	129	28%
Milk Shake	2 oz	8	250	29%
Milky Way	3.63 oz	18	470	35%
	2.2 oz	11	290	34%
Fun Size	1 bar	4	110	33%
Mint Non Pariels	1 oz	9	150	54%
Mints-(Kraft)-Butter	1	–	8	–
Party	1	–	8	–
Mounds Bar-(Peter Paul)	1 oz	7	135	47%
Mr. Goodbar	1.75 oz	19	290	59%
My Buddy	1.8 oz	13	250	47%
Nestle Chunky Bar	1.4 oz	12	210	51%
Nestle Crunch Bar	1.4 oz	10	210	43%
Snack Size	2 bars	5	100	45%
Nutcracker	1 oz	10	161	56%
Oh Henry! (Nestle)	2 oz	14	280	45%
PB Max	1.48 oz	16	240	60%
(Panda)-Licorice	3.5 oz	< 1	340	1%
Raspberry-Flavored Chew	3.5 oz	< 1	340	1%
Pay Day	1.9 oz	12	250	43%
Park Avenue	1.8 oz	9	230	35%
Peanut Brittle-(Estee)	¼ oz	1	35	26%
(Kraft)	1 oz	5	130	35%
Peanut Butter Cups-(Estee)	1	3	40	68%
(Reese's)	1.8 oz/			
	2 cups	17	280	55%
	2 cups	15	250	54%
miniatures	6 cups	14	230	55%
Snack Size	1 bar	6	100	54%

Food and Description	Amount	Fat Grams	Total Calories	% Fat Calories
Peanuts-yogurt covered	1 oz	9	125	65%
(Pearson's)-Carmel Nip	4 pieces	3	120	23%
Chocolate Parfait	4 pieces	3	120	23%
Coffee Nip	4 pieces	3	120	23%
Licorice Nip	4 pieces	3	120	23%
Penuchi	1 oz	4	120	30%
(Planters)-Old Fashioned				
Peanut Candy	1	9	140	58%
Peanut Bar	1.6 oz	11	230	43%
Honey Roasted	1.6 oz	13	230	51%
Sweet'N Crunchy	1.6 oz	15	250	54%
Peppermint Patties-(Nabisco)	1 oz	1	110	8%
(York)	1 oz	3	120	23%
Pom Poms	1 oz	3	100	27%
Power House	1 oz	5	130	35%
	2 oz	11	260	38%
Pralines	1 oz	3	90	30%
Raisinets-(Nestle)				
milk chocolate covered	1⅜ oz	6	180	30%
	1 oz	5	130	35%
Reese's Peanut Butter Cups/Crunchy	1.8 oz/ 2 cups	18	200	81%
Reese's Pieces-(Hershey)	1.95 pkg	11	270	37%
Rolo chocolate caramels (Hershey)	9 pieces	12	270	
Skittles	2 oz	5	320	14%
Fruit	2 oz	2	230	8%
Skor Toffee Bar	1.4 oz	14	220	57%
Slo Poke	1 sucker	2	124	15%
Snickers-peanut butter	1.75 oz	18	280	58%
plain	Fun Size	5	110	41%
	2.07 oz	14	280	45%
	3.7 oz	24	510	42%
Sno Caps-sweet chocolate nonpareils				
(Nestle)	2.3 oz	13	320	37%
(Sorbee)-sour lemon	1	–	12	–
wintergreen	1	–	12	–
Starbar	1 oz	7	140	45%
Starburst Fruit Chews	2 oz	5	240	19%
Sugar Babies	1 pkg	2	180	10%
Sugar Daddy	1	1	150	6%
Sugar Mama	¾ oz	3	90	30%
Summit	.76 oz	6	100	54%
Symphony-(Hershey)-milk chocolate	1.4 oz	13	220	53%
	1.75 oz	16	270	53%

Food and Description	Amount	Fat Grams	Total Calories	% Fat Calories
milk choc w/almonds & toffee chips	1.4 oz	14	220	57%
	1.75 oz	17	280	54%
Taffy	1 oz	1	100	9%
Thin Mint (Nabisco)	1	1	42	21%
Thousand Grand	1.5 oz	8	200	36%
3 Musketeers	1 oz	4	120	30%
	2.13 oz	9	260	31%
Toffee-(Kraft)	1	1	30	30%
Tootsie Roll	1 small	–	28	–
	1 large	2.6	127	18%
Twix-Caramel	2 oz/2 bars	14	280	45%
Twix-Chocolate Fudge	1 bar	8	130	55%
Twix Cookies-n-Creme	1 bar	7	120	52%
Twix-Peanut Butter	1.71 oz/			
	2 bars	16	260	55%
Twizzlers-Strawberry (Y&S)	1 oz		100	5%
Vanilla Creams	1 oz	4.8	123	35%
Whatchamacallit	1.8 oz	13	260	45%
White Chocolate-(Nestle)				
Alpine w/almonds	1.25 oz	14	210	60%
Zagnut	1 oz	4	131	28%
Zero	2 oz	8	250	29%
CANNELLINI BEAN (See KIDNEY BEAN, WHITE)				
CANTALOUPE				
~ 9.5 oz wt	½ fruit	.7	94	7%
pieces	1 cup	< 1	57	8%
CAPOCOLLO (See LUNCHEON MEATS)				
CAPON				
giblets-simmered	5 oz	7.8	238	30%
meat and skin-roasted	~1.5 lb	74	1457	46%
	3.5 oz	11.7	229	46%
meat only-roasted	3.5 oz	8.8	178	44%
CARAWAY SEED	1 tsp	–	7	–
CARDOON				
cooked	3 oz	–	19	–
raw-shredded	1 cup	–	35	–
CARIBOU/raw-boneless	3 oz	5	159	28%
CAROB CHIPS	1 oz	7	140	45
Mint	1 oz	7	140	45%
CAROB POWDER				
Chatfield's	¼ cup	–	96	–
El Molino	¼ cup	–	110	–
CARDAMOM/ ground	1 tsp	–	6	–
CARISSA (Natal Plum)/ raw	1	–	12	–

Food and Description	Amount	Fat Grams	Total Calories	% Fat Calories
CARP				
cooked-dry heat	3 oz	6	138	39%
breaded & fried	3 oz	12	226	48%
raw	3 oz	4.76	108	40%
roe-raw	3 oz	1.7	111	14%
smoked	1 oz	1.8	50	32%
CARROT				
canned	½ cup	–	20	–
canned-fingerling (Thank You)	½ cup	–	30	–
canned-Julienne French Style				
Fancy (S&W)	½ cup	–	30	–
Whole Tiny Fancy (S&W)	½ cup	–	30	–
canned-sliced (Nutradiet)	½ cup	–	30	–
canned-sliced-Fancy (S&W)	½ cup	–	30	–
cooked-slices	½ cup	–	35	–
crinkle sliced (Freshlike)	½ cup	–	30	–
diced (S&W)	½ cup	–	30	–
diced, sliced, or whole (Del Monte)	½ cup	–	30	–
fresh-cooked	1	–	21	–
frozen-cooked	½ cup	–	26	–
Parisienne (C & W)	½ cup	–	37	–
raw	1	–	31	–
raw-shredded	½ cup	–	24	–
sliced (Pictsweet)	3.3 oz	–	40	–
sliced (Pictsweet) Express Microwave	2.5 oz	–	30	–
whole baby (Birds Eye)	½ cup	–	40	–
whole baby (Pictsweet)	2.5 oz	–	30	–
CARROT DISHES				
Glazed Carrots, frozen				
(Birds Eye) Specialty Classics	5 oz	9	180	45%
CARROT JUICE /canned	6 oz	–	73	–
CASABA MELON /~ 6 oz wt	1/10 fruit	–	43	–
pieces	1 cup	< 1	45	10%
CASHEW				
dry roasted	1 oz	13	163	72%
(Guy's) whole salted	1 oz	14	170	74%
honey roasted				
(Eagle)	1 oz	12	170	64%
lightly salted	1 oz	14	170	74%
mixed w/peanuts	1 oz	13	170	69%
(Planters)	1 oz	12	170	64%
honey roasted/peanut cashew mix	1 oz	13	170	69%
(Planters)	1 oz	12	170	64%
oil roasted	1 oz	13.69	163	76%

Food and Description	Amount	Fat Grams	Total Calories	% Fat Calories
(Planters)				
dry roasted	1 oz	13	160	73%
unsalted	1 oz	13	60	73%
oil roasted-fancy	1 oz	14	170	74%
oil roasted halves	1 oz	14	170	74%
unsalted	1 oz	14	170	74%
CASHEW BUTTER				
plain	1 oz	14	167	75%
	1 Tbs	8	94	77%
raw (Hain)	2 Tbs	15	190	71%
toasted (Hain)	2 Tbs	16	190	76%
CATFISH (*See also* SEAFOOD ENTREE/DINNER)				
baked or broiled	3 oz	7	149	42%
cooked-breaded & fried	3 oz	11	194	51%
raw	3 oz	3.6	99	33%
CATSUP/Ketchup	1 cup	1	290	3%
	1 Tbs	–	15	–
(Del Monte) tomato	¼ cup	–	60	–
(Hain)natural or no salt	1 Tbs	–	16	–
(Heinz)				
Hot tomato	1 Tbs	–	18	–
Lite tomato	1 Tbs	–	8	–
Low Sodium tomato	1 Tbs	–	8	–
Regular tomato	1 Tbs	–	18	–
(Hunt's)-tomato	1 Tbs	–	16	–
(Smucker's) tomato	1 tsp	–	8	–
(Weight Watchers) tomato	1 Tbs	–	15	–
CAULIFLOWER				
fresh-cooked	½ cup	–	15	–
frozen-cooked	½ cup	–	17	–
frozen				
(Birds Eye)	½ cup	–	25	–
(Green Giant)	½ cup	–	12	–
(Freshlike)	3.3 oz	–	25	–
(Pictsweet)	3.3 oz	–	25	–
florets	3.2 oz	–	20	–
Hot & Spicy (Vlasic)	1 oz	–	4	–
raw	½ cup	–	12	–
sweet (Vlasic)	1 oz	–	35	–
CAULIFLOWER DISHES				
Cauliflower Crisp, frozen (Ore Ida)	3 oz	9	150	54%
Cauliflower in butter sauce (Green Giant)	½ cup	1	30	30%
Cauliflower in cheese flavored sauce				
frozen (Green Giant)	½ cup	2	60	30%

Food and Description	Amount	Fat Grams	Total Calories	% Fat Calories
Cauliflower in cheese sauce, frozen				
(Birds Eye)	5 oz	6	110	49%
(Freshlike) Micro Quick	4.5 oz	3	70	39%
Cauliflower in cheese sauce one serving vegetables/frozen				
(Green Giant)	5.5 oz	2	80	23%
Cauliflower in cheese sauce Singles frozen (Stokely)	4 oz	3	70	39%
Cauliflower in White Cheddar cheese flavored sauce, frozen (Green Giant)	½ cup	2	50	36%
CAULIFLOWER SOUP (See SOUP)				
CAVIAR , Black & Red				
granular	1 Tbs	3	40	68%
	1 oz	5	71	63%
pressed	1 Tbs	2.8	54	47%
	1 oz	4.7	90	47%
CELERIAC ROOT (wild celery) raw	4 or 5	–	40	–
	½ cup	–	31	–
CELERY				
cooked	½ cup	–	11	–
frozen (Freshlike)	3.5 oz	–	14	–
raw	1 stalk	–	6	–
	½ cup	–	9	–
CELERY SEED	1 tsp	.5	8	56%
CELERY SOUP (See SOUP)				
CEREAL				

(NOTE: All cereals are either dry or prepared with water per directions on packaging. If milk is used, calorie and fat content increase accordingly. Data on milk is shown in the Quick Reference below. For additional information on milk, see MILK.)

QUICK REFERENCE: MILK	Amount	Fat Grams	Total Calories	% Fat Calories
Skim	¼ cup	–	23	–
	½ cup	–	45	1%
lowfat	¼ cup	0.5	26	17%
	½ cup	1	55	16%
2% lowfat	¼ cup	1	31	29%
	½ cup	2.5	61	37%
Whole	¼ cup	2	38	47%
	½ cup	4	75	48%

COOKED

CREAM OF RICE (Nabisco) Instant/dry	2½ Tbs	–	100	–
CREAM OF RYE (Roman Meal)	1 Serving	0.5	110	4%

Food and Description	Amount	Fat Grams	Total Calories	% Fat Calories
CREAM OF WHEAT (Nabisco)				
Instant/dry	2½ Tbs	–	100	–
Mix & Eat/prepared				
Original	1 serving	–	100	–
Apple cinnamon	1 serving	–	130	–
Brown sugar/cinnamon	1 serving	1	130	7%
Maple/brown sugar	1 serving	–	130	–
Mixed fruit	1 serving	1	140	6%
Regular	1 serving	0.5	133	3%
FARINA				
(Pillsbury)	1 serving	< 1	80	6%
(Quaker) Quick Creamy wheat	1 serving	–	100	–
FIBER CEREAL-HOT (Golden Harvest)				
Maple/brown sugar	⅓ cup	2	100	18%
HOMINY GRITS (*See* CORN GRITS)				
MALTEX	1 serving	1	180	5%
MALT-O-MEAL				
Plain and chocolate	1 serving	–	122	–
Plus 40% Oat Bran	1 serving	1	120	8%
Wheat with oat bran	1 serving	1	120	8%
(MAYPO)				
30-second maple	1 serving	1	100	9%
Vermont Style	1 serving	1	105	9%
w/added oat bran	1 serving	2	130	14%
OAT BRAN				
(Health Valley)				
Apples/cinnamon	1 serving	1	100	9%
Raisin /spice	1 serving	1	100	9%
(Mother's)	1 serving	2	90	20%
(Nabisco) Wholesome'N Hearty	1 serving	2	90	20%
Instant				
Apple Cinnamon	1 package	2	130	14%
Apple/spice	1 package	2	120	15%
Honey	1 package	2	110	16%
Oat	1 package	2	80	23%
Raisin/cinnamon	1 package	2	120	15%
Regular	1 package	2	80	23%
(Quaker)	1 serving	2	90	20%
(Roman Meal)	1 serving	3	115	24%
(Skinner's)	1 serving	2	110	16%
(Stone-Buhr)	1 serving	2	108	17%
OATMEAL				
(General Mills)/Oatmeal Swirlers				
Apple cinnamon/raspberry	1 package	2	160	11%

Food and Description	Amount	Fat Grams	Total Calories	% Fat Calories
Cherry/strawberry	1 package	2	150	12%
Cinnamon spice/maple brown sugar	1 package	2	160	11%
Milk chocolate	1 package	2	170	11%
OATMEAL, Instant				
(General Mills)/Undercover Bears Instant Oatmeal				
Apple Cinnamon	1 package	3	170	16%
Fruit Punch	1 package	3	170	16%
Maple & Brown Sugar	1 package	3	170	16%
Strawberry	1 package	3	170	16%
Honey Nut	1 package	3	130	21%
Regular	1 package	2	90	20%
w/apples and cinnamon	1 package	1	120	8%
w/bananas and cream	1 package	3	160	45%
w/blueberries and cream	1 package	3	160	45%
w/bran and raisins	1 package	1.9	158	11%
w/cinnamon and spice	1 package	2	160	11%
w/cinnamon/raisins/almonds	1 package	4	150	24%
w/honey and graham	1 package	1.7	136	11%
w/maple	1 package	2	150	12%
w/maple and brown sugar	1 package	2	150	12%
w/peaches and cream	1 package	2	130	14%
w/raisins and spice	1 package	2	150	12%
w/raisins/dates/walnuts	1 package	4	140	26%
w/strawberries and cream	1 package	2	130	14%
(Quaker), Extra-fortified Instant				
Apples & spice w/raisins/ cinnamon	1 package	1	130	7%
Regular	1 package	2	100	18%
Quick & Old Fashioned	1 serving	2	100	18%
(Rogers)/Micro Quick				
Apples/cinnamon	1 package	2	142	13%
Maple/brown Sugar	1 package	2	157	12%
Regular-unsweetened	1 package	2	120	15%
Sure Brunet d'Erable	1 package	2	157	12%
Tropical Fruit	1 package	3	164	17%
(Roman Meal)				
Quick cooking	1 serving	2	100	18%
Oats/wheat/dates/raisins/almonds	1 serving	3	140	19%
Oats/wheat/honey/coconut/almonds	1 serving	6	150	36%
Oats/wheat/rye/bran/flax	1 serving	2	120	15%
Old fashioned oats	1 serving	2	100	18%
plain	1 serving	0.7	111	6%
Total, Instant				
Apple cinnamon	1 package	2	130	14%

Food and Description	Amount	Fat Grams	Total Calories	% Fat Calories
Cinnamon raisin	1 package	2	170	11%
Maple brown sugar	1 package	2	160	11%
Mixed nut	1 package	4	140	26%
Quick	1 serving	2	90	20%
Regular	1 package	2	100	18%
(PRITIKIN) HEARTY HOT CEREAL				
Apple Raisin Spice	1 package	2	160	11%
Multi grain	1 package	1	150	6%
(RALSTON), High Fiber 100% wheat				
recipe	1 serving	1	90	10%
plain	1 serving	0.6	100	5%
(STONE-BUHR)				
4 Grain Cereal Mates	1 serving	2	210	9%
Hot Apple Granola	1 serving	2	200	9%
7 Grain Cereal	1 serving	3	200	14%
WHEAT HEARTS (General Mills)	1 serving	1	110	8%
WHEAT, RYE, BRAN, FLAX				
(Roman Meal)	1 serving	0.5	80	6%
WHEATENA	1 serving	1	100	9%
WHOLE WHEAT HOT NATURAL CEREAL				
(Mother's)	1 serving	1	100	9%
(Quaker's)	1 serving	1	90	10%
READY-TO-EAT				
AGAIN & AGAIN (Arrowhead Mills)	2 oz	2	220	8%
ALMOND DELIGHT				
w/almonds/pecans/walnuts	1 oz/1 cup	1.6	110	13%
ALPEN MUESLI RAISINS & NUTS	½ cup	3	220	12%
ALPHA-BITS	1 cup	0.7	110	6%
w/marshmallows	1 cup	1	110	8%
AMARANTH CRUNCH				
w/raisins (Health Valley)	1 oz	3	110	25%
AMARANTH FLAKES (Health Valley)	1 oz	1	110	8%
AMARANTH 100% NATURAL				
SPROUTED w/bananas	½ cup	2	100	18%
APPLE JACKS	1 cup	–	110	–
ARROWHEAD CRUNCH	1 oz	3	120	23%
BABY FOOD (See BABY FOOD)				
BASIC 4 (General Mills)	¾ cup	2	130	14%
BATMAN CEREAL (Ralston)	1 oz	1	110	8%
BENEFIT				
Regular	¼ cup	1	90	10%
w/raisins	1 cup	1	120	8%
BIGG MIX	½ cup	2	110	16%

Food and Description	Amount	Fat Grams	Total Calories	% Fat Calories
BODY BUDDIES				
Brown sugar and honey	1 cup	1	110	8%
Natural fruit flavor	1 cup	1	110	8%
BOOBERRY	1 cup	1	110	8%
BRAN				
All Bran				
Original	⅓ cup	0.5	71	6%
Fruit and almonds	⅓ cup	2	100	18%
w/Extra Fiber	½ cup	1	50	18%
Bran Buds	⅓ cup	0.7	73	9%
Bran Chex	⅔ cup	0.7	90	8%
Bran Flakes				
(Arrowhead Mills)	1 oz	1	100	9%
(Kellogg's)	¾ cup	0.5	93	5%
(Post)	⅔ cup	–	90	–
Bran Muffin Crisp	⅔ cup	1	130	7%
Bran News	1 oz	–	100	–
40+ Bran Flakes	⅔ cup	0.5	90	5%
40% Bran Flakes	⅔ cup	1	106	9%
Fruitful Bran	⅔ cup	–	110	–
Health Valley Bran Cereal				
w/apple cinnamon	1 oz	1	109	8%
w/raisins	1 oz	1	105	9%
Honey Bran	⅞ cup	0.6	97	6%
La Loma Bran Cereal	1 oz	1	90	10%
Mueslix	½ cup	2	140	13%
100% Bran				
plain	⅓ cup	2	70	26%
w/oat bran	1 oz	1	80	11%
Unprocessed Bran (Quaker)	2 Tbs	–	8	–
BREAKFAST O'S w/oat bran				
(Barbara's)	1¼ cup	2	120	15%
BREAKFAST W/BARBIE	1 oz/1 cup	1	110	8%
BROWN RICE LITES (Health Valley)	½ cup	–	50	–
CAP'N CRUNCH				
Regular	¾ cup	2	120	15%
Crunchberries	¾ cup	2	120	15%
Peanut butter	¾ cup	3	120	23%
CHEERIOS				
Regular	1¼ cups	1.8	110	15%
Apple Cinnamon	1¼ cups	1.8	110	15%
CINNAMON MINI BUNS (Kellogg's)	¾ cup	1	110	8%
CINNAMON TOAST CRUNCH	¾ cup	3	120	23%
CIRCUS FUN	1 oz/1 cup	1	110	8%

Food and Description	Amount	Fat Grams	Total Calories	% Fat Calories
CLUSTERS				
Regular	⅓ cup	3	100	27%
w/almonds/walnuts/pecans	½ cup	3	100	27%
COCOA FLAKES	⅔ cup	–	110	–
COCOA FLAKES MAIZORO	1 oz	–	110	–
COCOA KRISPIES	¾ cup	–	110	–
COCOA PEBBLES	⅞ cup	1	110	8%
COCOA PUFFS	1 oz/1 cup	1	110	8%
COMMON SENSE OAT BRAN				
Regular	⅔ cup	1	100	27%
w/raisins	⅔ cup	–	120	–
COOKIE CRISP				
Chocolate chip	1 cup	1	110	8%
Vanilla wafer	1 cup	1	110	8%
CORN BRAN	⅔ cup	0.9	109	7%
CORN CHEX	⅔ cup	–	110	–
CORN FLAKES				
Arrowhead Mills	1 oz	1	110	8%
Barbara's Blue Corn Flakes	1 cup	–	110	–
(Health Valley)	½ cup	1	90	10%
Country (General Mills)	1 oz/1 cup	–	110	4%
Featherweight	1 oz	–	110	–
Kellogg's	1¼ cup	–	100	–
Post Toasties (Post)	1 oz/1 cup	–	108	–
Total (General Mills)	1 oz/1 cup	1	110	8%
CORN POPS	1 cup	–	110	–
COUNT CHOCULA	1 cup	1	110	8%
CORN TOTAL	1 oz/1 cup	1	110	8%
CRAKLIN BRAN	⅓ cup	4	108	33%
CRACKLIN OAT BRAN	¼ cup	4	110	33%
CRISPIX	¾ cup	–	110	–
CRISPY CRITTERS	1 cup	–	110	–
CRISPY OATMEAL & RAISIN CHEX	¾ cup	0.5	140	3%
CRISPY RICE	1 oz/1 cup	–	112	–
(Grainfield's)	1 oz	< 1	100	5%
CRISPY WHEATS & RAISINS	¾ cup	1	110	8%
CRUNCHY BRAN	1 oz	1	90	10%
CRUNCHY RICE BRAN (Quaker)	⅔ cup	1	100	9%
CRUNCHY STARS	1 cup	1	111	8%
DINERSAURS (Ralston)	1 oz/1 cup	1	110	8%
DINO PEBBLES (Post)	1 oz/⅞ cup	1	110	8%
DOUBLE CHEX (Ralston)	¾ cup	–	100	–
DUNKIN' DONUTS (Ralston)	1 oz	1	120	8%
FIBER ONE	½ cup	1	60	15%

Food and Description	Amount	Fat Grams	Total Calories	% Fat Calories
FIBER 7 FLAKES (Health Valley)	½ cup	1	100	9%
FORTIFIED OAT FLAKES	⅔ cup	1	110	8%
FRANKENBERRY	1 oz/1 cup	1	110	8%
FROOT LOOPS	1 oz/1 cup	0.5	111	4%
FROSTED MINI WHEATS (Kellogg's)	4 biscuits	–	100	–
FROSTED RICE KRINKLES	⅞ cup	–	109	–
FROSTED WHEAT SQUARES	½ cup	–	100	–
FRUIT & FIBRE (Post)				
Dates/raisins/walnuts	⅔ cup	2	120	15%
Peaches/raisins/almonds	⅔ cup	2	120	15%
Tropical Fruit w/oat clusters	⅔ cup	3	120	23%
FRUIT & FITNESS (Health Valley)	2 oz	4	190	19%
FRUIT LITES (Health Valley)				
Corn	.5 oz	–	45	–
Rice	.5 oz	–	45	–
Wheat	.5 oz	–	45	–
FRUIT'N OAT BRAN CRUNCH (Kolln)	1 oz	1	100	9%
FRUIT WHEATS				
Apple	½ cup	–	100	–
Blueberry	½ cup	–	100	–
Raisin	½ cup	–	100	–
Raspberry	½ cup	–	90	–
Strawberry	½ cup	–	100	–
FRUITY MARSHMALLOW KRISPIES	1 oz	–	140	–
FRUITY PEBBLES	⅞ cup	1	110	8%
FRUITY YUMMY MUMMY	1 oz/1 cup	1	110	8%
GHOST BUSTERS	1 oz/1 cup	1	110	8%
GOLDEN CORN LITES (Health Valley)	½ cup	–	50	–
GOLDEN GRAHAMS	¾ cup	1	110	8%
GOLDEN RICE LITES (Health Valley)	½ cup	–	50	–
GOLDEN WHEAT LITES(Health Valley)	½ cup	–	50	–
GRAHAM CRACKOS	¾ cup	–	102	–
GRANOLA				
(Arrowhead Mills)				
Apple amaranth	2 oz	6	225	24%
Maple nut	2 oz	11	260	38%
Bread Shop Granola Super Natural	⅓ cup	5	120	38%
(C. W. Post) Hearty Granola				
Plain	¼ cup	4	130	28%
w/raisins	¼ cup	4	123	29%
(Health Valley)-Real Granola				
Almond Crunch	1 oz	3	120	23%
Raisins & Nuts	1 oz	3	120	23%

Food and Description	Amount	Fat Grams	Total Calories	% Fat Calories
(Nature Valley)				
Cinnamon & raisin	⅓ cup	4	120	30%
Fruit & nut	⅓ cup	5	130	35%
(Nectar Sweet) Granola				
Blueberry'N Cream	⅓ cup	4	110	33%
Raspberry'N Cream	⅓ cup	4	110	33%
Strawberry'N Cream	⅓ cup	4	110	33%
Standard Home Recipe (USDA)	¼ cup	7.7	138	50%
(Sunbelt)				
Banana almond	1 oz	4	130	28%
Fruit & nut	1 oz	5	120	38%
(Sun Country)				
w/almonds	¼ cup	5	130	35%
w/raisins	¼ cup	5	130	35%
w/raisins and dates	¼ cup	4	130	28%
GRAPE-NUTS				
Flakes	⅞ cup	1	100	9%
Original	¼ cup	–	110	–
Raisin	¼ cup	–	98	–
GREAT GRAINS (Post)				
Double Pecan	⅓ cup	3	120	23%
Raisin, date, and pecan	⅓ cup	3	130	21%
HEALTHY CRUNCH (Health Valley)				
Cinnamon	1 oz	3	110	25%
w/almonds and dates	1 oz	3	110	25%
HEARTLAND NATURAL (Pet)				
Plain	¼ cup	4	130	28%
w/coconut	¼ cup	4.5	130	31%
w/raisins	¼ cup	4	130	28%
HEARTWISE FLAKES (Kellogg's)	1 oz	1	90	10%
HEARTWISE NUGGETS w/prunes (Kellogg's)	1 oz	1	110	8%
HONEY & NUT CORN FLAKES	¾ cup	1.5	113	12%
HONEY & NUT TOASTY O'S	¾ cup	1	110	8%
HONEY BUC WHEAT CRISP	¾ cup	1	110	8%
HONEY BUNCHES OF OATS				
Regular	⅔ cup	2	114	16%
w/almonds	⅔ cup	3	118	23%
HONEY GRAHAM CHEX	⅔ cup	1	110	8%
HONEY NUT CHEERIOS				
Regular	¾ cup	1	110	8%
w/almonds	⅔ cup	3	120	23%
HONEY NUT OAT CHEX	½ cup	1	110	8%
HONEY SNACKS	¾ cup	1	110	8%

Food and Description	Amount	Fat Grams	Total Calories	% Fat Calories
HONEYCOMB	1⅓ cups	–	110	–
ICE CREAM CONES/all flavors	¾ cup	2	110	16%
JETSONS	¾ cup	1	110	8%
JUST RIGHT				
w/Fiber nuggets	⅔ cup	1	100	9%
w/Fruits & nuts	¾ cup	1	140	6%
KABOOM	1oz/1cup	1	110	8%
KASHI/puffed	1 cup	0.5	74	6%
KELLOGG'S SQUARES				
Apple Cinnamon	½ cup	–	90	–
Raisin	½ cup	–	90	–
Strawberry	½ cup	–	90	–
KENMEI (Kellogg's)				
Plain	1 oz	1	100	9%
w/almonds & raisins	1 oz	2	140	13%
KING VITAMIN	1¼ cups	1	112	8%
KIX	1½ cups	1	110	8%
LIFE				
Cinnamon	⅔ cup	1.6	110	13%
plain	⅔ cup	1.8	111	15%
w/raisins	⅔ cup	1.8	105	15%
LUCKY CHARMS	1 oz/1 cup	1	110	8%
MORNING FUNNIES	1 oz/1 cup	1	110	8%
MOST	⅔ cup	–	95	–
MULTI BRAN CHEX	⅔ cup	–	90	–
MUESLI, FRUIT (Ralston)				
Dates/almonds	1 oz	2	140	13%
Raisins/peaches/pecans	1 oz	3	150	18%
Raisins/walnuts/cranberries	1 oz	3	150	18%
MUESLIX				
Crispy Blend	⅔ cup	2	160	11%
5 Grain	½ cup	1	140	6%
Golden Crunch				
w/apples and almonds	½ cup	2	120	15%
NATURE O's (Arrowhead Mills)	1 oz	1	110	8%
NATURE VALLEY 100% Oat Cereal				
w/fruit and nuts	⅓ cup	5	130	35%
NECTAR SWEET CRUNCH OAT BRAN	⅓ cup	5	110	41%
NINTENDO CEREAL SYSTEM	1 oz/1 cup	1	110	8%
NUT & HONEY CRUNCH	⅔ cup	1	110	8%
NUT & HONEY CRUNCHO'S	⅔ cup	2	110	16%
NUTRIFIC OATMEAL FLAKES	1 oz	2	120	15%
NUTRI-GRAIN				
Almond & Raisins	¾ cup	2	140	13%

Food and Description	Amount	Fat Grams	Total Calories	% Fat Calories
Barley	½ cup	–	106	–
Corn	½ cup	0.7	108	6%
Raisin Bran	⅔ cup	1	130	7%
Rye	⅔ cup	–	102	–
Wheat	⅔ cup	–	102	–
Wheat & Raisin	⅔ cup	–	130	–
NUTRI-GRAIN BISCUITS	1 oz	–	90	–
NUTRI-GRAIN NUGGETS	¼ cup	–	110	–
OATBAKE				
Honey Bran	1 oz	3	110	25%
Raisin Nut	1 oz	3	110	25%
OAT BRAN				
Crunch (Kolln)	1 oz	2	120	15%
Flakes (Health Valley)				
plain	1 oz	0.8	110	7%
Wheat Free	½ cup		100	5%
w/almonds and dates	1 oz	0.8	100	7%
w/raisins	1 oz	0.8	100	7%
(Health Valley)				
Almond Crunch	1 oz	3	110	25%
Raisin Nut	1.2 oz	3	130	21%
(Health Valley)-O's				
Plain	1 oz	1.6	90	16%
Fruits and Nuts	1 oz	2	90	20%
Options (Ralston)	1.45 oz	–	130	–
(Quaker)	1 oz	2	100	18%
Raisin Fruit Wheats	½ cup	–	90	–
OAT CHEX (Ralston)	1 oz	1	100	9%
OAT FLAKES (Post)	⅔ cup	1	110	8%
OAT SQUARES	1 oz	1.6	105	14%
OATIOS				
Honey Almond	1.1 oz	2	120	15%
Oat Bran	1 oz	2	110	16%
OATMEAL CRISP	½ cup	2	110	16%
OATMEAL RAISIN CRISP	½ cup	2	110	16%
OH'S				
Apple Cinnamon	1 oz/1 cup	2	120	15%
Crunchy Nut	1 oz	4	130	28%
Honey Graham	1 oz	3	120	23%
ORANGEOLA (Health Valley)				
Almonds & Dates	¼ cup	4	120	30%
OUTRAGEOUS FRUIT & GRAINS	¼ cup	6	130	42%
PAC MAN	1 oz/1 cup	1	110	8%
POPEYE SWEET CRUNCH CEREAL	1 cup	2	120	15%

Food and Description	Amount	Fat Grams	Total Calories	% Fat Calories
PRODUCT 19	1 oz/1 cup	–	100	–
PUFFED CORN (El Molino)	¾ cup	–	50	–
PUFFED MILLET (El Molino)	¾ cup	–	50	–
PUFFED RICE (El Molino)	¾ cup	–	50	–
PUFFED WHEAT (El Molino)	¾ cup	–	50	–
QUAKER 100% NATURAL				
plain	¼ cup	5.6	130	39%
w/apples & cinnamon	¼ cup	5	133	34%
w/raisins & dates	¼ cup	5	120	38%
QUAKER OAT SQUARES	½ cup	2	100	18%
QUISP	1 oz/1 cup	2	117	15%
RAISIN BRAN				
(Health Valley) Flakes	1 oz	–	100	–
(Grainfield's)	1 oz	–	110	–
(Kellogg's)	¾ cup	1	120	8%
(Post)	¾ cup	1	120	8%
(Ralston Purina)	¾ cup	–	120	–
(Skinner's)	½ cup	1	100	9%
RAISIN DATE NATURAL	1 oz	5	123	37%
RAISIN NUT BRAN	½ cup	3	110	25%
REAL 100% NATURAL				
Almond & Crunch	¼ cup	3	120	23%
RICE BRAN (Quaker)				
Crunchy	⅔ cup	1	100	9%
Honey Crunch	¼ cup	5	100	45%
RICE CHEX	1⅛ cups	–	110	–
RICE KRISPIES				
Regular	1 oz/1 cup	–	110	–
Frosted	1 oz/1 cup	–	109	–
RICE TOASTIES	¾ cup	–	108	–
ROCKY ROAD	⅔ cup	2	120	15%
RUSKETS BISCUITS (La Loma)	~ 1 oz	–	110	–
7 GRAIN (La Loma)	1 oz	1	110	8%
Crunchy	1 oz	2	110	16%
S. W. GRAHAM				
Cinnamon	½ cup	–	100	–
plain	½ cup	–	100	–
SHREDDED WHEAT				
Bite size				
(Kellogg's)	½ cup	–	100	–
(Sunshine)	⅔ cup	1	110	8%
Original rectangles				
(Nabisco)	1 biscuit	1	90	10%
(Quaker)	2 biscuits	1	130	7%

Food and Description	Amount	Fat Grams	Total Calories	% Fat Calories
(Sunshine)	1 biscuit	1	90	10%
Spoon size (Nabisco)	1 oz	1	90	10%
w/oat bran (Nabisco)	1 oz	1	100	9%
SHREDDED WHEAT'N Bran	1 oz	1	90	10%
SHREDDED WHEAT SQUARES				
All flavors	½ cup	–	90	–
S'MORES CRUNCH	¾ cup	2	120	15%
SMURF BERRY CRUNCH	1 oz	1	110	8%
SMURF MAGIC BERRIES	1 oz/1 cup	1	110	8%
SPECIAL K	1⅓ cups	–	110	–
SPROUTS 7 (Health Valley) w/raisins	¼ cup	1	90	10%
STONE BUHR 4 Grain Cereal Mates	2 oz	2	210	9%
STONED WHEAT FLAKES				
(Health Valley)	1 oz	–	100	–
SUGAR CORN POPS	1 oz/1 cup	–	108	–
SUGAR FROSTED FLAKES	¾ cup	–	110	–
SUGAR PUFFS	⅞ cup	1	110	8%
SUGAR SMACKS	¾ cup	1	110	8%
SUGAR SPARKLED FLAKES	¾ cup	–	108	–
SUN FLAKES				
Corn & Rice	1 oz/1 cup	0.9	110	7%
Wheat & Rice	1 oz/1 cup	3	135	20%
SUPER GOLDEN CRISP	1 oz	–	110	–
SUPER SUGAR CRISP	⅞ cup	–	106	–
SWISS BREAKFAST (Health Valley)				
Raisin nut	1 oz	3	100	27%
Tropical fruit	1 oz	3	100	27%
TASTEEOS	1¼ cups	0.8	111	7%
TEAM FLAKES	1 oz/1 cup	0.5	110	4%
TEDDY GRAHAMS BREAKFAST BEARS				
Chocolate	⅓ cup	3	120	23%
Cinnamon	⅓ cup	3	120	23%
Honey	⅓ cup	3	120	23%
TEENAGE MUTANT NINJA TURTLES	1 oz	1	110	8%
TINY TOON (Quaker)	1 oz	1	110	8%
TOASTED WHEAT AND RAISINS	1 oz	1	100	9%
TOASTED WHEAT BRAN	⅓ cup	2	60	30%
TOASTY O'S	1¼ cups	2	110	16%
TOTAL				
Corn Flakes	1 oz/1 cup	1	100	9%
Raisin Bran	1.5 oz	1	130	7%
Whole Wheat	1 oz	1	110	8%
TRIPLES (General Mills)	1 oz/¾ cup	1	110	8%
TRIX	1.5 oz	–	109	–

Food and Description	Amount	Fat Grams	Total Calories	% Fat Calories
UNCLESAM	1oz	1	110	8%
WAFFELOS	1.5 oz	1	115	8%
WEETABIX Whole Wheat	2 oz	1	120	8%
WHEAT BRAN				
Arrowhead Mills	2 oz	2	200	9%
Millers Flakes (Health Valley)	1 oz	2	70	26%
Toasted (Health Valley)	⅓ cup	2	60	30%
WHEAT'N BRAN (Nabisco)	1 oz	–	90	–
WHEAT'N RAISIN CHEX	¾ cup	–	130	–
WHEAT CHEX	⅔ cup	0.7	100	6%
WHEAT GERM				
Arrowhead Mills	2 oz	6	210	26%
Kretschmer				
Plain	¼ cup	3	110	25%
Honey crunch	¼ cup	3	110	25%
Toasted, w/brown sugar				
w/honey	¼ cup	2	100	18%
WHEAT GERM & FIBER (Health Valley)				
w/almonds and dates	1 oz	1	100	9%
WHEATIES	1 oz/1 cup	.5	99	5%
CHARD				
fresh-cooked	½ cup	–	18	–
raw-chopped	½ cup	–	3	–
CHARLOTTE RUSSE w/lady fingers				
(whipped cream filling)	4 oz	16.6	326	46%
CHAYOTE				
(tropical American perennial)	1 medium	–	56	–
boiled	½ cup	–	19	–
CHEESE				
American				
(Alpine Lace)-past. Processed	1 oz	7	90	70%
50% less sodium	1 oz	7	90	70%
(Borden)-processed slices	1 oz	9	110	74%
Light 15% milkfat	1 oz	5	70	64%
processed cheese food				
singles	1 oz	7	90	70%
(Harvest Moon)	1 oz	4	70	51%
(Nucoa)-Heart Beat-sandwich slices	1 oz	2	50	36%
(Kraft)-cheese food	1 oz	7	90	70%
Deluxe-loaf	1 oz	9	110	74%
Deluxe-slices	1 oz	9	110	74%
grated-cheese food	1 oz	7	130	49%
Light singles	1 oz	4	70	51%
white-cheese food	1 oz	7	90	70%

Food and Description	Amount	Fat Grams	Total Calories	% Fat Calories
(Land O'Lakes)-process	1 oz	9	110	74%
& Swiss-process	1 oz	8	100	72%
Sharp-process	1 oz	9	100	81%
(Light N'Lively)-cheese food	1 oz	4	70	51%
(Lite-Line) 8% milkfat	1 oz	2	50	36%
15% milkfat	1 oz	4	70	51%
(Old English)-loaf	1 oz	9	110	74%
slices	1 oz	9	110	74%
(Sargento)-Hot Pepper	1 oz	9	110	74%
Pimento	1 oz	9	110	74%
Snack-pasteurized/process	1 oz	9	110	74%
(Weight Watchers)	1 oz	2	50	36%
Dijon	1 oz	2	50	36%
American-Swiss				
(Formagg)	¾ oz	5	70	64%
(Land O'Lakes)	1 oz	9	100	81%
Babybel (Fromageries Bel)	1 oz	7	91	69%
	8 oz	57	726	71%
mini	¾ oz	6	74	73%
Blue	1 oz	8	100	72%
	1 cup	38.8	477	73%
(Kraft)	1 oz	9	100	81%
(Sergento)	1 oz	8	100	72%
Bonbel (Fromageries Bel)	1 oz	8	100	72%
	8 oz	65	790	74%
mini	¾ oz	6	74	73%
Bonbino (Fromageries Bel)	1 oz	9	103	79%
	8 oz	68	822	75%
Brick	1 oz	9	110	74%
(Kraft)	1 oz	9	110	74%
natural (Land O'Lakes)	1 oz	8	110	66%
(Sargento)	1 oz	8	105	69%
snack-pasteurized process	1 oz	9	100	81%
Brie	1 oz	7.85	95	74%
(Corneville)-soft ripened	1 oz	7.5	90	75%
(Fromageries Bel)	1 oz	8	90	80%
(Sargento)	1 oz	8	95	76%
Burger Cheese (Sargento)	1 oz	8.86	106	75%
Cajun (Sargento)	1 oz	9	110	74%
Camembert	1 oz	6.9	85	73%
(Corneville)-soft ripened	1 oz	7.5	90	75%
Cream Cheese-The Little Cheeserie (Fleur De Lait)				
Chunky Spreadables				
Bay Shrimp	1 oz	5	70	64%

Food and Description	Amount	Fat Grams	Total Calories	% Fat Calories
Italian Garlic	1 oz	5	65	69%
Plump Strawberry	1 oz	5	80	56%
Zesty Salsa	1 oz	5	60	56%
Danish (Sargento)	1 oz	7	90	70%
(Fromagerie)	1 oz	8	90	80%
Caraway	1 oz	8	107	67%
(Kraft)-natural	1 oz	8	100	72%
Cheddar, breaded/frozen (Banquet)	3 oz	30	414	65%
Chedda Delite Deli Light (Dorman's)	1 oz	7	90	70%
Extra Sharp-(Land O'Lakes)process	1 oz	9	100	81%
Imitation/Golden Image-mild				
cheddar (Kraft)	1 oz	9	110	74%
(Sargento)	1 oz	6	90	60%
(Weight Watchers)				
shredded-part skim milk	1 oz	5	80	56%
Cheddar, Mild	1 oz	9	114	71%
(Formagg)-cheese food	1 oz	5	70	64%
(Fromageries Bel)	1 oz	9	110	74%
	8 oz	73	883	74%
wedges-process cheese	1 oz	6	72	75%
wedges reduced calorie	¾ oz	2	35	51%
(Land O'Lakes)-La Chedda				
cheese food	1 oz	7	90	70%
(Light Naturals)-reduced fat	1 oz	5	80	56%
(Sargento)	1 oz	9	110	74%
shredded	1 cup	37	455	73%
(Weight Watchers)	1 oz	5	80	56%
Natural-(Kraft)	1 oz	9	110	74%
Light Naturals reduced fat	1 oz	5	90	50%
(Land O'Lakes)	1 oz	9	110	74%
(Lifetime)-Lite	1 oz	3	55	49%
(Weight Watchers)	1 oz	5	80	56%
New York-(Sargento)	1 oz	9	110	74%
Semi-soft (Alpine Lace) part skim	1 oz	8	100	72%
Sharp/with wine	1 oz	6.9	93	67%
cheese ball w/almonds	1 oz	6	90	60%
(Light N'Lively)	1 oz	4	70	51%
(Lite-Line) 8% milkfat	1 oz	2	50	36%
Nut Log (Sargento)	1 oz	7	100	63%
singles-cheese food				
(Kraft)	1 oz	8	100	72%
(Weight Watchers)	1 oz	2	50	36%
Smokey w/almonds-log	1 oz	6	90	60%
Cheddar Cheese Soup (See SOUP)				

Food and Description	Amount	Fat Grams	Total Calories	% Fat Calories
Cheddarella/(Land O'Lakes)-natural	1 oz	8	100	72%
(Lake to Lake)	1 oz	8	100	72%
Cheese Food Pasteurized Process Misc.-				
Cheddar & Bacon-(Land O'Lakes)	1 oz	9	110	74%
Jalapeno-(Kraft)	1 oz	7	90	70%
Non-fat				
(Alpine Lace)-Free N'Lean	1 oz	–	35	–
(Kraft)-Free	1 oz	–	45	–
Port Wine-(Wispride)-cold pack	1 oz	7	100	63%
Sharp Cheddar-(Wispride)				
cold pack	1 oz	7	100	63%
Slices (Land O'Lakes)	⅔ oz	4	60	60%
w/Bacon (Kraft)	1 oz	7	90	70%
w/Garlic (Kraft)	1 oz	7	90	70%
Cheese Sauce/canned	2 oz	4	60	60%
mix	4 oz	18	225	72%
Cheese Souffle/homemade (8" square)	~ 4 oz	18.8	240	71%
collapsed	1 cup	16	207	70%
	1 oz	4.8	62	70%
Cheese Spreads/with bacon (Kraft)	1 oz	6	80	68%
with garlic (Kraft)	1 oz	6	80	68%
(Alouette)-spreadable				
French Onion	1 oz	9	95	85%
Garlic & Spices	1 oz	9	95	85%
Zesty Pepper	1 oz	9	90	90%
American Pasteurized (Kraft)	1 oz	6	80	68%
American Sharp Pasteurized Processed				
(Sargento)	1 oz	9	110	74%
(Cheez Whiz)-hot Mexican	1 oz	5.7	80	64%
mild Mexican	1 oz	5.7	80	64%
pimento	1 oz	5.7	80	64%
plain	1 oz	5.7	80	64%
w/jalapeno pepppers	1 oz	5.7	80	64%
Country Crock (Shedds)-				
Fresh Cheddar	1 oz	4	70	51%
Fresh Cheddar-Mexican style	1 oz	4	70	51%
Fresh French Onion	1 oz	7	70	90%
Fresh Garden Vegetable	1 oz	7	70	90%
Fresh Herb & Garlic	1 oz	7	70	90%
Crockery (Kraft)				
Classic Ranch	1 oz	7	70	90%
French Onion	1 oz	6	70	77%
Garden Vegetable	1 oz	6	70	77%
Garlic & Herb	1 oz	7	70	90%

Food and Description	Amount	Fat Grams	Total Calories	% Fat Calories
Medium Cheddar	1 oz	4	70	51%
Port Wine	1 oz	4	70	51%
Easy Cheese (Nabisco)-				
American	1 oz	6	80	68%
Cheddar	1 oz	6	80	68%
Cheddar'n Bacon	1 oz	6	80	68%
Nacho	1 oz	6	80	68%
Sharp Cheddar	1 oz	6	80	68%
(Fromageries Bel)-Price's-				
Pimento Spread	1 oz	6	80	68%
(Fromageries Bel)-The Laughing Cow-				
Cheezbits	⅙ oz	1	13	69%
Lite soft cheese spread	1 oz	2	45	40%
Regular cheese spread	1 oz	6	70	77%
Golden Velvet (Land O'Lakes)	1 oz	6	80	68%
Imperial) Ala Mode Gourmet	1 Tbs	7	70	90%
(Italian Rose)-Garlic Spread	1 Tbs	6.9	60.9	68%
Jalapeno Pasteurized-loaf	1 oz	6	80	68%
Jalapeno Pepper (Kraft)	1 oz	5	70	64%
Limburger (Mohawk Valley)	1 oz	6	70	77%
(Old English) Sharp	1 oz	7	80	79%
Olives & pimento (Kraft)	1 oz	5	60	75%
-soft	1 oz	8	90	80%
Pimento (Kraft)	1 oz	5	70	64%
Pineapple (Kraft)	1 oz	5	70	64%
Roka Blue (Kraft)	1 oz	6	70	77%
Spreadery (Kraft)				
Classic Ranch	1 oz	7	70	90%
French Onion	1 oz	6	70	77%
Garden Vegetable	1 oz	6	70	77%
Garlic & Herb	1 oz	7	70	90%
Squeeze-A-Snack (Kraft)-				
Garlic	1 oz	7	80	79%
Hickory Smoke	1 oz	7	80	79%
w/ Bacon	1 oz	7	80	79%
Jalapeno Pepper	1 oz	6	80	68%
Sharp	1 oz	7	80	79%
Velveeta Spread (Kraft)	1 oz	6	80	68%
Mexican Hot	1 oz	6	80	68%
-shredded	1 oz	7	100	63%
Mexican Mild	1 oz	6	80	68%
-shredded	1 oz	7	100	63%
Pimento	1 oz	6	80	68%
Slices	1 oz	6	90	60%

Food and Description	Amount	Fat Grams	Total Calories	% Fat Calories
Cheez'N Bacon singles cheese food				
(Kraft)	1 oz	7	90	70%
Cheshire	1 oz	8.68	110	71%
Colbi-Lo (Alpine Lace)-low sodiium	1 oz	5	80	56%
Colby	1 oz	9	110	74%
Cheese Alternative				
(Dorman's)-Lo-Chol	1 oz	6	90	60%
Golden Image-Imitation Colby(Kraft)	1 oz	9	110	74%
(Kraft)-natural	1 oz	9	110	74%
Light Naturals	1 oz	5	80	56%
(Land O'Lakes)-natural	1 oz	9	110	74%
(Sargento)	1 oz	9	112	72%
(Weight Watchers)-natural	1 oz	5	80	56%
Colby-Jack (Sargento)	1 oz	9	109	74%
Colby Longhorn/(Delcia)-imitation	1 oz	6	80	68%
(Cracker Barrel)-Cheese Ball				
sharp cheddar w/almonds	1 oz	6	90	60%
Cheese Log-port wine cheddar				
w/almonds	1 oz	6	90	60%
Cheese Log-sharp cheddar				
w/almonds	1 oz	6	90	60%
Cheese Log-Smokey cheddar				
w/almonds	1 oz	6	80	60%
Cold Packs-Extra Sharp Cheddar	1 oz	7	90	70%
Port Wine Cheddar	1 oz	7	90	70%
Sharp Cheddar	1 oz	7	90	70%
W/Bacon	1 oz	7	90	70%
Diet Snack/(Weight Watchers)-				
sharp cheddar flavor	1 oz	3	70	39%
port wine flavored	1 oz	3	70	39%
Edam	1 oz	7.88	101	70%
(Fromageries Bel)	1 oz	8	100	72%
	8 oz	66	800	74%
(Kraft)-natural	1 oz	7	90	70%
(Land O'Lakes)-natural	1 oz	8	100	72%
(May-Bud)	1 oz	8	100	72%
(Sargento)	1 oz	8	101	71%
Farmer's/(May-Bud)-semisoft				
part skim	1 oz	7	90	70%
(Sargento)	1 oz	8	102	71%
Feta	1 oz	6	75	72%
(Churny)-Natural	1 oz	6.5	75	78%
(Sargento)	1 oz	6	80	68%
Fontina (Sargento)	1 oz	8.8	110	72%

Food and Description	Amount	Fat Grams	Total Calories	% Fat Calories
Gjetost	1 oz	8	132	55%
(Sargento)	1 oz	8	130	55%
(Ski Queen)	1 oz	9	130	62%
Gorgonzola (Sargento)	1 oz	8	100	72%
Gouda	1 oz	7.78	101	69%
(Fromageries Bel)	1 oz	9	110	66%
	8 oz	73	880	75%
mini	¾ oz	6	80	68%
mini red bottle container				
processed	1 oz	6	80	68%
Nacho Cheese Sauce	1 oz	6	80	68%
Neufchatel Spread				
garlic & herb	1 oz	7	80	79%
garden veg	1 oz	7	80	79%
Port Wine Cheddar	1 oz	7	90	70%
Sharp Cheddar	1 oz	6	90	60%
Lite spread	1 oz	4	70	51%
Sharp Cheddar Log w/almonds	1 oz	7	100	63%
Sharp Lite	1 oz	4	70	51%
Smoky Sharp Cheddar	1 oz	7	90	70%
(Kaukauna) Microwave spreadable cheese				
Cheddar	1 oz	6	80	68%
Jalapeno	1 oz	6	80	68%
Limburger	1 oz	7.7	93	75%
Little Gem Size				
(Mohawk Valley)	1 oz	8	90	80%
(Sargento)	1 oz	8	90	80%
Macaroni Cheese Loaf (Eckrich)	1 oz	6	75	72%
Monterey	1 oz	8.58	106	73%
Monterey Jack	1 oz	9	110	74%
(Formagg)-cheese food	1 oz	5	70	64%
Jalapeno Flav	1 oz	5	70	64%
(Kraft)-natural	1 oz	9	110	74%
cheese food singles	1 oz	7	90	70%
Lite (Lifetime)	1 oz	3	55	49%
(May-Bud)	1 oz	9	110	74%
Natural (Land O'Lakes)	1 oz	9	110	74%
reduced fat (Light Naturals)	1 oz	5	80	56%
(Sargento)	1 oz	9	110	74%
(Weight Watchers)	1 oz	5	80	56%
with jalapeno peppers-mild (Kraft)	1 oz	9	110	74%
Monti-Jack-Lo (Alpine Lace)	1 oz	5	80	56%
Mozzarella/breaded-frozen (Banquet)	2.6 oz	12	220	49%
(Formagg)	1 oz	5	70	64%

Food and Description	Amount	Fat Grams	Total Calories	% Fat Calories
Imitation (Sargento)	1 oz	6	80	68%
(Lite-Line) 8% milkfat				
pasteurized process	1 oz	2	50	36%
low moisture	1 oz	7	90	70%
Natural (Land O'Lakes)				
low moisture part skim	1 oz	5	80	56%
(Weight Watchers)	1 oz	4	70	51%
shredded	1 oz	4	70	51%
part skim	1 oz	5	85	53%
Alpine Lace part skim and low				
moisture	1 oz	5	70	64%
(Sargento) part skim and low				
moisture	1 oz	5	80	56%
string	1 oz	5	80	56%
(Precious)	1 oz	6	88	61%
string w/jalapeno peppers–(Kraft)	1 oz	5	80	56%
strip (Arpin)				
real cheese snacks	1 oz	6	85	64%
w/pizza spices (Sargento)	1 oz	5	79	57%
whole milk	1 oz	6	80	68%
Whole milk (Sargento)	1 oz	7	90	70%
Muenster	1 oz	8.5	104	74%
(Alpine Lace)	1 oz	8	100	72%
(Dorman's)-Lo-Chol	1 oz	7	100	63%
(Kraft)	1 oz	9	110	74%
Natural (Land O'Lakes)	1 oz	9	100	81%
Red Rind (Sargento)	1 oz	9	100	81%
Nacho (Sargento)	1 oz	9	106	76%
Nacho Cheese Dip, Premium (Kraft)	2 Tbs	4	50	72%
(New Holland)-Caraway	1 oz	8	90	80%
Garlic & Herb	1 oz	8	90	80%
Hot Jalapeno	1 oz	8	90	80%
Natural-part skim-semi-soft	1 oz	8	90	80%
Neufchatel	1 oz	7	80	79%
Nippy (Kraft)	1 oz	7	90	70%
Norwegian Jarlsbery-Sliced				
(Sargento)	1 oz	7	100	63%
Nuggets-Breaded Cheese				
(Schwan's)-frozen	3.5 oz	19	360	48%
Onion (Land O'Lakes)-cheese food	1 oz	7	90	70%
Parmesan/fresh (Sargento)	1 oz	7	111	57%
grated	1 Tbs	1.5	23	59%
	1 oz	8.5	129	59%
(Sargento)	1 oz	9	130	55%

Food and Description	Amount	Fat Grams	Total Calories	% Fat Calories
hard	1 oz	7	111	57%
natural (Kraft)	1 oz	7	110	57%
Parmesan & Romano (Sargento)				
grated	1 oz	7	110	57%
Parmesan Wedge (Frigo)	1 oz	7	110	57%
Pepperoni (Land O'Lakes)				
cheese food	1 oz	7	90	70%
Pimento/pasteurized	1 oz	8.8	106	75%
pasteurized process slices (Kraft)	1 oz	8	100	72%
singles cheese food (Kraft)	1 oz	7	90	70%
snack (Sargento)-pasteurized				
process	1 oz	9	110	74%
Pizza Topper (Formagg)	1 oz	5	70	64%
Pizza Topping (Lunch Wagon)	1 oz	6	80	68%
Port du Salut	1 oz	8	100	72%
Port Wine Nut Log (Sargento)	1 oz	7	100	63%
Pot				
(Land O'Lakes)	4 oz	5	120	38%
(Sargento)	1 oz	–	25	–
Provo-Lo (Alpine Lace)	1 oz	5	72	63%
Provolone	1 oz	7.55	100	68%
(Formagg)-cheese food	1 oz	5	70	64%
(Kraft)	1 oz	7	100	63%
Natural (Land O'Lakes)	1 oz	8	100	72%
(Sargento)	1 oz	8	100	72%
Pub Cheese -soft w/Garlic & Herbs	1 oz	8	90	80%
Queso Blanco (Sargento)	1 oz	9	100	81%
Queso de Papa (Sargento)	1 oz	9	110	66%
Ricotta				
(Frigo)				
Low-fat	1 oz	1	30	30%
Part skim	1 oz	3	40	68%
Whole milk	1 oz	5	60	75%
(Formagg)-cheese food	1 oz	5	130	35%
Lite (Sargento)	1 oz	1	23	39%
Low-fat (Frigo)	1 oz	1	20	45%
part skim milk	½ cup	9.8	171	52%
	1 oz	3	42	64%
(Sargento)	1 oz	2	30	60%
whole milk	½ cup	16	216	67%
(Sargento)	1 oz	4	40	90%
Romano	1 oz	7.6	110	62%
grated (Kraft)	1 oz	9	130	62%
(Sargento)	1 oz	8	110	66%

Food and Description	Amount	Fat Grams	Total Calories	% Fat Calories
Romano-Flavored Spagetti Topping				
Grated	1 oz	3	80	34%
(Rondele') soft spreadable cheese				
Fine Herbs	1 oz	9	100	81%
Garlic & Harbs	1 oz	9	100	81%
Jardiniere-Garden Vegetables	1 oz	9	100	81%
Roquefort	1 oz	8.69	105	75%
Salami Cheese Food (Land O'Lakes)	1 oz	7	90	70%
Sandwich Slices (Lunch Wagon)	1 oz	7	90	70%
Smokelle (Kraft)-cheese food	1 oz	7	90	70%
Smokestick (Sargento)	1 oz	7	100	63%
(Squeeze Cheese)/bacon	1 oz	6	82	66%
Jalapeno	1 oz	6	82	66%
Mild Cheddar	1 oz	6	82	66%
(Stella)				
Fontinella	1 oz	9	110	74%
Italian Sharp	1 oz	9	110	74%
Kasseri	1 oz	9	110	74%
Provolone	1 oz	7	100	63%
String Cheese/(Sargento)	1 oz	5	80	56%
(Sargento)-Smoked	1 oz	5	80	56%
Swiss	1 oz	7.78	107	65%
aged (Kraft)	1 oz	8	110	66%
almond nut log (Sargento)	1 oz	7	90	70%
(Alpine Lace)-Swiss-Lo	1 oz	7	100	63%
(Borden)	1 oz	8	100	72%
(Cache Valley)-natural	1 oz	8	100	72%
(Dorman's)-Deli Light				
90% less salt	1 oz	8	100	72%
(Kraft)-Deluxe				
slices				
cheese food	1 oz	7	90	70%
Light singles	1 oz	3	70	39%
Singles				
cheese food	1 oz	7	90	70%
Very Low Sodium	1 oz	8	110	66%
(Land O'Lakes)-natural	1 oz	8	110	66%
(Lifetime)-Lite	1 oz	3	55	49%
(Light N'Lively)	1 oz	4	70	51%
(Lite-Line)	1 oz	2	50	36%
pasteurized	1 oz	7	95	66%
processed	1 oz	7	95	66%
reduced fat (Light Naturals)	1 oz	5	90	50%
(Sargento)-natural	1 oz	8	110	66%

Food and Description	Amount	Fat Grams	Total Calories	% Fat Calories
cheese food	1 oz	7	95	66%
sliced Finland	1 oz	8	110	66%
snack-pasteurized process	1 oz	7	100	63%
(Weight Watchers)	1 oz	2	50	36%
natural	1 oz	5	80	56%
Taco/(Sargento)	1 oz	9	110	74%
shredded (Kraft)	1 oz	9	110	74%
Tilsit	1 oz	7	96	66%
Tilsiter/(Dorman's)-natural	1 oz	11	120	83%
(Sargento)	1 oz	7	100	63%
Tybo-Red Wax (Sargento)	1 oz	7	100	63%
(Velveeta) light	1 oz	4	70	51%
Welsh Rarebit (also Rabbit)				
homemade	1 cup	32	415	69%
CHEESE SNACKS				
(Cheetos)				
Crunchy	1 oz	10	150	60%
Light Cheese Flavored				
Crunchy	1 oz	6	120	45%
Puffed Balls	1 oz	10	160	56%
Puffs	1 oz	10	160	56%
(Cheetos)				
Cheddar Valley	1 oz	9	160	51%
(Eagle)				
Cheese Crunch	1 oz	10	160	56%
(Featherweight)				
Cheese Curls	1 oz	9	150	54%
(Laura Scudder)				
Crunchy Cheese-Flavored Snacks	1 oz	10	160	56%
Puffed Cheese-Flavored Snacks	1 oz	9	150	54%
(Planter's)				
Cheez Balls	1 oz	11	160	62%
Cheez Curls	1 oz	11	160	62%
(Health Valley)				
Cheese Puffs				
Cheddar Light	¼ oz	2	40	45%
Cheddar Lites w/green onion	¼ oz	1	40	23%
(Wise)				
Cheez Doodles				
Crunchy	1 oz	10	160	56%
Puffed	1 oz	9	150	54%
Cheez Waffles	1 oz	8	140	51%
CHEESE SOUP (*See* SOUP)				

Food and Description	Amount	Fat Grams	Total Calories	% Fat Calories
CHEESE SUBSTITUTE				
CHEESE-FLAVORED SPRINKLE PRODUCTS				
Best of Butter-cheddar cheese	½ tsp	< 1	6	75%
Molly McButter	½ tsp	–	4	–
(Cheeztwin)Singles:	½ tsp	6	90	60%
(Delica)-American pasteurized				
process	½ tsp	6	80	68%
American & Caraway				
pasteurized process	½ tsp	6	80	68%
American & Hot Pepper				
pasteurized process	½ tsp	6	80	68%
American & Salami				
pasteurized process	½ tsp	6	80	68%
American-Hickory Smoked				
pasteeurized process	½ tsp	6	80	68%
(Fisher Ched-O-Mate)-cheddar				
shredded	½ tsp	7	90	70%
(Fisher Pizza-Mate)-Mozzarella				
shredded	½ tsp	7	90	70%
(Fisher Sandwich-Mate)-singles	½ tsp	6	90	60%
(Formagg)-no lactose - lower in saturated fat - made w/canola oil				
American				
white	½ tsp	5	70	64%
yellow	½ tsp	5	70	64%
cheddar	½ tsp	5	70	64%
cream cheese style	½ tsp	5	70	64%
cottage-flavored	½ tsp	5	70	64%
jalapeno	½ tsp	5	70	64%
mild cheddar	½ tsp	5	70	64%
monterey jack	½ tsp	5	70	64%
mozzarella-shredded	½ tsp	5	70	64%
parmesan-shredded	½ tsp	5	70	64%
pasta topping-grated	½ tsp	5	70	64%
pizza topper-shredded	½ tsp	5	70	64%
provolone	½ tsp	5	70	64%
ricotta	½ tsp	.85	35	22%
salad topper-shredded	½ tsp	5	70	64%
sour cream style	½ tsp	5	70	64%
Swiss	½ tsp	5	70	64%
(Lite-Line) Low Cholesterol				
Singles	½ tsp	7	90	70%
CHERIMOYA				
raw-5" dia.	1	2	459	4%

Food and Description	Amount	Fat Grams	Total Calories	% Fat Calories
CHERRY				
Maraschino	10 large	–	97	–
	1 large	–	10	–
with liquid	1 oz	–	33	–
Royal Anne				
canned (World Classic)	½ cup	–	90	–
Sour-Red	1 cup	< 1	51	9%
canned				
in water	1 cup	< 1	87	5%
in light syrup	1 cup	< 1	188	2%
in heavy syrup	1 cup	< 1	232	2%
in xtra heavy syrup	1 cup	< 1	296	2%
frozen				
no sugar	1 cup	.7	72	9%
	3.5 oz		50	3%
sweetened	1 cup	.7	224	3%
Sweet	1 cup	1	104	9%
	10	.7	49	13%
candied				
whole	10	< 1	119	4%
	1 oz	< 1	96	5%
canned				
in water	1 cup	< 1	114	4%
in juice	1 cup	< 1	136	3%
in light syrup	1 cup	< 1	170	3%
in heavy syrup	1 cup	< 1	213	2%
in xtra heavy syrup	1 cup	< 1	266	2%
canned (Del Monte)				
dark sweet				
w/pits	½ cup	< 1	90	5%
w/o pits	½ cup	< 1	90	5%
light sweet				
w/pits	½ cup	< 1	100	5%
frozen				
sweetened	1 cup	< 1	232	2%
unsweetened	3.5 oz	< 1	60	8%
CHERRY DRINK				
(Hi-C)	6 oz	–	100	–
(Juice Works)	6 oz	–	96	–
(Kool-Aid Kooler)	8.45 oz	–	140	–
Squeezit (Betty Crocker)	6.75 oz	–	110	–
(Tang) Fruit Box	8.45 oz	–	120	–
BLACK CHERRY DRINK				
Black Cherry Cooler (Health Valley)	13 oz	1	144	6%

Food and Description	Amount	Fat Grams	Total Calories	% Fat Calories
Black Cherry Drink	8 oz	–	117	–
CHERRY FRUIT JUICE COCKTAIL				
(Welch's)	6 oz	–	110	–
frozen	6 oz	–	90	–
CHERRY JUICE				
Cherry Delight Nectar	6 oz	–	80	–
Cherry-Juicy Juice (Libby's)	6 oz	–	90	–
MOUNTAIN CHERRY JUICE				
(Dole) Pure & Light	6 oz	–	90	–
CHERVIL				
dried	1 tsp	–	1	–
raw	4 oz	–	65	–
CHESTNUT				
Chinese				
boiled-steamed	1 oz	–	44	–
dried	1 oz	.5	103	4%
roasted	1 oz	–	68	–
European				
boiled-steamed	1 oz	–	37	–
dried	1 oz	1	106	8%
roasted	1 oz	.6	70	8%
Japanese				
boiled-steamed	1 oz	–	16	–
dried	1 oz	–	102	–
roasted	1 oz	–	57	–
CHESTNUT FLOUR	4 oz	4	410	9%
CHICKEN				
Chicken, broilers or fryers				
flesh, skin, giblets, & neck 1 chicken				
batter dipped/fried	~ 2¼ lb	180	2987	54%
flour coated/fried	~ 1½ lb	108	1928	50%
roasted	~ 1½ lb	90	1598	51%
stewed	~ 1½ lb	92.9	1625	52%
Chicken, broilers or fryers-flesh & skin ½ chicken				
batter dipped/fried	~ 1 lb	80.8	1347	54%
flour coated/fried	~ ¾ lb	46.8	844	50%
roasted w/skin	~ ¾ lb	40.67	715	51%
stewed w/skin	~ ¾ lb	41.96	730	52%
Chicken, broilers or fryers-flesh only				
fried	~ 5 oz	12.77	307	37%
roasted w/skin	~ 5 oz	10	266	34%
stewed w/skin	~ 5 oz	9	248	33%
Chicken-Dark Meat w/skin				
battered dipped/fried	~ 9.5 oz	51.8	828	56%

Food and Description	Amount	Fat Grams	Total Calories	% Fat Calories
flour coated/fried	~6.5 oz	31	523	53%
roasted	~6 oz	26	423	55%
stewed	~6.5 oz	26.97	428	57%
Chicken-Light Meat w/skin				
batter dipped/fried	~7 oz	29	520	50%
flour coated/fried	~5 oz	15.7	320	44%
roasted	~5 oz	14	293	43%
stewed	~5 oz	14.95	302	45%
Chicken-Dark Meat w/o skin				
fried	~5 oz	16	334	43%
roasted	~5 oz	13.6	286	43%
stewed	~5 oz	12.57	269	42%
Chicken-Light Meat w/o skin				
fried	~5 oz	7.76	268	26%
roasted	~5 oz	6	242	22%
stewed	~5 oz	5.58	223	23%
Chicken Giblets				
flour coated/fried	1 cup	19.5	402	44%
simmered	1 cup	6.9	228	27%
Chicken Gizzard/simmered	1 cup	5	222	20%
Chicken Heart/simmered	3 oz	5	158	29%
Chicken Liver/simmered	~5 oz	7.6	219	31%
Individual Pieces of broilers or fryers				
Chicken Backs/meat & skin				
batter coated/fried	~4 oz	26	397	59%
flour-coated/fried	~2.5 oz	14.9	238	56%
roasted	~2 oz	11	159	62%
stewed	~2 oz	11	158	63%
Chicken Backs/meat only				
fried	~2 oz	8.88	167	48%
roasted	~1.5 oz	5	96	47%
stewed	~1.5 oz	4.7	88	48%
Chicken Breast/meat & skin				
battered dipped/fried	~5 oz	18.5	364	46%
flour-coated/fried	~3.5 oz	8.69	218	36%
roasted	~3.5 oz	7.6	193	35%
stewed	~4 oz	8	202	36%
Chicken Breast/meat only				
fried	~3 oz	4	161	22%
roasted	~3 oz	3	142	19%
stewed	~3 oz	2.88	144	18%
Chicken Breast/smoked				
(Butterball)-97% fat free	¾ oz	1	25	36%
(Eckrich)-Lite	1 oz	1	30	30%

Food and Description	Amount	Fat Grams	Total Calories	% Fat Calories
Chicken Drumstick/meat & skin				
batter dipped/fried	~ 2.5 oz	11	193	51%
flour-coated/fried	~ 2 oz	6.7	120	50%
roasted	~ 2 oz	5.8	112	47%
stewed	~ 2 oz	6	116	47%
Chicken Drumstick/meat only				
fried	~ 1.5 oz	3	82	33%
roasted	~ 1.5 oz	2	76	24%
stewed	~ 1.5 oz	2.6	78	30%
Chicken Leg/meat & skin				
batter dipped/fried	~ 5.5 oz	25.55	431	53%
flour-coated/fried	~ 4 oz	16	285	51%
roasted	~ 4 oz	15	265	51%
stewed	~ 4 oz	16	275	52%
Chicken Leg/meat only				
fried	~ 3 oz	8.76	195	40%
roasted	~ 3 oz	8	182	40%
stewed	~ 3.5 oz	8	187	39%
Chicken Thigh/meat & skin				
batter dipped/fried	~ 3 oz	14	238	53%
flour-coated/fried	~ 2 oz	9	162	50%
roasted	~ 2 oz	9.6	153	56%
stewed	~ 2 oz	10	158	57%
Chicken Thigh/meat only				
fried	~ 2 oz	5	113	40%
roasted	~ 2 oz	5.66	109	47%
stewed	~ 2 oz	5	107	42%
Chicken Wing/meat & skin				
batter dipped/fried	~ 2 oz	10.68	159	61%
flour-coated/fried	~ 1 oz	7	103	61%
roasted	~ 1.5 oz	6.6	99	60%
stewed	~ 1.5 oz	6.7	100	60%
Chicken Wing/meat only				
fried	~ 1 oz	1.8	42	39%
roasted	~ 1 oz	1.7	43	36%
stewed	~ 1 oz	1.7	43	36%
Chicken, Roasting/roasted				
meat & skin	~ 5 oz	9	233	35%
light meat/meat only	~ 5 oz	5.7	214	34%
Chicken, Stewing				
meat, skin, & giblets				
stewed 1 chicken	~ 1 ¼ lb	106.9	1636	59%
meat & skin, no giblets	~ 9 oz	49	744	59%
meat only	~ 5 oz	16.6	332	45%

Food and Description	Amount	Fat Grams	Total Calories	% Fat Calories
light meat w/o skin	~ 5 oz	11	298	33%
dark meat w/o skin	~ 5 oz	21	361	52%
giblets-simmered	~ 5 oz	1		
CHICKEN ENTREE/DINNER (*See also* FROZEN ENTREE/DINNER)				
Chicken A la king/canned	~ 5 oz	11.7	182	58%
(Swanson)	5.25 oz	12	180	60%
frozen (Banquet) Cookin'Bags	4 oz	5	110	41%
homemade	1 cup	34	468	65%
Chicken Almond, w/rice				
(Van de Kamp's)	11 oz	15	440	31%
Chicken Applause! Oven Bake Dinners (Kraft) - box				
Barbeque & scalloped potatoes	1 Serving	7	380	17%
Mushroom & rice	1 Serving	6	380	14%
Three Cheese & rice	1 Serving	15	430	31%
Chicken Cacciatore/frozen				
(Lean Cuisine)	~ 11 oz	10	280	32%
/homemade	1 cup	32	525	55%
Chicken Cordon Bleu/homemade	8 oz	13	335	35%
(Swift) International Entree	6 oz	17	360	43%
Chicken/(Country Pride)-frozen -				
Chicken Chunks	3 oz	15	238	57%
Chicken Patties	3 oz	16	245	59%
Chicken Sticks	3 oz	14	233	54%
Southern Fried Chicken Chunks	3 oz	20	276	65%
Southern Fried Chicken Patties	3 oz	15	232	58%
Chicken - creamed/homemade	½ cup	12	208	52%
Chicken Creole/no rice/homemade	~ 6.5 oz			
	(¾ cup)	3	137	20%
Chcicken Croissant/frozen (Sara Lee)	1	17	340	45%
Chicken/Egg noodles w/chicken dinner				
(Kraft) box mix	¾ cup	9	240	34%
Chicken Fiesta/(International Lites)				
microwavable - box prepared	10 oz	3	220	12%
Chicken Fricassee				
Standard Home Recipe (USDA)	1 cup	22	386	51%
Chicken, Glazed Breast of (Top Shelf)				
microwavalbe - box prepared	10 oz	3	210	13%
Chicken Hash/homemade	1 cup	11	239	41%
Chicken Helper - (Betty Crocker) Box mix - prepared				
Chicken Tetrazzini	1 serving	12	320	34%
Crispy Chicken & Biscuits	1 serving	42	710	53%
Crispy Chicken & Seasoned Rice	1 serving	38	690	50%
Mushroom Chicken	1 serving	25	470	48%
Stuffing	1 serving	32	570	51%

Food and Description	Amount	Fat Grams	Total Calories	% Fat Calories
Chicken/(Hunt's Minute Gourmet) - Box mix				
Barbeque Chicken	6.8 oz	4	320	11%
Chicken Cacciatore	~ 8 oz	6	280	19%
Chicken Italian Style/frozen				
(Weaver)	3 oz	11	205	48%
Chicken Kiev/(Swift)				
International Entree	6 oz	24	420	51%
Chicken Marsala, Breast of				
frozen (Lean Cuisine)	8.5 oz	5	190	24%
Chicken & Noodles/frozen (Swanson)	9 oz	16	400	36%
Chicken w/noodles/homemade	1 cup	18	365	44%
Chicken Pie/frozen (Stouffer's)	10 oz	33	530	56%
Chicken Pot Pies				
Standard Home Recipe (USDA)- 9"dia	⅓ serving/ ~ 8 oz	31	545	51%
frozen (Banquet)	7 oz	35	540	58%
frozen-(Banquet)				
supreme microwave	7 oz	27	429	57%
(Morton)	7 oz	27	415	59%
(Swanson)	7 oz	22	370	54%
(Swanson) Homestyle Recipe	8 oz	19	380	45%
(Swanson) Hungry Man	16 oz	41	740	50%
Chicken & Rice/box-mixes prepared				
Almond Chicken-Wild Rice				
(Savory Classics)	1 serving	4	140	26%
Chicken-Broc-Dijon/				
(Savory Classics)	1 serving	5	160	28%
Chicken Flavor/(Rice-A-Roni)	1 serving	1	130	7%
Chicken Florentine/				
(Savory Classics)	1 serving	.8	108	7%
Chicken Mushroom/(Rice-A-Roni)	1 serving	1	129	7%
Chicken-peas & Carrots				
(Minute Microwave)	½ cup	1	130	7%
Chicken Rice & Sauce/(Lipton)	½ cup	4	150	24%
Chicken & Vegtables/				
(Rice-A-Roni)	1 serving	3	140	19%
Chicken-Vermicelli/				
(Rice-A-Roni)	1 serving	5	170	27%
Chicken Salad				
Standard Home Recipe (USDA)	½ cup	8	121	60%
Chicken Stew/canned				
(Chef Boyardee)	7 oz	5	140	32%
(Heinz)-w/dumplings	7.5 oz	9	210	39%
(Swanson)	7⅝ oz	7	170	37%

Food and Description	Amount	Fat Grams	Total Calories	% Fat Calories
Chicken Supreme/frozen				
(Lite Pockets)	1	5	240	19%
Chicken Tetrazzini/frozen	11.5 oz	14	320	39%
Chicken Tortellini Alfredo (International Lites)				
microwave box mix	10 oz	13	290	40%
Chicken & Vegetable Stew/(Bounty)	7.5 oz	7	166	38%
Chunk Style Mixin' Chicken				
canned (Swanson)	2½ oz	8	130	55%
Great Beginnings (Hormel)-Box mix				
w/chunky chicken	5 oz	8	147	49%
w/chunky turkey	5 oz	8	138	52%
(Hormel) Chicken By George Gourmet Entree-found in the grocery meat case				
Cajun	5 oz	9	200	41%
Country Mustard & Dill	5 oz	7	180	35%
For Fajitas	5 oz	4	170	21%
Italian Blue Cheese	5 oz	8	190	40%
Lemon Herb	5 oz	4	150	24%
Mesquite Barbeque	5 oz	4	170	21%
Tomato Herb w/Basil	5 oz	7	190	33%
(Lean Cuisine)-chicken/frozen				
Breast of Chicken/				
Herb Cream Sauce	9.5 oz	10	260	35%
Breast of Chicken Parmasan	10 oz	8	250	29%
Chicken'a l' orange	~8 oz	5	260	17%
Glazed Chicken	8.5 oz	8	270	27%
Chicken & Vegetables	11.75 oz	8	270	27%
(Schwan's)-chicken/home delivery-frozen-partially or fully cooked, unless otherwise stated.				
BBQ Wings	3.5 oz	14	220	57%
Breaded Chicken	7.5 oz	14	250	50%
Breast Fillet-raw-unbreaded	3.25 oz	1	90	10%
Breast Patties	3 oz	14	210	60%
Breast Strips	3.5 oz	14	270	47%
Breast w/Asparagus & Cheese	6 oz	14	300	42%
Chicken Kiev	5 oz	24	360	60%
Chicken Marco Polo	5.3 oz	12	290	37%
Chicken Nuggets	3.5 oz	17	260	59%
Cordon Bleu	5 oz	14	290	43%
Diced Chicken Meat	3.5 oz	4	120	30%
Drummies	3.5 oz	15	260	52%
Golden Chicken Nuggets	3.5 oz/~ 7 nuggets	9	180	45%
Hot & Spicy Chicken Nuggets	3.5 oz/5-6 nuggets	19	320	53%

Food and Description	Amount	Fat Grams	Total Calories	% Fat Calories
Hot Wings	3.5 oz	14	220	57%
(Swanson)-frozen Plump & Juicy Chicken				
Chicken Dipsters	3 oz	14	220	57%
Chicken Drumlets	3 oz	14	220	57%
Chicken Nibbles	3¼ oz	20	300	60%
Chicken Nuggets	8¾ oz	25	460	49%
Fried Chicken-breast portion	4½ oz	22	360	55%
1 lb Take-Out pre-fried chicken	3¼ oz	17	270	57%
Take-Out fried chicken	3¼ oz	17	270	57%
Thighs and Drumsticks	3¼ oz	19	280	61%
(TastyBird Foods)-chicken/frozen-raw-ready to cook				
Breast Fillet Pattie	3.5 oz	14	229	55%
Breast Fillet Pattie				
hoagie shaped	3.5 oz	10.8	211	46%
Breast Strip	1 oz	2.8	54	47%
Breast Tenderloins	3.5 oz	8.7	189	41%
Chicken Delites	3.5 oz	19	252	68%
Chicken Nuggets	3.5 oz	13.8	215	58%
Hi-Pro Chicken Patties	3.5 oz	19	252	68%
Natural Breast Fillet	3.5 oz	8.6	187	41%
Spicy Breast Tenderloins	3.5 oz	7	170	37%
Tastybird Breaded Breast				
Quarters	3.5 oz	11	192	52%
Tastybird Breaded Leg Quarters	3.5 oz	11.7	199	53%
(Tyson)				
Chicken/frozen				
Boneless				
Breast Chunks	3 oz	17	240	64%
Breast Fillets	3 oz	9	190	43%
Breast Patties	2.6 oz	15	220	61%
Breast Patties-southern fried	2.6 oz	15	220	61%
Breast Tenders-southern fried	3 oz	11	220	45%
Chick'n Cheddar	2.6 oz	15	220	61%
Chick'n Chunks	2.6 oz	15	220	61%
Chunk'n Chunks-southern fried	2.6 oz	15	220	61%
Cornish Game Hens	3.5 oz	14	240	57%
Diced Meat	3 oz	5	150	30%
Thick & Crispy Patties	2.6 oz	14	220	57%
Flyers (wings) -				
Barbecue	3.5 oz/6-7 wings	14	220	57%
Hot & Spicy	3.5 oz/6-7 wings	14	220	57%

Food and Description	Amount	Fat Grams	Total Calories	% Fat Calories
Italian	3.5 oz/6-7 wings	14	220	57%
Roasted	3.5 oz/6-7 wings	14	220	57%
Gourmet Selection Entrees				
A L'Orange	9.5 oz	8	300	24%
Chicken & Beef Luau	10.5 oz	10	330	30%
Dijon	8.5 oz	17	310	49%
Francais	9.5 oz	12	280	39%
Kiev	9.25 oz	33	520	57%
Lasagna	11.5 oz	14	380	33%
Marsala	10.5 oz	13	300	39%
Mesquite	9.5 oz	11	320	31%
Parmigiana	11.25 oz	12	330	33%
Picatta	9 oz	10	240	38%
Marinated Chicken Breast				
Barbecue	3.75 oz	2	120	15%
Butter Dill	3.75 oz	2	130	14%
Butter Garlic	3.75 oz	7	160	39%
Dijon	3.75 oz	2	130	14%
Italian	3.75 oz	2	130	14%
Lemon Pepper	3.75 oz	2	120	15%
Savory	3.75 oz	2	130	14%
Microwave				
Breast Sandwich	1	12	275	39%
Chicken Corn Dogs	3.5 oz	14	280	45%
Chunks	4.5 oz	15	220	61%
Mini Sandwich	1	5	230	20%
Nuggets	4 oz	15	220	61%
Tenders	4 oz	11	230	43%
(Weaver)-chicken/frozen				
Battered Dipped Fried Chicken				
Breasts	3.5 oz	16	250	58%
Thighs & Drums	3.5 oz	15.5	245	57%
Wings	3.5 oz	18.5	270	62%
Breast Fillet Strips	3.5 oz	9	200	41%
Breast Fillets	3.5 oz	10	195	46%
Breast Pattie	3.5 oz	10	185	49%
Cheese Rondelet	3 oz	12.5	215	52%
Chicken AuGratin	1 serving	6.5	140	42%
Chicken Nuggets	3.5 oz	16	255	57%
Crisp Mini Drums	1 serving	11	205	48%
Crispy Dutch Frye Fried Chicken				
Breasts	3.5 oz	17.5	285	55%

Food and Description	Amount	Fat Grams	Total Calories	% Fat Calories
Thighs & Drums	3.5 oz	20	295	61%
Wings	3.5 oz	25	360	63%
Assorted	3.5 oz	19.5	300	59%
Crispy Light Fried Chicken	1 serving	8.5	160	48%
Croquettes	3.5 oz	14.5	245	53%
Gravy	1 serving	2	50	36%
Herbs'N Spice Mini Drums	1 serving	11	205	48%
Homestyle Rondelt	3 oz	10	185	49%
Italian Rondelet	3 oz	11	200	50%
Mini Drums	3 oz	12	210	51%
Original Rondelet	3 oz	9.5	185	46%
Spicy Herb Fried Chicken				
Assorted	3.5 oz	21.5	310	62%
Tenders	1 serving	8.5	170	45%
Honey Battered	1 serving	9	180	45%
Zesty Wings	3.5 oz	16	245	59%
(Weight Watchers)-chicken/frozen				
A la King	9 oz	8	220	33%
Cordon Bleu	8 oz	11	230	45%
Fettucini	8.25 oz	10	290	31%
Imperial Chicken	9.25 oz	4	220	16%
Nuggets	5.9 oz	12	270	40%
CHICKEN PRODUCTS (*See also* LUNCHEON MEATS)				
Chicken/canned-boned w/broth	2.5 oz	5.6	117	43%
(Hormel)-Chunk Breast of	6¾ oz	20	350	51%
Chunk Dark Meat	6¾ oz	18	327	50%
Chunk White & Dark	6¾ oz	20	340	53%
Chunk White & Dark				
no salt	6¾ oz	18	330	49%
(Swanson)-Premium Chunk White	2½ oz	4	100	36%
(Swanson)-Premium Chunk				
White & Dark	2½ oz	4	100	36%
Chicken Frankfurter	1 (1.5 oz)	8.8	116	68%
Chicken Liver-canned	1 oz	3.7	57	58%
Chicken Roll/light	2½ oz	4	90	40%
Chicken Spread/chunky/canned				
(Underwood)	½ can/ 2.25 oz	11	150	66%
CHICKEN SEASONING				
(French's) Microwave Mixes				
Barbecue Chicken	¼ pkg	2	50	36%
Garlic Butter Chicken	¼ pkg	1	50	36%
Italian Parmesan Chicken	¼ pkg	2	50	36%
(Lipton) Microeasy Family Favorites - dry				

Food and Description	Amount	Fat Grams	Total Calories	% Fat Calories
Barbeque Style Chicken	¼ pkg	.5	108	4%
Country Style Chicken	¼ pkg	.6	78	7%
(McCormick/Schilling)				
Bag'N Season - dry				
Chicken	1 pkg	1.5	177	8%
Italian Herb	1 pkg	–	94	–
Chicken Sauce Blends - dry				
Cacciatore	1 pkg	4.8	132	33
Creole	1 pkg	4.8	140	31%
CHICKEN SOUP (*See* SOUP)				
CHICORY/ raw	8 oz	–	15	–
CHILI (*See* MEXICAN FOOD and SOUP)				
CHILI SAUCE (*See* SAUCE)				
CHINESE FOOD (*See* ORIENTAL FOOD)				
CHIVES				
freeze-dried	1 Tbs	–	1	–
raw	1 Tbs	–	1	–
	¼ cup	–	2	–
CHOCOLATE, BAKING				
Baker's				
Semi-sweet bar	1 oz	9	140	58%
Sweet German	1 oz	10	140	64%
Unsweetened	1 oz	15	140	96%
Hershey's	1 oz	16	190	76%
Nestles				
Premier white	1 oz	5	80	56%
Semi-sweet	1 oz	9	160	51%
Unsweetened	1 oz	14	180	70%
Pre-melted-Choco Bake	1 oz	16	190	76%
CHOCOLATE CHIPS				
Baker's				
Milk chocolate	1 oz	8	140	51%
Big Chips	¼ cup	13	220	53%
Chocolate-flavored	¼ cup	9	200	41%
	½ cup	18	380	43%
Big Chips	¼ cup	13	240	49%
Semi-sweet	¼ cup	11	200	50%
	½ cup	24	400	54%
Hershey's				
Milk chocolate	1 oz	8	150	48%
Semi-sweet Big Chips	¼ cup	12	220	49%
CHOCOLATE MORSELS				
Nestles				
Butterscotch	1 oz	8	150	48%

Food and Description	Amount	Fat Grams	Total Calories	% Fat Calories
Chocolate	1 oz	7	150	42%
Semi-sweet	1 oz	8	150	48%
CHOCOLATE NAPS (Champion)	1 oz	14	140	90%
CHOCOLATE SYRUP (Hershey's)	2 Tbs	1	80	11%
CHOCOLATE TREASURES				
(Nestles)				
Milk	1 oz	9	150	54%
Premier White	1 oz	10	160	56%
Semi-sweet chocolate	1 oz	8	150	48%
CHUB/raw	3 oz	7.5	124	54%
CINNAMON/ground	1 tsp	–	6	–
CITRON				
candied	1 oz	–	89	–
	3 oz	–	270	–
CLAM (*See also* SEAFOOD ENTREE/DINNER)				
breaded & fried	3 oz	9	171	47%
	20 Small	20.96	379	50%
canned	3 oz	1.65	126	12%
canned-chopped				
(Doxsee)				
liquid & solids	6.5 oz	.5	90	5%
(S&W)				
Fancy	2 oz	< 1	28	16%
canned-minced				
(Doxsee)				
liquid & solids	6.5 oz	.5	90	5%
(S&W)				
Fancy	2 oz	< 1	28	16%
canned-minced & chopped				
(Gorton's)	½ can	1	70	13%
canned-whole baby chowder				
(S&W)	2 oz	< 1	33	14%
raw	3 oz	.8	63	11%
steamed	3 oz	1.65	126	12%
	20 Small	1.75	133	12%
	1 cup	3	235	12%
CLAM CHOWDER (*See* SOUP)				
CLAM JUICE				
Clam (Doxsee)	3 oz	–	4	–
Clamato (Mott's)	6 oz	–	90	–
CLAM SAUCE (*See* SAUCE)				
CLOVE				
ground	1 tsp	–	7	–
CLUB SODA (*See* SODA)				

Food and Description	Amount	Fat Grams	Total Calories	% Fat Calories
COCKTAIL SAUCE (*See* SAUCE)				
COCKTAILS AND MIXERS:				
Alexander	2.5 fl oz	1.8	179	9%
Bacardi	2.5 fl oz	–	118	–
Black Russian	3 fl oz	–	255	–
Bloody Mary	5 fl oz	–	116	–
Bloody Mary Mix (Libby's)	6 fl oz	–	40	–
Bourban & Soda	4 fl oz	–	105	–
Brandy	1 fl oz	–	75	–
Collins Mixer	6 fl oz	–	70	–
Daiquiri	2 fl oz	–	111	–
Daiquiri Mixer (*See* Holland House)				
Gibson	2.5 fl oz	–	158	–
Gimlet	2.5 fl oz	–	132	–
Gin Rickey	7 fl oz	–	114	–
Gin & Tonic	7.5 fl oz	–	171	–
Gold Cadillac	4.5 fl oz	3.6	394	8%
Grasshopper	2.25 fl oz	3.6	164	20%
Grenadine Mixer (bottled)	1 fl oz	–	64	–
High Ball	8 fl oz	–	165	–
Holland House Mixers				
Bloody Mary (bottled)	1 fl oz	–	1	–
Daiquiri				
Plain				
(pouch)	1	–	4	–
(bottled)	1 fl oz	–	31	–
Strawberry (bottled)	1 fl oz	–	27	–
Mai Tai				
(bottled)	1 fl oz	–	29	–
(pouch)	1	–	4	–
Margarita (pouch)	1	–	4	–
Manhattan (bottle)	1 fl oz	–	27	–
Old Fashioned (bottle)	1 fl oz	–	33	–
Sweet & Sour Drink (bottle)	1 fl oz	–	29	–
Lemon Sour Mixer	6 fl oz	–	75	–
Mai Tai	4.5 fl oz	–	310	–
Manhattan	2.5 fl oz	–	128	–
Margarita	3 fl oz	–	170	–
Martini	2.5 fl oz	–	156	–
Mint Julep	10 fl oz	–	215	–
Old Fashioned	4 fl oz	–	180	–
Pina Colada				
Canned	4.5 fl oz	11	347	29%
Standard Home Recipe	4.5 fl oz	2.6	262	9%

Food and Description	Amount	Fat Grams	Total Calories	% Fat Calories
Rum (hot-buttered)	9 fl oz	11.9	317	34%
Screwdriver	7 fl oz	–	174	–
Singapore Sling	8 fl oz	–	228	–
Sloe Gin Fizz	8 fl oz	–	121	–
Sour Mixer				
Canada Dry	12 fl oz	–	135	–
Schweppes	12 fl oz	–	149	–
Stinger	3 fl oz	–	282	–
Tequila Sunrise	5.5 fl oz	–	189	–
Tom Collins	7.5 fl oz	–	121	–
	10 fl oz	–	180	–
Tom Collins Mix (bottled)	1 fl oz	–	42	–
Vodka Mixer (Schweppes)	12 fl oz	–	139	–
Whiskey Sour	3 fl oz	–	123	–
Whiskey Sour Mix				
(bottled)	2 fl oz	–	55	–
Prepared w/whiskey	3.5 fl oz	–	158	–
(powder)	1 packet	–	64	–
White Russian	3.5 fl oz	1	268	3%
COCOA (See also MILK, Mixes)				
	1 Tbs	1	14	6%
	⅓ cup	4	120	30%
	½ cup	5	173	26%
(Baker's)	3.5 oz	13	220	53%
(Hershey's)	⅓ cup	3.5	115	27%
(Nestles)	½ cup	6	180	30%
COCONUT				
(Baker's) Angel Flake				
Canned	⅓ cup	9	110	74%
Package	⅓ cup	8	120	60%
Premium Shred	⅓ cup	9	140	58%
Toasted	⅓ cup	17	200	77%
Durkee-shredded	1 cup	28	277	91%
COCONUT, CREAM OF				
(Coco Lopez)	2 Tbs	5	120	38%
COCONUT MEAT				
dried-shredded				
unsweetened	1 oz	18	187	87%
sweetened	4 oz	40	570	63%
dried-canned-flakes				
sweetened	4 oz	36	505	64%

Food and Description	Amount	Fat Grams	Total Calories	% Fat Calories
dried-packaged flakes				
sweetened	4 oz	36.56	539	61%
	1 cup	23.8	351	61%
raw-shredded	½ cup	13.39	141	86%
toasted	1 oz	13	168	70%
COCONUT MILK/raw	1 Tbs	3.58	35	92%
	1 cup	57	552	93%
canned	1 Tbs	3	30	90%
COCONUT-PINEAPPLE JUICE				
Nectar (Kern's)	6 oz	–	120	–
COCONUT WATER	1 cup	.5	46	10%
COD (*See also* SEAFOOD ENTREE/DINNER)				
Atlantic & Pacific				
raw	3 oz	.57	70	7%
breaded & fried	3 oz	9	175	46%
canned	3 oz	.7	89	7%
cooked-dry heat	3 oz	.7	89	7%
dried	3 oz	2	246	7%
frozen				
(Gorton's)	5 oz	1	110	8%
Roe	3 oz	1.7	111	14%
smoked	3 oz	< 1	87	5%
COFFEE AND COFFEE-LIKE BEVERAGES				
Brewed	6 oz	–	4	–
(Yuban)	6 oz	–	2	–
Brewed-Decaf	6 oz	–	4	–
(Brim)	6 oz	–	2	–
(Maxwell House)	6 oz	–	2	–
(Sanka)	6 oz	–	2	–
(Yuban)	6 oz	–	2	–
Espresso	2 oz	–	1	–
Instant/flavored -				
W/Cappuccio powder				
2 round tsp	6 oz	2	62	29%
W/Chicory powder				
1 round tsp	6 oz	–	6	–
W/French Flavor powder				
2 round tsp	6 oz	3	57	47%
(General Foods) International Coffees				
Cafe Amaretto powder				
2 round tsp	6 oz	2	50	36%
sugar-free	6 oz	2	35	51%
Cafe Francais	6 oz	3	60	45%
sugar-free	6 oz	2	55	33%

Food and Description	Amount	Fat Grams	Total Calories	% Fat Calories
Cafe Irish Creme	6 oz	2	50	36%
sugar-free	6 oz	2	30	60%
Cafe Vienna	6 oz	2	60	30%
sugar-free	6 oz	2	30	60%
Double Chocolate Mint	6 oz	2	50	36%
Double Dutch Chocolate	6 oz	2	50	36%
Irish Mocha Mint	6 oz	2	50	36%
sugar-free	6 oz	2	25	72%
Orange Cappuccio	6 oz	2	60	30%
sugar-free	6 oz	2	30	60%
Suisse Mocha	6 oz	2	55	33%
sugar-free	6 oz	2	30	60%
(Hills Bros)				
Cafe Vienna	6 oz	2	60	30%
Dutch Chocolate	6 oz	2	60	30%
Orange Capri	6 oz	2	60	30%
Swiss Mocha	6 oz	2	60	30%
sugar free	6 oz	2	40	45%
(MJB)-Banana Nut Mocha				
sugar-free	6 oz	2	40	45%
Cafe Mocha	6 oz	1	50	18%
Cherry Mocha	6 oz	1	50	18%
Fudge Mocha-sugar-free	6 oz	2	40	45%
Mint Mocha	6 oz	1	50	18%
sugar-free	6 oz	1	35	26%
Vanilla Mocha-sugar-free	6 oz	2	40	45%
Instant/regular	6 oz	–	4	–
(Brim)	6 oz	–	4	–
(KAVA)	1 tsp	–	2	–
(Maxwell House)	6 oz	–	2	–
(Nescafe)-Brava	6 oz	–	4	–
Classic	6 oz	–	4	–
Decaf	6 oz	–	4	–
Silka	6 oz	–	4	–
(Sanka)-1.7 grams pkg	6 oz	–	2	–
decaffeinated	6 oz	–	4	–
1.5 grams pkg	6 oz	–	2	–
(Taster's Choice)	6 oz	–	4	–
decaffeinated	6 oz	–	4	–
(Yuban)	6 oz	–	4	–
Kaffree Roma (Worthington)				
caffeine free	1tsp	–	6	–
(PERO)-non-caffeinated Hot Beverage				
Drink w/malt & barley	6 oz	–	4	–

Food and Description	Amount	Fat Grams	Total Calories	% Fat Calories
(Postum)-coffee-flavored grain				
beverage	6 oz	–	12	–
w/whole milk + 1 tsp pdr.	6 oz	6	123	44%
coffee-flavored-no caffeine	6 oz	–	12	–
Turkish	4 oz	–	45	–
COLD CUTS (See LUNCHEON MEATS)				
COLLARDS				
canned-chopped, seasoned				
w/pork (Luck's)	7.5 oz	7	90	70%
fresh-cooked	½ cup	–	13	–
frozen-cooked	½ cup	–	31	–
(Pictsweet)	3.3 oz	–	25	–
raw-chopped	½ cup	–	18	–
COOKIE (See also BROWNIE)				
Animal (Sunshine)	14 cookies	3	120	23%
(Archway)				
Apple Filled	1 cookie	3	100	27%
Date Filled Oatmeal	1 cookie	3	100	27%
Frosty Lemon	1 cookie	5	120	38%
Ginger Snaps	1 cookie	1	35	28%
Molasses	1 cookie	3	110	25%
Old Fashion Windmill	1 cookie	3	90	30%
Oatmeal	1 cookie	3	110	25%
Oatmeal Raisin	1 cookie	4	120	30%
Ruth's Oatmeal	1 cookie	4	120	30%
Soft Sugar	1 cookie	3	90	30%
Arrowroot	1 cookie	1	25	36%
(Bakery Wagon)				
Apple Cinnamon	1 cookie	3	96	28%
Apple Filled Oatmeal	1 cookie	4	90	40%
Apple Raisin	1 cookie	3	97	28%
Date Filled Oatmeal	1 cookie	3	94	29%
Honey Fruit Bar	1 cookie	3	95	28%
Iced Molasses	1 cookie	4	100	36%
Lemon Filled Pudding Cookies	1 cookie	3	87	31%
Peanut Jumble	1 cookie	7	112	56%
Raspberry Filled	1 cookie	3	92	29%
Soft Oatmeal	1 cookie	5	104	43%
(Break Cake) Cookies				
Brownie Creme	1-2 oz	8	240	30%
Chocolate Chip	2-2.5 oz	12	310	35%
Chocolate Sugar Wafer	4 wafers	9	200	41%
Coconut Macaroons	2-2 oz	14	270	47%
Frosty Coconut Macaroon	2-2 oz	13	260	45%

Food and Description	Amount	Fat Grams	Total Calories	% Fat Calories
Fruit 'N Honey Bar	1 bar	3	90	30%
Hermit	1-2 oz	7	230	27%
Marshmallow Pie/Banana	1-1.2 oz	5	150	30%
Marshmallow Pie/Chocolate	1-1.2 oz	5	150	30%
Marshmallow Pie/Devil's Food	1-1.2 oz	4	140	26%
Marshmallow Pie/Double Decker Chocolate	3 oz	11	360	28%
Marshmallow Pie/Double Decker Vanilla	3 oz	11	360	28%
Peanut Butter Wafer	1 wafer	9	180	45%
Spice Bar	1-2 oz	7	230	27%
Strawberry Wafer	4 wafers	11	220	45%
Striper Wafer	1 wafer	10	180	50%
Vanilla Sugar Wafer	4 wafers	11	220	45%
Chocolate Chip				
box mix				
(Big Batch)	2 cookies	6	120	45%
(Duncan Hines)	2 cookies	5	130	35%
commercial (2-¼"dia)	4 cookies	9	180	45%
homemade (2-1/3" dia)	4 cookies	12	206	52%
packaged (Archway)	1 cookie	3	50	54%
packaged (Duncan Hines)	2 cookies	5	110	41%
refrigerated dough (2-¼" dia)	4 cookies	11	225	44%
Chocolate Chip Cheese Cake (Formagg)	1 cookie	2	49	37%
Chocolate Creme-filled (Little Debbie)	1.8 oz	12	250	43%
Coconut Bars	1 cookie	5	110	41%
Coconut Macaroons	2 cookies	5	100	45%
Date Bar-box mix (Classics Dessert)	2 bars	4	120	30%
Date Pecan Fancy Fruit (Health Valley)	2 cookies	2	70	26%
(Estee)				
Assorted Creme Filled Wafers	1 wafer	2	30	60%
Chocolate	1 wafer	1	20	45%
Vanilla	1 wafer	1	20	45%
Cookies	1 cookie	1	30	30%
Sandwich Cookies	1 cookie	2-3	45-50	50%-54%
Snack Wafers				
Chocolate, Vanilla, & Strawberry	1 wafer	4	80	45%
Snack Wafers/Chocolate coated	1 wafer	7	130	49%
(FFV)				
Animal	9 cookies	4	130	28%

Food and Description	Amount	Fat Grams	Total Calories	% Fat Calories
Dinosaurs	10 cookies	5	130	35%
Ginger Boy	7 cookies	4	120	30%
Praline Pecan	1 cookie	2	40	45%
(Famous Amos)				
chocolate chip-no nuts				
extra chips	1 oz	8	147	49%
chocolate chip w/macadamias	1 oz	9	152	53%
chocolate chip w/pecans	1 oz	8	151	48%
oatmeal w/cinnamon & raisins	1 oz	6	133	41%
(Featherweight)				
Chocolate Chip	1 cookie	2	40	45%
Lemon	1 cookie	2	40	45%
Vanilla	1 cookie	2	40	45%
Vanilla Wafers	1 cookie	2	30	60%
Fig Bars	4 bars	4	210	17%
Figaroos (Little Debbie)	1.5 oz	4	160	23%
(Frookie)				
Apple Cinnamon Oat Bran	1 cookie	2	45	40%
Chocolate Chip	1 cookie	2	45	40%
Ginger Spice	1 cookie	2	45	40%
Mandarin Orange Chocolate Chip	1 cookie	2	45	40%
Oat Bran Muffin	1 cookie	2	45	40%
Oatmeal Raisin	1 cookie	2	45	40%
Fruit & Honey (Entenmann's)				
fat free	2 cookies	–	80	–
Fruit Jumbos (Health Valley)				
Almond date	1	3	70	39%
Oat Bran	1	2	70	26%
Raisin nut	1	3	70	39%
Tropical Fruit	1	3	70	39%
Grahamy Bears (Sunshine)	9 cookies	5	130	35%
(Grandma's)				
Candied Animal Cookies	1 oz	6	140	39%
Chocolate Chip Big Cookies	2 cookies	17	370	41%
Chocolate Sandwich Cookies	1.8 oz	12	260	42%
Fudge Choc Chip Big Cookies	2 cookies	13	350	33%
Glazed Gingerbread Soft Cookies	1 oz	3	120	23%
Oatmeal Apple Spice Big Cookies	2 cookies	12	330	33%
Old Time Molasses Big Cookies	2 cookies	9	320	25%
Peanut Butter Big Cookies	2 cookies	30	410	66%
Peanut Butter Sandwich Creme	1.8 oz	13	260	45%
Rich'N Chewey-Chocolate Chip	1 oz	6	140	39%
Soft Raisin Big Cookies	2 cookies	10	320	28%
Vanilla-Flavored Sandwich Creme	1.8 oz	12	260	42%

Food and Description	Amount	Fat Grams	Total Calories	% Fat Calories
(Health Valley)				
Amaranth Jumbo	1 cookie	3	70	39%
Crisp cinnamon Jumbo	1 cookie	2	70	26%
Fat Free fruit	3 cookies	< 1	75	6%
Fruit Bars				
Apple Bakes	2 bars	4	164	22%
Raisin Bakes	2 bars	4	160	23%
Fruit & Fitness	2 oz	4	200	18%
Oat Jumbo	2 cookies	4	130	28%
Oat Bran Animal Cookies	1 oz	3	90	30%
Oat Bran Fruit Cookies	1 cookie	4	110	33%
Oat Bran Honey Jumbos	1 cookie	2	60	30%
Peanut Butter Jumbo	1 cookie	2	70	26%
Tofu	~ 1 oz	5	130	35%
Wheat-Free	1.5 oz	6	160	34%
(Keebler)				
Baby Bear	3 cookies	3	70	39%
Bite Size				
Chips Deluxe	4 cookies	5	80	56%
Pecan Sandies	4 cookies	5	90	50%
Chips Deluxe	1 cookie	4	80	45%
Deluxe Grahams-Fudge Covered	1 cookie	2	40	45%
E.L. Fudge Sandwich	1 cookie	3	70	39%
Elfkins				
Butter w/fudge filling	4 cookies	3	70	39%
Fudge w/fudge filling	4 cookies	3	70	39%
Fudge Cremes	1 cookie	3	60	45%
Fudge Stripes	1 cookie	3	50	54%
French Vanilla Creme	1 cookie	4	80	45%
Magic Middles/all flavors	1 cookie	5	80	56%
Mini Middles				
Chocolate Chip	4 cookies	4	80	45%
Oatmeal	4 cookies	5	80	56%
Shortbread	4 cookies	4	80	45%
Pecan Chips Deluxe	1 cookie	4	70	51%
Pecan Sandies	1 cookie	5	80	56%
Playland	3 cookies	2	60	30%
Oatmeal Cremes	1 cookie	3	80	34%
Old Fashioned Oatmeal	1 cookie	3	80	34%
Pitter Patter	1 cookie	4	90	40%
Rainbow Chips Deluxe	1 cookie	3	80	34%
Rich'n Chips	1 cookie	4	80	45%
Soft Batch				
Chocolate Chip	1 cookie	4	80	45%

Food and Description	Amount	Fat Grams	Total Calories	% Fat Calories
Peanut Butter Choc Chip	1 cookie	5	80	56%
Peanut Butter Nut	1 cookie	4	80	45%
Walnut Chocolate Chip	1 cookie	4	80	45%
Thin Bits				
Choc-covered graham snacks	12 pieces	3	70	39%
Vanilla Wafers	5 cookies	5	100	45%
Lady Fingers	1 cookie	–	40	–
	4 cookies	3	158	17%
(Lance)-packaged				
Apple Oatmeal Bar	1 pkg	7	190	33%
Apple Cinnamon	1 pkg	5	120	38%
Blueberry	1 pkg	4	120	30%
Bonnie	1 pkg	4	100	36%
Chocolate Chip	1 pkg	7	135	47%
Chocolate Chip Fudge	1 pkg	5	130	35%
Fig Bar	1	1	71	13%
Malt	1	10	190	47%
Oatmeal	1 pkg	5	130	35%
Peanut Butter Creme Filled	1 pkg	10	240	38%
Strawberry	1 pkg	4	120	30%
Lemon Ohs! (Austin)	1.8 oz	9	240	34%
(Lu)				
Chips Chocolate	1 cookie	4.6	85	49%
Craquelin	2 cookies	4.5	100	41%
Crokine	2 cookies	–	37	–
Gaufretts	2 cookies	4	85	42%
Little School Boy	1 cookie	3.5	65	49%
Marie LU	2 cookies	3.6	101	32%
Marie LU Whole Wheat & Cinnamon	2 cookies	2	95	19%
Natalu	3 cookies	6.8	112	55%
Petit Beurre	1 cookie	1	40	23%
Pims	2 cookies	2.5	97	23%
Prince	2 cookies	5.9	135	39%
Schoks, Chocolate	2 cookies	6	104	52%
Sirtaki	3 cookies	6	125	43%
Macaroons				
homemade (2-¾" dia, ¼" thick)	2 cookies	8.8	181	44%
Marshmallow Pies				
Banana (Little Debbie)	1 pkg/1.4 oz	6	170	32%
	1 pkg/3 oz	12	360	30%
Chocolate (Little Debbie)	1 pkg/1.38 oz	6	170	32%
	1 pkg/3 oz	13	370	32%
Milk Chocolate (Duncan Hines)	2 cookies	5	110	41%

Food and Description	Amount	Fat Grams	Total Calories	% Fat Calories
(Mother's)				
Almond Shortbread	2 cookies	7	120	53%
Apple Filled Oatmeal	1 cookie	4	90	40%
Butter-Flavored	4 cookies	5	97	46%
Checkerboard Wafer	5 cookies	4	86	42%
Chocolate Chip	1 cookie	5	79	57%
(bag)	4 cookies	7	124	51%
Chocolate Chip Angel	2 cookies	8	120	60%
Chocolate Creme Sandwich	2 cookies	7	109	58%
Chocolate Mint Creme Sandwich	2 cookies	7	109	58%
Circus Animal	4 cookies	6	107	51%
Cocadas Coconut	4 cookies	6	123	44%
Date Filled Oatmeal	1 cookie	3	94	29%
Dinosaur Grrrahams -original	1 cookie	2	72	25%
chocolate	1 cookie	3	76	36%
cinnamon	1 cookie	3	77	35%
Double Fudge Sandwich	2 cookies	4	98	37%
Duplex Sandwich	2 cookies	5	104	43%
English Tea Sandwich	1 cookie	4	99	36%
Fig Bars	2 bars	2	112	16%
Flaky Flix Fudge Wafer	2 cookies	9	131	62%
Flaky Fix Vanilla Wafer	2 cookies	5	116	39%
Frosted Holiday	6 cookies	6	107	51%
Fudge'N Chips	4 cookies	7	118	53%
Fudge Swirl	1 cookie	6	74	73%
Gaucho Peanut Butter Sandwich	1 cookie	5	90	50%
Iced Molasses	1 cookie	4	100	36%
Iced Oatmeal	1 cookie	3	72	38%
Iced Raisin	1 cookie	4	79	46%
Macaroon	1 cookie	6	85	64%
Mint Patties	2 cookies	5	118	38%
Oatmeal	1 cookie	4	65	55%
Oatmeal Chocolate Chip	1 cookie	3	66	41%
Oatmeal Raisin	4 cookies	7	121	52%
Oatmeal Walnut Chocolate Chip	1 cookie	3	70	39%
Royal Grahams	1 cookie	4	69	52%
Striped Shorbread	2 cookies	5	101	45%
Sugar	1 cookie	4	65	55%
Taffy Sandwich	1 cookie	6	97	56%
Vanilla Wafer	4 cookies	4	93	39%
Walnut Fudge	1 cookie	4	70	51%
Whole Wheat Fig Bars	2 bars	2	122	15%
(Nabisco) Almost Home				
Fudge Chocolate Chip	2 cookies	5	130	35%

Food and Description	Amount	Fat Grams	Total Calories	% Fat Calories
Oatmeal Raisin	2 cookies	5	130	35%
Old Fashioned Sugar	2 cookies	5	130	35%
Peanut Butter Fudge	2 cookies	7	140	45%
Real Chocolate Chip	2 cookies	5	130	35%
Walnut Chocolate Chip	2 cookies	7	140	45%
Bakers Bonus Oatmeal	2 cookies	5	130	35%
Bakers Own				
Apple filled	1 cookie	2	70	26%
Blueberry filled	1 cookie	2	70	26%
Raspberry filled	1 cookie	2	70	26%
Barnum's Animal Crackers	11 cookies	4	130	28%
Biscos Sugar Wafers	8 wafers	7	150	42%
Biscos Waffle Cremes	3 pieces	7	150	42%
Brown Edge Wafers	5 wafers	6	140	39%
Bugs Bunny Graham Cookies	9 cookies	4	120	30%
Cameo Creme Sandwich	2 cookies	5	140	32%
Chips Ahoy				
Chewy Chocolate Chip	2 cookies	6	130	42%
Mini Chocolate chip	6 cookies	3	70	39%
Pure Chocolate Chp	2 cookies	7	140	45%
Chips Ahoy-Selctions				
Chocolate Chocolate Chunk	2 cookies	9	150	48%
Chocolate Chocolate Walnut	1 cookie	6	95	57%
Chocolate Chunk Pecan	2 cookies	10	160	56%
Chunky Chocolate Chip	2 cookies	8	150	48%
Health Toffee Chunk	1 cookie	5	90	50%
Oatmeal chocolate chunk	1 cookie	5	95	47%
Chips Ahoy-Sprinkled	1 cookie	2	50	36%
Chocolate Chip Snaps	6 cookies	4	130	28%
Chocolate Grahams	3 pieces	7	150	42%
Chocolate Snaps	7 cookies	4	140	28%
Cookie Break				
Vanilla Creme Sandwich	3 cookies	6	140	39%
Cookies'N Fudge				
Party Grahams	3 cookies	7	140	45%
Striped Chocolate Chip	3 cookies	8	150	48%
Striped Peanut Butter Nut	3 cookies	8	150	48%
Striped Shortbread	3 cookies	7	150	42%
Striped Wafers	2 wafers	8	150	48%
Famous Chocolate Wafers	5 wafers	4	130	28%
Famous Cookie Assortment				
Baronet Creme Sdw	3 cookies	6	140	39%
Biscos Sugar Wafers	3 wafers	7	150	42%
Butter-Flavored	6 cookies	5	130	35%

Food and Description	Amount	Fat Grams	Total Calories	% Fat Calories
Cameo Creme Sandwich	2 cookies	5	140	31%
Kettle Cookies	4 cookies	5	130	35%
Lorna Doone Shortbread	4 cookies	7	140	45%
Oreo Choc Sandwich	3 cookies	6	140	39%
Giggles Sandwich				
chocolate	2 cookies	6	140	39%
vanilla	2 cookies	6	140	39%
Heyday Bars				
fudge, caramel, & peanut	1 bar	8	140	51%
Ideal Bars /chocolate peanut	2 bars	8	150	48%
Imported Danish	5 cookies	8	150	48%
Lorna Doone Shortbread	4 cookies	7	140	45%
Mallomars Chocolate Cakes	2 pieces	6	130	42%
Marshmallow Puffs	1 piece	4	120	30%
Marshmallow Twirls Cakes	1 piece	5	130	35%
Mystic Mint Sandwich	2 cookies	8	150	48%
National Arrowroot Biscuit	6 biscuits	4	130	28%
Newtons Fruit Chewy Cookies				
Apple, Blueberry, Raspberry, and Strawberry Newtons	1½ cookies	2	110	16%
Cinnamon Raisin	1 cookie	2	60	30%
Fig Newtons	2 cookies	2	100	18%
Nilla Wafers	7 cookies	4	130	28%
Nutter Butter Peanut Butter Sdw	2 cookies	6	140	39%
Creme Patties	4 patties	8	150	48%
Old Fashion Ginger Snaps	4 cookies	3	120	23%
Oreo Big Stuf Chocolate Sdw	1 cookie	12	250	43%
Oreo Chocolate Sandwich	3 cookies	6	140	39%
Oreo Double Stuf Chocolate Sdw	2 cookies	7	140	45%
Oreo Fudge Covered Chocolate Sdw	2 cookies	8	150	48%
Pantry Molasses cookies	2 cookies	4	130	28%
Pecan Shortbread	2 cookies	6	110	49%
Pinwheels Choc & Marshmallow cakes	1	5	130	35%
Pure Chocolate Middles	2 cookies	8	150	48%
Social Tea Biscuits	6 biscuits	4	130	28%
Striped Chips Ahoy-Choc Chip	2 cookies	8	150	48%
Suddenly S'Mores	1 cookie	4	100	36%
White Fudge-covered Oreos	1 cookie	6	110	49%
Oatmeal-homemade	1 cookie	3	65	42%
Oatmeal-packaged-(Little Debbie)	1 pkg/ 2.75 oz	12	340	32%
Oatmeal Chocolate Chip/homemade	1 cookie	3	60	45%
Oatmeal Creme Pies (Little Debbie)	1.33 oz	6	160	34%
	2.75 oz	14	350	36%

Food and Description	Amount	Fat Grams	Total Calories	% Fat Calories
Oatmeal w/raisins (2-5/8" dia 1/4" thick)	4 cookies	10	245	37%
box mix-(Duncan Hines)	2 cookies	6	130	42%
homemade	4 cookies	10	245	37%
packaged				
(Duncan Hines)	2 cookies	5	110	41%
(Entenmann's) Fat Free	2 cookies	–	89	–
Peanut Butter				
box mix (Duncan Hines)	2 cookies	7	140	45%
homemade (2-5/8"dia)	4 cookies	14	245	51%
Peanut Butter Bars (little Debbie)	2.5 oz	18	370	44%
	1.83 oz	13	260	45%
(Pepperidge Farm)				
American Collection Cookies				
Beacon Hill Brownie Nut	1	7	120	52%
Chesapeake Chocolate Chunk				
Pecan	1	7	130	49%
Nantucket Chocolate Chunk	1	7	120	52%
Sante Fe Oatmeal Raisin	1	4	110	33%
Sausalito Milk Choc Macadamia	1	7	110	57%
Distinctive Box Cookies				
Champagne	3 cookies	5	95	47%
Choc Laced Pirouettes	2 cookies	4	70	51%
Monte Carlo	2 cookies	5	90	50%
Original Pirouettes	3 cookies	7	110	57%
Paris	2 cookies	5	100	45%
Seville	2 cookies	5	100	45%
Southport	2 cookies	8	150	48%
Distinctive Cookies				
Bordeaux	3 cookies	5	110	41%
Brussels	3 cookies	8	160	45%
Brussels Mint	3 cookies	10	200	45%
Cappucino	3 cookies	9	160	51%
Capri	2 cookies	9	160	51%
Chessmen	3 cookies	6	130	42%
Geneva	3 cookies	11	190	52%
Lido	2 cookies	11	190	52%
Linzer	1 cookie	4	120	30%
Milano	3 cookies	10	180	50%
Mint Milano	3 cookies	13	230	51%
Nassau	2 cookies	10	170	53%
Orange Milano	3 cookies	13	230	51%
Orleans	3 cookies	6	90	60%
Orleans Sandwich	3 cookies	12	180	60%
Tahiti	2 cookies	11	170	58%

Food and Description	Amount	Fat Grams	Total Calories	% Fat Calories
Fruit Cookies				
Apricot-Raspberry	3 cookies	6	150	36%
Strawberry	3 cookies	7	150	42%
Kitchen Hearth Cookies				
Date Pecan, Raisin Bran	3 cookies	8	160	45%
Old Fashioned Cookies				
Brownie Chocolate Nut	3 cookies	10	160	56%
Chocolate Chip	3 cookies	8	150	48%
Chocolate Chocolate Chip	3 cookies	9	160	51%
Gingerman	3 cookies	4	100	36%
Hazelnut	3 cookies	9	170	48%
Irish Oatmeal	3 cookies	7	140	45%
Lemon Nut Crunch	3 cookies	10	170	53%
Molasses Crisps	3 cookies	5	100	45%
Oatmeal Raisin	3 cookies	8	170	42%
Shortbread	2 cookies	8	150	48%
Sugar	3 cookies	8	150	48%
Special Collection				
Almond Supreme	2 cookies	10	140	64%
Chocolate Chunk Pecan	2 cookies	7	130	49%
Milk Chocolate Macadamia	2 cookies	8	140	51%
Wholesome choice				
Apple Oatmeal Tart	1 cookie	2	0	25%
Carrot Walnut	1 cookie	1	60	15%
Cranberry Honey	1 cookie	2	60	30%
Date Walnut	1 cookie	2	60	30%
Raspberry Tart	1 cookie	2	70	25%
Pumpkin Bar-homemade	1.5 oz	11	190	52%
Ready-To-Bake (Nestle Toll House)				
Chocolate Chip	2 cookies	7	150	42%
Chocolate Chip w/nuts	2 cookies	8	160	45%
Double Chocolate Chip	2 cookies	7	150	42%
Oatmeal Raisin	2 cookies	5	130	35%
Refrigerated (Pillsbury)				
Chocolate Chip	1	3	70	39%
Choc Chocolate Chip	1	3	70	39%
Oatmeal Rasin	1	3	70	39%
Peanut Butter	1	3	70	39%
Sugar	1	3	70	39%
Sandwich (Estee)	1	2	45	40%
Sandwich type				
(choc or vanilla) 1-¾"dia	4 cookies	8	195	37%
Shortbread				
commercial-small	4 cookies	8	155	47%

Food and Description	Amount	Fat Grams	Total Calories	% Fat Calories
homemade-large	2	8	145	50%
(Stella D'Oro)				
Almond Toast	1 piece	1	58	16%
Angel Bars	1	4.7	74	57%
Angel Puffs	1 cookie	–	13	–
Angel Wings	1 cookie	4.7	74	57%
Angelica Goodies	1 cookie	4	104	35%
Anginetti	1 cookie	1	31	29%
Anisette Sponge	1 cookie	.8	51	14%
Anisette Toast	1 cookie	.6	46	12%
Anisette Toast-Jumbo	1 cookie	1	109	8%
Breakfast Treats	1 piece	3.6	101	32%
Castelets				
chocolate	1 piece	2.8	64	39%
vanilla	1 piece	3	72	38%
Chinese Dessert	1 cookie	8.9	169	47%
Coconut Macaroons	1 cookie	3	60	45%
Coconut, Dietetic	1 cookie	2	50	36%
Como Delight	1 cookie	7	145	43%
Dietetic Egg Biscuits	1 piece	1	43	21%
Dutch Apple Bars	1 piece	3	112	24%
Egg Jumbo	1 piece	.7	47	13%
Fruit Slices	1	2	60	30%
Golden Bars	1	4	109	33%
Holiday Trinkets	1	1.9	38	45%
Hostess Assortment	1 cookie	2	42	43%
Lady Stella Assortment	1 cookie	2	42	43%
Love, Dietetic	1 cookie	5	106	43%
Margherite, chocolate	1 cookie	3	72	38%
Margherite, vanilla	1 cookie	2.8	72	35%
Peach Apricot Pastry	1 cookie	3.8	93	37%
Pfeffernusse	1 cookie	.8	35	20%
Roman Egg Biscuits	1 piece	5	137	33%
Royal Nuggets	1 piece	–	1	–
Sesame	1 piece	2	48	38%
Sesame, Dietetic	1 piece	2	43	42%
Sugared Egg Biscuits	1 piece	1	75	12%
Swiss Fudge	1 piece	3	68	40%
Sugar				
homemade	1 cookie	3	90	30%
refrigerated dough				
(2½"dia¼"thick)	4 cookies	12	235	46%
Sugar, Golden-box mix (Duncan Hines)	2 cookies	6	130	42%

Food and Description	Amount	Fat Grams	Total Calories	% Fat Calories
(Sunshine)				
Butter Flavored	4 cookies	5	120	38%
Chip-A-Roos	2 cookies	7	130	49%
Chip-o-lotomus	2 cookies	7	120	53%
Chips'n Middles	2 cookies	6	140	39%
Chocolate Fudge Sandwich	2 cookies	7	150	42%
Cup Custard	2 cookies	6	130	42%
Family Bears				
Chocolate	2 cookies	7	140	45%
Peanut butter	2 cookies	6	140	39%
Vanilla	2 cookies	6	130	42%
Fig Bars	2 cookies	2	90	20%
Ginger Snaps	5 cookies	3	90	30%
Golden Fruit Cookie	2 cookies	3	150	18%
Hydrox	3 cookies	7	160	39%
Lemon Coolers	5 cookies	6	140	39%
Mallowpuffs	2 cookies	4	140	26%
Oat Bran w/nuts & raisins	2 ookies	6	120	45%
Oatmeal	2 cookies	5	110	41%
Oatmeal Peanut Sdw	2 cookies	6	140	39%
Peanut Butter Wafers	3 wafers	6	120	45%
School House	15 pieces	4	120	30%
Sprinkles	2 cookies	3	130	42%
Sugar Wafers	3 wafers	6	130	42%
Vanilla Wafers	6 wafers	6	130	42%
Vienna Fingers	2 cookies	6	140	39%
(Sweet Pretenders)				
Choc Flavored Chip	1	2	45	40%
Lemon	1	2	45	40%
Oatmeal Raisin	1	2	45	40%
Vanilla	1	2	45	40%
Peanut Butter	1	2	40	45%
Vanilla Wafers (1-¾" dia)	10 cookies	7	185	34%
COOKING SPRAY, NO STICK				
(Mazola)	2 second spray	.8	6	100%
(Pam)				
Butter Flavor	⅓ of 10" Skillet	1	2	100%
Olive Oil	⅓ of 10" Skillet	1	2	100%
Original	¼ second spray	1	7	100%
CORIANDER/raw	¼ cup	–	1	–

Food and Description	Amount	Fat Grams	Total Calories	% Fat Calories
CORIANDER LEAF/dried	1 tsp	–	2	–
CORIANDER SEED	1 tsp	–	5	–
CORN				
Sweet-white or yellow				
cooked	½ cup	1	89	10%
cooked	1 ear	.98	89	10%
cabbed-Baby Corn On Cob				
(Bristol)	4 ears/			
	½ oz	–	12	–
canned-cream style	½ cup	.5	93	5%
(Green Giant)	½ cup	1	100	9%
(Nutradiet)	½ cup	1	100	9%
canned				
cream Premium Homestyle				
(S&W)	½ cup	1	120	8%
cream-golden				
(Del Monte)	½ cup	1	90	10%
cream-white				
(Del Monte)	½ cup	–	90	–
canned				
golden whole kernels				
(Del Monte)	½ cup	1	70	13%
canned-kernels				
golden vacuum packed				
(Del Monte)	½ cup	1	90	10%
canned-kernels				
(Green Giant)	½ cup	–	80	–
(Nutradiet)	½ cup	1	80	11%
canned-kernels				
50% Less Salt (Green Giant)	½ cup	–	70	–
canned-kernels in brine				
(Festal)	½ cup	1	90	10%
canned-kernels w/peppers				
(Freshlike)	½ cup	1	90	10%
(Mexicorn)	½ cup	1	80	11%
canned-kernels				
(Niblets)	½ cup	–	80	–
canned-young, tender whole kernel				
Premium (S&W)	½ cup	1	90	10%
canned-white whole kernels				
(Del Monte)	½ cup	–	70	–
frozen				
cob corn				
(Ore Ida)	1 ear	1	150	6%

Food and Description	Amount	Fat Grams	Total Calories	% Fat Calories
cream style	½ cup	.6	120	5%
cut (Pictsweet)	3.2 oz	1	80	11%
kernels				
(Birds Eye)	3.3 oz	1	80	11%
(Health Valley)	5.8 oz	–	134	–
frozen-On-The-Cob,				
BIG EARS (Birds Eye)	1 ear	1	160	6%
frozen-On-The-Cob,				
LITTLE Ears (Birds Eye)	2 ears	1	130	7%
frozen-on-the-cob	1 ear	1	150	6%
(Pictsweet)				
3"	1 ear	–	50	–
6"	1 ear	1	110	8%
(Pictsweet)				
Express microwave	1 ear	–	50	–
frozen-(Niblets)	½ cup	1	80	11%
frozen-(Niblets)				
Corn-on-the-Cob (pkg of 4)	1 ear	1	150	6%
Corn-on-the-Cob (pkg of 6)	2 ears	1	150	6%
White Shoepeg				
canned				
(Green Giant)	½ cup	–	90	–
frozen	½ cup	1	70	13%
frozen				
(Harvest Fresh)	½ cup	1	90	10%
(Green Giant) microwaveable				
Pantry Express	½ cup	1	80	11%
CORN AND MOLASSES				
(Pepperidge Farm)	1 slice	.5	70	6%
CORN CHIPS (*See also* MEXICAN FOOD, TORTILLA)				
(Fritos)				
Bar-B-Q	1 oz	9	150	54%
Chili Cheese Flavored	1 oz	10	160	56%
Crisp'N Thin	1 oz	10	160	56%
Dip Size	1 oz	9	150	54%
Regular	1 oz	9	150	54%
(Health Valley)				
Cheese	1 oz	10	160	56%
No Salt	1 oz	11	160	62%
Plain	1 oz	11	160	62%
(Keebler)				
Hooplas				
Nacho	1 oz	8	140	51%
Original	1 oz	8	140	51%

Food and Description	Amount	Fat Grams	Total Calories	% Fat Calories
(Old Vienna)				
Plain	1 oz	6	140	39%
(Planters)				
plain	1 oz	10	160	56%
(Pringles)				
Fresh Roasted	1 oz	7	140	45%
Tangy Cheese	1 oz	7	140	45%
(Weight Watchers)				
Corn Snackers	.5 oz	2	60	30%
Nacho Cheese Flavor	.5 oz	2	60	30%
(Wise)				
Corn Chips/Corn Crunchies	1 oz	10	160	56%
Corn Spirals-Crispy Corn Twists, Nacho Cheese	1 oz	11	160	62%
Toasted Corn Spirals-Crispy Corn Twists	1 oz	11	160	62%
CORN CHOWDER (*See* SOUP)				
CORN DISHES				
Corn on the Cob in butter sauce				
frozen				
(Green Giant)	1 ear/ 2 half ears	2	150	12%
Corn Pudding				
homemade	½ cup	6.6	136	44%
Delicorn				
canned				
(Green Giant)	½ cup	1	80	11%
Fritters				
homemade	1 oz	2	62	29%
frozen				
(Pepperidge Farm)	2	12	250	43%
Mexican Style Corn in Mild Red Chile Sauce				
microwave Veg. Classics				
(Del Monte)	½ cup	4	90	40%
Micro Quick				
(Freshlike)				
frozen Corn in Butter Sauce	5 oz	2	130	14%
(Niblets) in butter sauce	½ cup	2	100	18%
(Niblets) in butter sauce				
one serving vegetables, frozen	4.5 oz	2	110	16%
Scalloped/homemade	½ cup	7	250	25%
White Shoepeg Corn in butter sauce				
(Green Giant)	½ cup	2	100	18%
CORN FLAKE CRUMBS (Kellogg's)	¼ cup	–	110	–

Food and Description	Amount	Fat Grams	Total Calories	% Fat Calories
CORN GRITS				
Albers	1 serving	–	150	–
Instant/White Hominy	1 serving	–	82	–
Quick/yellow Hominy/dry	3 Tbs	–	101	–
Regular and quick	1 Serving	0.5	146	3%
w/cheddar cheese flavor	1 serving	1	104	9%
w/cheese flavor	1 serving	0.9	107	8%
w/imitation bacon bits	1 serving	0.5	104	4%
w/imitation ham bits	1 serving	–	103	–
Quaker-Instant				
Real Butter Flavor	1 packet	1	100	9%
CORN PONE				
w/whole ground cornmeal (9" dia)	⅛ pone	3	122	22%
(Country Hearth)				
European Butter Sesame	1 slice	1	70	13%
Grainola	1 slice	1	75	12%
Honey Nugget	1 slice	1	70	13%
Indian	1 slice	1	100	9%
Old Fashioned Buttermilk	1 slice	1	70	13%
Old Fashioned Wheat	1 slice	1	70	13%
Old Fashioned Sandwich	1 slice	1	75	12%
7 Whole Grain	1 slice	1	80	11%
Stone Ground Whole Wheat	1 slice	1	70	13%
Wheat Berry	1 slice	1	70	13%
Wheat Sandwich	1 slice	1	70	13%
CORN PUDDING (*See* PUDDING)				
CORN STARCH	1 Tbs	–	30	–
	1 cup	–	463	–
CORNBREAD				
box mix (Aunt Jemima) Easy mix	⅙ pkg	7	210	30%
box mix (Ballard)	⅛ pkg	3	140	19%
box mix (Dromedary)	2"x2" sq.	5	130	35%
box mix-Cotton Pickin (Martha White)	¼ pan	3	170	16%
box mix-honey cornbread (Krusteaz)	1/16 pkg	3	120	23%
box mix-Light Crust - homemade-3" sq.	1 piece	3	122	22%
pouch mix (Robin Hood/Gold Medal)- southern style w/degermed cornmeal	~ 3 oz	5	186	24%
white or yellow	⅙ mixture	5	50	30%
w/whole-ground cornmeal	~3 oz	6	161	34%
yellow (Martha White)	2 oz mix	4	140	26%

Food and Description	Amount	Fat Grams	Total Calories	% Fat Calories
CORNED BEEF (*See also* LUNCHEON MEAT)				
Briscut	3 oz	16	213	68%
Canned	1 oz	4	71	51%
(Hormel)-12 oz	2 oz	8	130	55%
Jellied loaf	1 oz	1.9	46	37%
CORNED BEEF HASH				
Canned				
(Armour)	7.5 oz	27	390	62%
(Libby's)	7.5 oz	27	400	61%
	8 oz	28	420	60%
(Mary Kitchen)	7.5 oz	24	360	60%
	8⅓ oz	27	400	61%
Standard Home Recipe (USDA)	1 cup	21.5	344	56%
W/potatoes	7.8 oz	24.9	399	56%
CORNMEAL				
Albers-yellow or white	1 oz	–	100	–
Aunt Jemima-yellow or white				
Enriched/unenriched	3 Tbs	1	100	9%
Blue (Arrowhead Mills)	2 oz	3	210	13%
Degermed	1 cup	1.7	502	3%
Self-rising Whole ground				
Yellow or white	1 cup	4	465	8%
Degermed	1 cup	1.6	491	3%
Whole-ground				
Bolted	1 cup	4	442	8%
Unbolted	1 cup	4.8	433	10%
CORNMEAL MIX				
Aunt Jemima				
Bolted white	3 Tbs	1	100	9%
Buttermilk self-rising				
White	3 Tbs	1	100	9%
Self-rising				
White enriched bolted	3 Tbs	1	100	9%
Yellow	3 Tbs	1	100	9%
COTTAGE CHEESE				
Creamed	4 oz	5	117	39%
(Borden) 4% milkfat	4 oz	5	120	38%
(Carnation)-Slender-1-½% milkfat	4 oz	2	90	20%
(Knudsen)-4% milkfat	4 oz	5	120	38%
(Land O'Lakes) 2%	4 oz	2	100	18%
(Lite-Line) low-fat 1-½%	4 oz	2	90	20%
(Lite N' Lively)	4 oz	1	80	11%
low-fat (2%)	4 oz	2	101	18%

Food and Description	Amount	Fat Grams	Total Calories	% Fat Calories
low-fat (1%)	4 oz	1	82	11%
(Weight Watchers)				
1%	4 oz	1	90	10%
2%	4 oz	2	100	18%
Dry Curd (Borden).5% milkfat	4 oz	1	80	11%
COTTAGE CHEESE FRUIT SALAD				
(Lucerne)	4 oz	4	130	28%
COWPEA (*See* BLACK-EYED PEA)				
CRAB (*See also* SEAFOOD ENTREE/DINNER)				
Alaska King				
cooked-moist heat	3 oz	1	82	11%
	1 Leg	2	129	14%
raw	3 oz	1	71	13%
	1 Leg	1	145	6%
Blue				
raw	3 oz	.9	74	11%
canned	3 oz	1	84	11%
Dungeness				
canned				
(S&W)	3.25 oz	2	81	22%
Imitation				
(from surimi)	3 oz	1	87	10%
(Louis Kemp)-King				
chunks style	2 oz	< 1	60	8%
flake style	2 oz	< 1	60	8%
Soft Shell				
fried	1	13	213	55%
Queen				
raw	3 oz	1	76	12%
CRAB SALAD				
homemade	5.5 oz	10.7	205	47%
CRAB SOUP (*See* SOUP)				
CRACKERS				
(Austin)				
Cheese on Cheese	.93 oz	5	130	35%
Cheese and Peanut Butter	1.4 oz	11	200	50%
Rye Cheese w/zesty cheese	1.4 oz	10	200	45%
Toasty Peanut Butter	.93 oz	5	130	35%
Wheat'N Cheddar	.93 oz	7	140	45%
Cheddar Cheese Lights (Old Brussels)	1 oz	10	167	54%
Cheese (Ritz)	10	6	140	39%
Chowder and Oyster (O.T.C.)	1	1	25	36%
Cracker Bread				
100% Stoneground Armenian (AK-MAK)	1	1	117	8%

Food and Description	Amount	Fat Grams	Total Calories	% Fat Calories
Extra Crisp (Wasa)	1	1	25	33%
Cracker crumbs				
(Nabisco)	2 Tbs	1	60	15%
(Sunshine)	½ cup	7	275	23%
Cracker meal-(Nabisco)	2 Tbs	–	50	–
CrackerDiles-(Delicious)	13	3	70	39%
Crisp Bakes, Dutch (Hans Boersma)	1	–	29	–
(Eagle) Snack Crackers				
Bacon Flavor Cheese	1 oz	6	140	39%
Cheese Flavor	1 oz	6	130	42%
Honey Roasted Peanut Butter	1.8 oz	16	280	51%
Crispbread (See CRISPBREAD)				
(Estee)				
6-Calorie Wafer	1	–	6	–
Cheddar Crackers	½ oz	4	70	51%
Party Crackers	½ oz	4	70	51%
Sesame	½ oz	4	70	51%
Fiber bread (Bran-A-Crisp)	1	–	22	–
Flat Bread				
Fiber w/sesame seeds (Ideal)	2	–	40	–
Extra Thin (Wasa)	3	–	48	–
Whole Grain, No Salt (Ideal)	2 slices	–	43	–
Graham Crackers				
(Health Valley)				
Amaranth	7	3	110	25%
Fancy Honey Graham	1 oz	4	100	36%
Oat Bran Graham	7	3	120	23%
(Honey Maid)	2	1	60	15%
Cinnamon	2	1	60	15%
Honeycomb Graham Snacks				
Apple Cinnamon	11	2	60	30%
Brown Sugar'N Spice	11	2	60	30%
Honey'N Oat Bran	11	2	60	30%
Raisin	2	1	60	15%
(Keebler)				
Cinnamon Crisp	1	2	70	26%
Honey	1	2	70	26%
Thin Bits				
Cinnamon	12	3	70	39%
Chocolate	12	3	70	39%
(Nabisco)	2	1	60	15%
(Sunshine)				
Cinnamon	1	3	70	39%
Grahamy Bears	9	5	130	35%

Food and Description	Amount	Fat Grams	Total Calories	% Fat Calories
Honey	1	2	60	30%
(Hain)				
Cheese Crackers	1 oz	6	130	42%
Crackerbread				
Hearts	2	–	28	–
Rounds				
Hors d'oeuvre size	1	1	28	32%
Luncheon size (5")	1	1	70	13%
Small	1	1	28	32%
Whole Wheat (5")	1	.8	66	11%
Onion	1 oz	6	130	42%
Pumpernickel	10	6	130	42%
Rich (salted or unsalted)	1 oz	5	130	35%
Sesame (salted or unsalted)	1 oz	7	140	45%
Sour Cream and Chives				
(salted or unsalted)	1 oz	6	130	42%
Stoneground				
Cheese	6	3	65	42%
Rye (salted or unsalted)	11	4	120	30%
Sour Dough (salted)	6	3	65	42%
Sour Dough (low salt)	1 oz	5	130	35%
Wheat Vegetable	6	3	65	42%
(Health Valley)				
Cheese Wheels	1 oz	9	140	48%
Garden Vegetable	1 oz	5	120	38%
Herb	1 oz	6	120	45%
7 Grain Vegetable	1 oz	5	130	35%
Sesame	1 oz	6	130	42%
Stoned Wheat	1 oz	6	120	38%
Hi-Ho (Sunshine)				
Original	10	10	180	50%
Whole Wheat	4	3	65	42%
Honey Bran (El Molino)	2	1	40	23%
(Keebler)				
Club	4	3	60	45%
Clubettes	22	4	70	51%
Harvest Wheats	3	4	70	51%
Munch ems				
Cheddar	½ oz	3	70	39%
Original	½ oz	3	70	39%
Sour Cream & Onion	½ oz	3	70	39%
Onion Toast	5	3	60	45%
Sun Toasted Wheats	10	4	70	51%
Toasted Poppy Seed	5	3	60	45%

Food and Description	Amount	Fat Grams	Total Calories	% Fat Calories
Toasted Rye	5	3	60	45%
Toasted Sesame	5	4	80	45%
Toasted Wheat	5	4	80	45%
Town House	5	5	80	56%
Town House Jrs, Cheddar Cheese	8	4	80	45%
Wheatables	12	3	70	39%
White Cheddar	11	4	70	51%
Whole Wheat	12	3	70	39%
Zesta Saltines	5	2	60	30%
(Lance)				
Bonnie	1 5/16 oz	6	160	34%
Captain Wafers	2	1	30	30%
Captain's Wafers w/cream cheese	1 5/8 oz	9	170	48%
Cheese On Wheat	1 5/16 oz	9	180	45%
Gold-N-Chee, Spicy	15	3	70	39%
Lanchee	1 1/4 oz	10	180	50%
Nip-Chee	1 5/16 oz	9	180	45%
Oyster	1/2 oz	2	70	11%
Peanut Butter Wheat	1 5/8 oz	10	190	47%
Rye Twins	2	1	30	30%
Rye-Chee	1 7/16 oz	9	190	43%
Saltines	2	1	25	36%
Sesame Twins	2	1	40	23%
Thin Wheat Snacks	7	4	80	45%
Toastchee	1 3/8 oz	10	190	47%
Toasty	1 1/4 oz	10	180	50%
Wheat Twins	2	1	30	30%
Wheatswafer	4	2	60	30%
Melba Toast (*See* MELBA TOAST)				
(Nabisco)				
American Classic Crackers Cracked Wheat, Dairy Butter, Golden Sesame, & Toasted Popp	4 crackers	3	70	39%
Bacon Flavored Thins	7 crackers	4	70	51%
Better Cheddars'N Bacon Thins	10 crackers	4	70	51%
Better Cheddars'N Onion Thins	10 crackers	3	70	39%
Better Cheddars Snack Thins	11 crackers	4	70	51%
Cheese Peanut Butter Sandwich	2 sandwiches	3	70	39%
Cheese Tid-Bits	16 crackers	4	70	51%
Chicken In a Biskit	7 crackers	4	70	51%
Crown Pilot Crackers	1 cracker	1	60	15%
Dandy Soup & Oyster	20 crackers	1	60	15%
Escort	3 crackers	4	80	45%

Food and Description	Amount	Fat Grams	Total Calories	% Fat Calories
Harvest Crisps				
–5-Grain	6 crackers	2	60	30%
Oat	6 crackers	2	60	30%
Rice	6 crackers	2	60	30%
Malted Milk Peanut Butter	2 sandwiches	3	70	39%
Meal Mates Sesame Bread Wafers	3 wafers	3	70	39%
Nips Cheese Snack	13 crackers	3	70	39%
Oat Thins	8 crackers	3	70	39%
Oysterettes Soup & Oyster	18 crackers	1	60	15%
Premium Bits	16 crackers	3	70	39%
Premium Saltine	5 crackers	2	60	30%
Fat free	5 crackers	–	50	–
unsalted tops	5 crackers	2	60	30%
Whole Wheat Premium Plus				
Saltines	5 crackers	2	60	30%
Quackers Crisp Snack				
Cheddar Chees	28 crackers	3	70	39%
Original	28 crackers	3	70	39%
Sour Cream & Onion	28 crackers	4	70	51%
Ritz (regular & low-salt)	4 crackers	4	70	51%
Ritz Bits Mini	22 crackers	4	70	51%
Ritz Bits - cheese	22 crackers	4	70	51%
Ritz Bits-cheese sandwiches	6 sandwiches	5	80	56%
Ritz Bits Peanut Butter				
Sandwiches	6 sandwiches	4	80	45%
Royal Lunch Milk Crackers	1 cracker	2	60	30%
Sea Round	1 cracker	2	60	30%
Sociable	6 crackers	3	70	39%
Swiss Cheese Snack	7½ crackers	3	70	39%
Toasted Bran Thins	7 crackers	3	60	45%
Toasted Peanut Butter Sandwich	2 sandwiches	4	70	51%
Teddy Grahams-chocolate, cinnamon, & honey	11 crackers	2	60	30%
Triscuit-Deli Style Rye	3 wafers	2	60	30%
Triscuit Wafers				
(regular & low-salt)	3 crackers	2	60	30%
Triscuit Bits	8 crackers	2	60	30%
Wheat'n Bran Triscuit	3 crackers	2	60	30%
Twigs - sesame & cheese	5 pieces	4	70	51%
Uneeda Biscuits-unsalted tops	3 biscuits	2	60	30%
Vegetable Thins	7 crackers	4	70	51%
Waverly (regular & low-salt)	4 crackers	3	70	39%
Wheat Thins				
Cheese	9 crackers	3	70	39%

Food and Description	Amount	Fat Grams	Total Calories	% Fat Calories
Low-salt	8 crackers	3	70	39%
Regular	8 crackers	3	70	39%
Nutty	8 crackers	4	70	51%
Wheatsworth Stone-ground Wheat	4 crackers	3	70	39%
Zings	15 pieces	3	70	39%
Zwieback Teething Toast	2 pieces	1	60	15%
Oat Bran Krisp	2 crackers	3	60	45%
Oyster	10 crackers	1	44	21%
Peanut Butter Cheese (Little Debbie)	.93	6	130	42%
Peanut Butter, Toasty (Little Debbie)	.93 oz	7	140	45%
	1.4 oz	12	200	54%
(Pepperidge Farm)				
Buttered Flavored	4 crackers	3	80	34%
Butter Thins	4 crackers	3	80	34%
Cracked Wheat	4 crackers	4	110	33%
English Water	4 biscuits	1	70	13%
Flutters				
Garden Herb	¾ oz	4	100	36%
Golden Sesame	¾ oz	5	110	41%
Original Butter	¾ oz	4	100	36%
Toasted Wheat	¾ oz	5	110	41%
Goldfish Cheese Thins	4 crackers	3	70	39%
Goldfish-Tiny				
Cheddar Cheese	45 crackers	6	140	39%
Original	45 crackers	7	140	45%
Parmesan Cheese	45 crackers	6	140	39%
Pizza Flavored	45 crackers	7	140	45%
Pretzel	40 crackers	3	120	23%
Hearty Wheat	4 crackers	4	100	36%
Sesame	4 crackers	3	80	34%
Symphony	4 crackers	3	80	34%
Three Cracker Asstmt	4 crackers	4	100	36%
Toasted Wheat w/onion	4 crackers	3	80	34%
(Planters)				
Round Toast Crackers	4 sandwiches	7	140	45%
Square Cheese Crackers	4 sandwiches	7	140	45%
Rusk (See CRISPBREAD)				
(Ry Krisp)				
Natural	2 crackers	–	40	–
Seasoned	2 crackers	1	45	20%
Sesame	2 crackers	2	50	36%
Saltines-regula	4 crackers	1	50	18%
(Sea Rounds)	½ oz	2	60	30%

Food and Description	Amount	Fat Grams	Total Calories	% Fat Calories
(Sunshine)				
Cheddar American Heritage	5 crackers	4	80	45%
Cheez-it	12 crackers	4	70	51%
Krispy saltines				
(regular & unslated tops	5 crackers	1	60	15%
Oyster	16 crackers	1	60	15%
Oyster & Soup	16 crackers	2	60	30%
Parmesan American Heritage	4 crackers	4	70	51%
Sesame American Heritage	4 crackers	4	70	51%
Wheat American Heritage	4 crackers	3	60	45%
Wheat Snack	8 crackers	4	70	51%
Wheat Wafers	8 wafers	4	80	45%
Tam Tams (Manischewitz)				
Garlic	10 pieces	8	153	47%
no salt	10 pieces	7	138	46%
Onion	10 pieces	8	150	48%
regular	10 pieces	8	147	49%
Wheat	10 pieces	8	150	48%
(Valley Lahvosh)				
Cracker Bread-Rounds white				
5"	1 piece	1	70	13%
Hors d'oeurve size	1 piece	.5	28	26%
whole wheat 5"	1 piece	.8	6	11%
Small Wheat Lahvosh	1 piece	1	28	32%
Small White Lahvosh	1 piece	1	28	32%
Wheat Wafers (Venus)	8 wafers	2	100	18%
Whole Wheat (Manischewitz)	10 crackers	1	90	10%
CRACKER CRUMBS-GRAHAM				
(Nabisco)	½ oz	1	60	15%
CRACKER MEAL (Nabisco)	½ oz	–	50	–
CRANBERRY/fresh				
chopped	1 cup	–	54	–
whole	1 cup	–	46	–
CRANBERRY-APPLE DRINK				
Cranapple Drink				
(Ocean Spray)	6 oz	–	130	–
–low-cal	6 oz	–	40	–
(Welch's)	6 oz	–	120	–
Cranberry-Apple	6 oz	–	123	–
(Seneca)	6 oz	–	110	–
–frozen	6 oz	–	110	–
Cranberry-Apple Cooler				
(Health Valley)	13 oz	1	144	6%
CRANBERRY-APRICOT JUICE	6 oz	–	118	–

Food and Description	Amount	Fat Grams	Total Calories	% Fat Calories
Cranicot Drink (Ocean Spray)	6 oz	–	110	–
CRANBERRY-BLUEBERRY JUICE				
(Ocean Spray)	6 oz	–	120	–
CRANBERRY DRINK				
Cranberry Juice Drink (Welch's)	6 oz	–	100	–
CRANBERRY-GRAPE JUICE				
Crangrape (Ocean Spray)	6 oz	–	130	–
CRANBERRY JUICE				
Cranberry Delight Nectar	6 oz	–	80	–
Cranberry Juice				
(Knudsen) Just Cranberry Juice	8 oz	–	40	–
(Smucker's)	8 oz	–	130	–
Cranberry Nectar (Knudsen)	8 oz	–	110	–
CRANBERRY JUICE COCKTAIL	8 oz	–	147	–
(Ocean Spray)	6 oz	–	110	–
low cal	6 oz	–	33	–
(Seneca)	6 oz	–	110	–
CRANBERRY JUICE COCKTAIL/FROZEN				
(Birds Eye)	6 oz	–	100	–
(Seneca)	6 oz	–	110	–
(Sunkist)	6 oz	–	110	–
CRANBERRY-ORANGE JUICE				
(Ocean Spray)	6 oz	–	100	–
(Tropicana)-single serve	10 oz	–	159	–
CRANBERRY-ORANGE RELISH				
canned	½ cup	–	246	–
uncooked	½ cup	–	245	–
CRANBERRY-RASPBERRY JUICE				
(Ocean Spray)	6 oz	–	110	–
low-cal	6 oz	–	40	–
CRANBERRY SAUCE				
Canned	1 cup	–	419	–
(Ocean Spray)				
Jellied	2 oz	–	90	–
Whole	2 oz	–	90	–
(S&W)				
Jellied	¼ cup	–	90	–
Old Fashioned-Whole Berry	¼ cup	–	90	–
CRAN-ORANGE SAUCE (Ocean Spray)	2 oz	–	100	–
CRAN-RASPBERRY SAUCE				
(Ocean Spray)	2 oz	–	90	–
CRAN-TASTIC BLENDED (Ocean Spray)	6 oz	–	110	–
CRAYFISH/mixed				
cooked-moist heat	3 oz	1	97	9%

Food and Description	Amount	Fat Grams	Total Calories	% Fat Calories
raw	3 oz	.9	76	11%
	8 fish	< 1	24	19%

CREAM (*See also* CREAM SUBSTITUTE, DESSERT TOPPING, SOUR CREAM, SOUR CREAM SUBSTITUTE, WHIPPED TOPPING)

Food and Description	Amount	Fat Grams	Total Calories	% Fat Calories
Coffee/Table light cream	1 Tbs	3	30	90%
	1 cup	46	469	90%
Coffee Lightener-non-dairy/liquid				
(Coffee Delight)	1 Tbs	2	20	90%
(Coffee Mate)	1 Tbs	1	16	56%
(Coffee Rich)	1 Tbs	1.6	22	66%
(Half & Half)	1 Tbs	1.7	20	77%
	½ cup	13	150	78%
(Maxwell House)	1 Tbs	1	12	75%
(Mocha Mix)	1 Tbs	2	20	90%
Lite	1 Tbs		10	45%
	1 cup	12	150	72%
Coffee Lightener-powdered-				
(Coffee-Mate)	1 tsp	1	10	90%
	1 pkt	1	16	56%
(Coffee-Mate)-Lite	1 tsp		8	56%
(Cremora)	1 tsp	1	12	75%
Lite	1 tsp		8	56%
(Maxwell House)	1 pkt	1	14	64%
(Weight Watchers)	1 pkt	–	10	–
Whipping Cream/fluid				
heavy	1 cup	88	820	100%
	1 Tbs	6	50	100%
heavy-whipped	2 cups	88	820	100%
(Land O'Lakes)				
Gourmet heavy	1 Tbs	6	60	100%
light	1 cup	73.88	704	100%
	1 Tbs	5	45	100%
light-whipped	2 cups	73.88	704	100%
(Land O'Lakes)-light	1 Tbs	5	45	100%

CREAM CHEESE (*See also* CHEESE)

Food and Description	Amount	Fat Grams	Total Calories	% Fat Calories
	1 oz	9.89	99	90%
Light (Philadelphia)	1 oz	5	60	75%
(Weight Watchers)	1 oz	2	35	51%
with chives	1 oz	9	90	90%
with herb & garlic	1 oz	9.9	103	87%
with fruit/all flavors	1 oz	8	90	80%
with honey	1 oz	8	100	72%
(soft)	1 oz	8	100	72%

Food and Description	Amount	Fat Grams	Total Calories	% Fat Calories
with olives & pimento	1 oz	8	90	80%
with onions & chives	1 oz	9	100	81%
with pimento	1 oz	9	90	90%
whipped-plain (Philadelphia)	1 oz	10	100	90%
w/bacon & horseradish	1 oz	9	90	90%
w/bleu cheese	1 oz	9	100	81%
w/chives	1 oz	8	90	80%
w/onions	1 oz	8	90	80%
w/smoked salmon	1 oz	8	90	80%
(soft)	1 oz	9	90	90%
(Woody's)-choc w/walnuts	1 oz	4	120	30%
choc mint fudge	1 oz	4	120	30%
maple walnut fudge	1 oz	4	120	30%
CREAM OF TARTAR	1 Tbs	–	23	–
	1 tsp	–	7	–
CREPE (Table de France)				
Fresh-Ready to use	1-9"	1	45	20%
CRISPBREAD (also referred to as snack bread)				
(Ideal)-Extra Thin Crispbread	3 slices	–	48	–
Whole Grain Crispbread	2 slices	–	43	–
w/sesame seeds	2 slices	–	40	–
(LU)-Crokine Crispbread	2 slices	–	37	–
(Kavli) Norwegian- rye-bran	2 slices	–	30	–
thick	1 slice	–	35	–
thin	2 slices	–	40	–
(Ryvita)-Dark	2 slices	–	38	–
Dark Rye	1 piece	–	26	–
Dark w/caraway seeds	2	–	38	–
High Fiber	1	–	14	–
Light Rye Hi-Fiber	1	–	35	–
Original Wheat	1	–	20	–
(Wasa) -Breakfast	1 slice	1	50	18%
Fiber Plus	1 slice	13	52	6%
Golden Rye	1 slice	–	35	–
Hearty Rye	1 slice	–	45	–
Lite Rye	1 slice	–	25	–
Sesame Wheat	1 slice	25	–	36%
(Weight Watchers)-all flavors	2 wafers	–	30	–
Rusk (Sweet hard crisp bread)-				
3⅜" dia ½" thick	1 piece	.8	38	19%
CROAKER				
breaded & fried	3 oz	10	188	48%
raw	3 oz	2.69	89	27%

Food and Description	Amount	Fat Grams	Total Calories	% Fat Calories
CROISSANT				
Croissant (recipe)	1/~ 2 oz	12	235	46%
(Pepperidge Farm) ready-to-serve				
all butter petite	1	7	120	53%
(Pepperidge Farm)-frozen				
all butter	1	14	240	53%
all butter-petite	1	8	140	51%
(Rainbo)-Wheat	1	19	300	57%
(Sara Lee)-frozen				
all butter	1	9	170	48%
all butter-petite	1	6	120	45%
CROUTON				
(Kellogg)-Croutettes	1 cup	–	144	–
(Pepperidge Farm)				
Cheddar & Romano Cheese	½ oz	2	60	30%
Cheese & Garlic, Onion & Garlic, Seasoned, Sour Cream & Chive	½ oz	3	70	39%
CROWDER PEA/canned				
Seasoned w/Pork (Luck's)	7.5 oz	7	200	32%
CUCUMBER (See also PICKLE)				
raw	1	–	29	–
slices	½ cup	–	7	–
CUMIN SEED	1 tsp	.5	8	56%
CUPCAKE (See CAKE, SNACK CAKE)				
CURRANT				
Black				
dried	½ cup	–	204	–
raw	½ lb	–	120	–
	½ cup	–	36	–
Red or White				
raw	½ lb	–	110	–
	½ cup	–	31	–
Zante				
(Del Monte)				
dried	½ cup	–	200	–
(Sun Maid)	½ cup	–	210	–
CURRANT JUICE				
Black	8 oz	–	138	–
CURRY POWDER	1 tsp	–	6	–
CURRY SAUCE (See SAUCE)				
CUSK				
raw	3 oz	1	74	12%

Food and Description	Amount	Fat Grams	Total Calories	% Fat Calories
steamed	1 lb	3	481	6%
	1 oz	< 1	30	15%
CUSTARD (See also PUDDING)				
homemade				
(baked)	1 cup	14.6	305	43%
(boiled)	½ cup	7	164	38%
mix				
(Jell-O)				
Americana Golden Egg				
prepared with whole milk	½ cup	5	160	28%
Flan-Spanish Style				
prepared with whole milk	½ cup	4	148	24%
Zabaglione/sauce topping for fruit				
homemade	¼ cup	4	80	45%
CUTTLEFISH/raw	3 oz	.6	67	8%

D

Food and Description	Amount	Fat Grams	Total Calories	% Fat Calories
DANDELION GREENS				
fresh-cooked	½ cup	–	17	–
raw-chopped	½ cup	–	13	–
DANISH (See CAKE AND CAKE PASTRY)				
DATE				
chopped	1 cup	.8	489	2%
(Dole)	½ cup	< 1	280	2%
(Dromedary)				
chopped	¼ cup	–	130	–
no pits	5 dates	–	100	–
	1 oz	–	100	–
natural & dry	10	–	228	–
(Sun Giant)				
chopped	1 cup	1	490	2%
pitted	10 dates	1	220	4%
DESSERT TOPPINGS (See ICE CREAM TOPPINGS)				
DIETING AIDS (See NUTRITIONAL SUPPLEMENTS)				

Food and Description	Amount	Fat Grams	Total Calories	% Fat Calories
DILL SAUCE (*See* SAUCE)				
DILL SEED	1 tsp	–	6	–
dried	1 tsp	–	3	–
DINNER (*See* FAST FOOD, FROZEN ENTREES/DINNER)				
DIP				
Sour Cream Dip				
(Dean's)/all flavors	1 Tbs	3	25	100%
(Kraft)				
Avocado (Guacamole)	2 Tbs	4	50	72%
Bacon & Horseradish	2 Tbs	5	60	75%
Clam	2 Tbs	4	50	72%
French Onion	2 Tbs	4	60	60%
Green Onion	2 Tbs	4	60	60%
Jalapeno Pepper	2 Tbs	4	50	72%
Premium Bacon & Horseradish	2 Tbs	4	50	72%
Premium Bacon & Onion	2 Tbs	5	50	90%
Premium Blue Cheese	2 Tbs	4	45	80%
Premium Clam	2 Tbs	4	45	80%
Premium Creamy Cucumber	2 Tbs	4	50	72%
Premium Cream Onion	2 Tbs	4	45	80%
Premium French Onion	2 Tbs	4	45	80%
Premium Jalapeno Pepper	2 Tbs	4	50	72%
(Slender Choice)				
French Onion	1 Tbs	1	14	64%
Green Onion	1 Tbs	1	16	56%
Jalapeno	1 Tbs	1	16	56%
Ranch Style	1 Tbs	1	16	56%
DISTILLED LIQUOR (All Scotch, Rye, Gin, Rum, Vodka, Whiskey, Tequila, Brandy, Etc.)				
NOTE: In all cases, the higher the proof (the % of alcohol), the higher the calories.				
80 proof	1 fl oz	–	67	–
84 proof	1 fl oz	–	70	–
86 proof	1 fl oz	–	72	–
86.8 proof	1 fl oz	–	72	–
90 proof	1 fl oz	–	75	–
90.4 proof	1 fl oz	–	75	–
94 proof	1 fl oz	–	78	–
94.6 proof	1 fl oz	–	79	–
97 proof	1 fl oz	–	81	–
100 proof	1 fl oz	–	83	–
DOCK				
cooked	3 oz	–	17	–
raw-chopped	3 oz	–	15	–

Food and Description	Amount	Fat Grams	Total Calories	% Fat Calories
DOGFISH/raw	3 oz	6.5	135	43%
DOLPHIN FISH	3 oz	.6	73	7%
DONUT				
(Break Cake)				
chocolate	1-1 oz	8	130	55%
cinnamon	1-1 oz	6	115	47%
powdered	1-1 oz	5	115	39%
Cake Type Donuts				
(3¼"dia. 1"high)	1	7.8	164	43%
(1½"dia. 1"high)	1	2.6	155	15%
(Dunkin' Donuts)				
apple filled w/cinnamon sugar	1	11	250	40%
bavarian filled w/choc frosting	1	14	226	56%
blueberry filled	1	11	240	34%
chocolate frosted yeast ring	1	8	210	34%
cookies				
chocolate chunk	1	10	200	45%
chocolate chunk w/nuts	1	11	210	47%
oatmeal bran raisin	1	9	200	41%
croissants				
almond	1	29	420	62%
chocolate	1	29	440	59%
plain	1	19	310	55%
glazed				
buttermilk ring	1	14	290	43%
chocolate ring	1	21	324	58%
coffee roll	1	12	280	39%
french cruller	1	8	140	51%
whole wheat ring	1	18	330	49%
yeast ring	1	9	200	41%
jelly filled	1	9	220	37%
lemon filled	1	12	260	42%
munchkin				
cake w/powdered sugar	1	4	69	52%
chocolate w/glaze	1	5	88	51%
yeast w/glaze	1	2	43	42%
plain cake ring	1	17	270	57%
(Earth Grains)				
cinnamon apple	1	17	310	49%
devil's food	1	21	330	57%
glazed (old fshnd)	1	18	310	52%
powdered (old fshnd)	1	19	290	59%
(Hostess) cake	1	7	115	55%
chocolate covered	1	7	130	49%

Food and Description	Amount	Fat Grams	Total Calories	% Fat Calories
cinnamon	1	6	110	49%
krunch	1	4	110	33%
old fashioned	1	10	180	50%
old fashioned				
glazed	1	12	230	47%
plain	1	7	110	57%
powdered sugar	1	4	110	33%
(Tastykake)				
cinnamon	1	10	195	46%
honey wheat				
mini	1	3	65	42%
plain	1	11	200	50%
powdered sugar	1	11	205	48%
mini	1	3	60	45%
premium				
fudge iced	1	18	340	48%
honey wheat	1	14	300	42%
orange glazed	1	16	335	43%
(Wenchell's)				
apple fritter	1	37	580	57%
cinnamon crumb	1	11	240	41%
cinnamon roll	1	21	360	53%
glazed jelly	1	13	300	39%
glazed round	1	12	210	51%
glazed twist	1	11	210	47%
iced chocolate bar	1	11	220	45%
iced chocolate cake	1	10	230	39%
iced chocolate devil's	1	12	240	45%
iced chocolate french	1	13	220	53%
iced chocolate raised	1	10	210	43%
plain	1	11	200	50%
plain donut hole	1	3	50	54%
Yeast-Leavened-Glazed Donuts				
(3¾" dia. 1¼" high)	1	13	235	50%
Yeast-Leavened-Jelly Filled Donuts	1	9	225	36%
DRUM/raw (freshwater)	3 oz	4	100	36%
DUCK				
Domestic				
liver-raw	1.5 oz	2	60	30%
meat & skin-roasted	~ ¾ lb	108	1287	76%
meat only-roasted	8 oz	24.75	445	50%
Wild				
breast meat only-raw	3 oz	35	102	31%
meat & skin-raw	9.5 oz	41	571	65%

E

Food and Description	Amount	Fat Grams	Total Calories	% Fat Calories
EEL				
cooked-dry heat	3 oz	12.7	200	57%
raw	3 oz	9.9	156	57%
smoked	~2 oz	16	188	77%
EGG (*See also* EGG SUBSTITUTE, MEAT SUBSTITUTE, VEGETARIAN FOOD)				
Chicken				
boiled, hard/soft	1 egg	5.6	79	64%
fried in butter	1	7	95	66%
hard boiled	1	5.6	79	64%
poached	1	5.6	79	64%
raw	1	5.6	79	64%
raw, yolk and white	1 egg	5.6	79	64%
raw, white only	1 egg	–	16	–
raw, yolk only	1 egg	5.6	63	64%
white	1	–	16	–
	1 cup	–	120	–
yolk	1	5.6	63	64%
Duck/raw	1	9.6	130	67%
Goose/raw	1	19	276	62%
Quail/raw	1	1	14	64%
Turkey/raw	1	9	135	60%
EGG MEALS (*See also* EGG, EGG SUBSTITUTE, FRENCH TOAST)				
Deviled	1 egg	13	145	81%
Egg Foo Yong-homemade	~ 5 oz	10	150	60%
Eggs on a biscuit - frozen				
Great Starts				
w/Canadian bacon & cheese	5¼ oz	22	420	47%
w/sausage & cheese	5½ oz	29	460	57%
Eggs on a muffin - frozen				
Great Starts				
w/beefsteak & cheese	4.9 oz	22	380	52%
w/Canadian bacon & cheese	4.1 oz	16	300	48%
Ham steak'n egg muffin - frozen				
Schwan's	1	17	340	45%

Food and Description	Amount	Fat Grams	Total Calories	% Fat Calories
Omelette				
Frozen Spanish Style				
(Swanson)	7¾ oz	16	240	60%
Standard home recipe (USDA) w/whole				
milk/cooked in butter	1 egg	7	95	66%
Quiche lorraine				
Standard home recipe (USDA)				
8" dia	⅛ quiche	48	600	72%
Scrambled eggs				
Frozen w/bacon and home fries				
(Swanson)	5¼ oz	28	360	70%
w/ham and hash browns				
(Downyflake)	6¼ oz	26	350	67%
w/ham and pecan twirls				
(Downyflake)	6¼ oz	28	470	54%
w/home fries				
(Swanson)	4⅜ oz	21	280	68%
w/mini oat bran muffins				
(Great Starts)	4¾ oz	12	250	43%
w/sausage and hash browns				
(Swanson)	6¼ oz	35	430	73%
Standard home recipe (USDA)				
w/whole milk/cooked in butter	1 egg	7	95	66%
EGG NOG				
Canned (Borden)	4 oz	9	160	51%
Commercial	8 oz	19	342	50%
(Land O'Lakes)	8 oz	15	123	11%
Lite (Carnation)	8 oz	8	320	23%
mix-dry	2 tsp	–	110	–
mix (2 heaping tsp) + whole milk	8 oz	8	260	28%
mix (PDQ)-⅔ tsp + whole milk	8 oz	5	230	20%
EGG SALAD-homemade	⅓ cup	19	205	83%
EGG SUBSTITUTE				
frozen	¼ cup	6.7	96	64%
(Healthy Choice)	¼ cup		30	15%
liquid	1½ oz	1.6	39	37%
powder	.35 oz	1	44	21%
BY BRAND NAME				
(Country Morning)	½ cup	12	173	62%
(Egg Beaters)	¼ cup	–	25	–
(Egg Beaters) w/cheese	½ cup	6	130	42%
(Egg Beaters)				
Veg. Omelette Mix	½ pkg	–	50	–
Egg Magic(Featherweight)	1 env =			
	2 eggs	8	120	60%

Food and Description	Amount	Fat Grams	Total Calories	% Fat Calories
(Egg Watchers)	2 oz =			
	1 egg	2	50	36%
(Scramblers)	¼ cup	3	60	45%
(Second Nature)	2 oz =			
	1 egg	2	60	30%
EGGPLANT				
fresh-boiled	½ cup	–	13	–
raw/sliced	½ cup	–	11	–
EGGPLANT DISHES				
Eggplant Parmigiana				
frozen				
(Celentano)	8 oz	15	280	48%
(Pepperidge Farm)	5 oz	17	260	59%
Eggplant Sticks				
fried				
frozen				
(Pepperidge Farm)	3½ oz	12	240	45%
ELDERBERRY/raw	½ lb	1	154	6%
	1 cup	.8	105	7%
ENCHILADA SAUCE (*See* SAUCE)				
ENDIVE/raw	½ cup	–	4	–
ESCAROLE/raw	4 oz	–	20	–
ESCAROLE SOUP (*See* SOUP)				
EXTRACTS & FLAVORS				
(Durkee)				
Almond pure extract	1 tsp	–	13	–
Anise extract	1 tsp	–	16	–
Banana flavor	1 tsp	–	15	–
Butter flavor	1 tsp	–	3	–
Brandy flavor	1 tsp	–	15	–
Black Walnut flavor	1 tsp	–	4	–
Chocolate flavor	1 tsp	–	7	–
Coconut flavor	1 tsp	–	8	–
Lemon extract	1 tsp	–	17	–
Malt extract-dried	1 oz	–	104	–
Maple extract	1 tsp	–	6	–
Orange extract	1 tsp	–	14	–
Peppermint extract	1 tsp	–	15	–
Pineapple flavor	1 tsp	–	6	–
Rum flavor	1 tsp	–	14	–
Strawberry extract	1 tsp	–	12	–
Vanilla-pure extract	1 tsp	–	8	–
Vanilla flavor	1 tsp	–	3	–

F

Food and Description	Amount	Fat Grams	Total Calories	% Fat Calories
FALAFEL				
homemade-pattied or balled	1 oz	6	115	47%
mix (Casbah)	1.33 oz	2	134	13%
FAT (*See also* LARD)				
Bacon fat	1 Tbs	14	126	100%
Beef fat/separable/raw	1 Tbs	12	108	100%
Chicken fat	1 Tbs	12	115	100%
Duck fat	1 Tbs	12	115	100%
Pork back fat/raw	2 oz	50	464	100%
FAT, COOKING/vegetable				
(Crisco) Regular & Butter	1 Tbs	12	113	100%
	1 cup	205	1810	100%
Snowdrift	1 Tbs	12	110	100%
Generic-Soybean/Cottonseed	1 Tbs	13	113	100%
	1 cup	205	1812	100%
FAVA BEANS/canned (Progresso)	8 oz	1	180	5%
FENNEL LEAVES/raw	2 oz	–	15	–
FENNEL SEED	1 tsp	–	7	–
FENUGREEK SEED	1 tsp	–	12	–
FIG				
canned	1 cup	–	228	–
(Del Monte)-whole	½ cup	–	100	–
(S&W)-fancy, whole kadota	½ cup	–	100	–
dried				
cooked	½ cup	–	140	–
	1 large	–	55	–
(Mariani) Calimyma	½ cup	2	250	7%
(Sun Maid)				
Calimyma	½ cup	2	250	7%
Mission	½ cup	1	210	4%
fresh	1 large	–	47	–
FILBERT OR HAZELNUT				
dried				
blanched	1 oz	17.8	179	90%
unblanched	1 oz	18.5	190	88%

Food and Description	Amount	Fat Grams	Total Calories	% Fat Calories
dry roasted	1 oz	18.8	188	90%
oil roasted	1 oz	18	187	87%
FISH (*See* individual listings)				
FISH CHOWDER (*See* SOUP)				
FISH ENTREE/DINNER (*See* SEAFOOD ENTREE/DINNER)				
FISH SEASONING				
(Durkee)				
Roastin' Bag Seasoning				
Creamy Dill Sauce for fish	1 pkg	14	153	82%
Lemon Butter for fish	1 pkg	.7	75	8%
(French's) Microwave Mixes				
Lemon Dill Fish	¼ pkg	1	45	20%
(McCormick/Schilling)				
Bag'N Season/dry				
Lemon & Dill	1 pkg	11	161	62%
(Shake & Bake) coating for fish				
Original	¼ pouch	1	70	13%
FLAN (*See* CUSTARD)				
FLATFISH				
cooked	3 oz	1	100	9%
raw	3 oz	1	80	11%
FLAVORS (*See* EXTRACTS & FLAVORS)				
FLOUNDER (*See also* SEAFOOD ENTREE/DINNER)				
baked w/butter	3 oz	7	171	37%
baked w/o butter	3 oz	1	80	11%
frozen-breaded	5 oz	15	300	45%
frozen-raw (Van de Kamp's)	4 oz	1	100	9%
FLOUR				
Amaranth	2 oz	1	190	5%
	1 cup	2	698	3%
(Arrowhead)	2 oz	3	200	14%
Arrowroot	1 Tbs	–	29	–
Barley	1 Tbs		28	16%
Bread				
(Gold Medal)-high protein	1 cup	1	400	2%
(Pillsbury's Best)	1 cup	2	400	5%
Brown Rice	2 oz	1	200	5%
Buckwheat, dark	1 cup	2	326	6%
Buckwheat, light	1 cup	1	340	3%
Buckwheat, whole grain	1 cup	2	335	5%
Cake or Pastry	4 oz	1	413	2%
Carob (St. John's Bread)	4 oz	3	420	6%
Corn	1 cup	3	430	6%
	1 Tbs	–	14	–

Food and Description	Amount	Fat Grams	Total Calories	% Fat Calories
Cottonseed				
Low-fat	1 oz	–	95	–
Partially defatted	2 Tbs	–	40	–
	1 cup	6	335	16%
Cracked Wheat (Krusteaz)	1 cup	2	320	6%
Drifted Snow (Pillsbury)	4 oz	1	400	2%
Ezekiel (Arrowhead Mills)	2 oz	1	200	5%
Garbanzo (Arrowhead Mills)				
Plain	2 oz	3	210	14%
Toasted	2 oz	4	210	18%
Graham (Krusteaz)	1 cup	2	320	6%
Gluten	1 cup	3	530	5%
La Pina	1 cup	1	400	2%
Millet	2 oz	2	185	10%
Oat (Arrowhead Mills)	2 oz	1	200	5%
Oat Flour Blend (Gold Medal)	4 oz/1 cup	3	390	7%
Peanut				
Defatted	1 oz	–	92	–
	2 Tbs	–	30	–
	1 cup	–	200	–
Low-fat	1 oz	6	120	45%
	1 cup	13	260	45%
Potato	1 cup	1.5	632	2%
Rice	2 oz	1	200	5%
	1 cup	1	398	2%
Rye (Fisher)	1 cup	2	450	4%
Rye, dark	1 cup	3	419	6%
Rye, light	1 cup	1	364	3%
Rye, medium (Pillsbury)	1 cup	2	400	5%
Rye & Wheat, Bohemian Style (Pillsbury)	1 cup	1	400	2%
Sesame-low-fat	1 cup	–	95	–
Shake & Blend (Pillsbury)	2 Tbs	–	50	–
Softasilk	¼ cup	–	100	–
Soy				
Gluten free	½ cup	< 1	180	3%
Whole grain (Arrowhead Mills)	2 oz	11	250	40%
Soybean, full fat				
Not stirred	1 cup	17.6	358	44%
Stirred	1 cup	14	295	43%
Soybean, defatted	1 cup	1	327	3%
Soybean, low-fat	1 cup	6	326	17%
Triticale	2 oz	1	200	5%
Wheat & Gluten	1 cup	3	530	5%

Food and Description	Amount	Fat Grams	Total Calories	% Fat Calories
White, all purpose	1 cup	1	401	2%
(Ballard & Pillsbury)	1 cup	1	400	2%
(Gold Medal)	1 cup	1	400	2%
(Mrs. Wright)	1 cup	1	400	2%
(Pillsbury's Best)	1 cup	1	400	2%
(Red Band)	1 cup	1	390	2%
Unbleached	1 cup	2	401	5%
(Pillsbury)	1 cup	1	400	2%
White, bread	1 cup	3	401	7%
White, cake	1 cup	1	430	2%
White, self-rising	1 cup	1	440	2%
(Gold Medal)	1 cup	1	380	2%
(Pillsbury & Ballard)	1 cup	1	380	2%
Whole Wheat	1 cup	2	400	5%
(Arrowhead Mills)	2 oz	1	200	5%
(Gold Medal)	1 cup	2	350	5%
(Krusteaz)	1 cup	2	450	4%
Self rising	1 cup	1	440	2%
Whole Wheat Blend				
(Gold Medal)	1 cup	2	370	5%
(Red Band)	1 cup	2	400	5%
Whole Wheat-stoneground	2 oz	1	200	5%
Wondra	1 cup	1	400	2%
FRANKFURTER	2 oz	16.8	183	83%
Beef frankfurters	1.6 oz	13	150	78%
Giant/all meat	1.6 oz	13	150	78%
Giant/beef	1	17	180	85%
Giant Great 8/all meat	2 oz	17	180	85%
Giant Great 8/beef	2 oz	17	180	85%
Jumbo Beef				
lower salt	2 oz	15	170	79%
regular	2 oz	18	190	85%
90% Fat free	2 oz	6	90	60%
Beef and Pork	2 oz	16.6	183	82%
	1.5 oz	13	144	81%
(Eckrich)				
1 lb pkg	1	14	160	79%
12 oz pkg	1	10	110	82%
Bunsize	1	17	190	81%
Bunsize-Lite	1	12	150	72%
Jumbo	1	17	190	81%
Lite	1	10	120	75%
(Hormel)				
12 oz pkg	1	10	110	82%

Food and Description	Amount	Fat Grams	Total Calories	% Fat Calories
1 lb pkg	1	13	140	84%
Light & Lean	1	5	70	77%
(Oscar Meyer)	~ 1.5 oz	13	145	81%
Bun Length	2 oz	17	180	85%
Jumbo	2 oz	17	185	83%
Little	9 grams	3	30	90%
Beef & turkey (Armour) 90% fat free	2 oz	6	90	60%
Cheese frankfurters				
(Eckrich)	1	16	180	80%
(Oscar Meyer) hot dogs	1	13	145	81%
hot dogs w/bacon & cheddar	1	13	145	81%
Franks	1	13	145	81%
(Wranglers)-smoked	1	16	180	80%
Chicken frankfurters	1.5 oz	8.8	116	68%
(Health Valley)	3.5 oz	26	290	81%
(Tyson)-corn dogs	1	14	280	45%
(Weaver)	1	10	115	78%
cheese	1	11	145	68%
Chili-Frank'n Stuff (Hormel)	1	15	165	82%
Cocktail-(Hormel)				
Smokie Cheezers	1 oz	8	90	80%
Smokies	1 oz	7	83	76%
Wieners	1 oz	7	80	79%
Corn Dogs-batter wrapped wieners				
(Hormel)-frozen	1	12	220	49%
Meatless frankfurters-(La Loma)-canned				
Big Franks	1.8 oz	6	110	49%
Linketts	2.5 oz	8	140	51%
Tater Dogs-batter wrapped wieners				
(Hormel)-frozen	1	14	210	60%
Turkey frankfurters	2 oz	8	110	66%
	1.5 oz	8	102	71%
w/cheese	1.5 oz	8.6	108	72%
(Butterball)-1 lb pkg	1	11	140	71%
(Health Valley)	3.5 oz	19.7	238	75%
(Louis Rich)	1.6 oz	9	103	79%
Bun Length	2 oz	11	130	76%
Cheese Franks	1.5 oz	9	110	74%
Franks	1.6 oz	8	105	69%
	1.5 oz	8	100	72%
	2 oz	11	130	76%
Weiners				
(Ball Park)				
beef	1	16	175	82%

Food and Description	Amount	Fat Grams	Total Calories	% Fat Calories
regular	1	16	167	86%
Beef	2 oz	16.77	184	82%
	1.5 oz	13	144	81%
(Best's)-Kosher Lower Fat	1	8	110	66%
(Eckrich)				
1 lb pkg	1	14	150	84%
12 oz pkg	1	10	110	82%
Bunsize	1	17	190	81%
Jumbo	1	17	190	81%
(Health Valley)	3.5 oz	25	288	78%
(Hebrew National)-Franks				
beef	1.7 oz	14	149	85%
Collagen	3 oz	19	204	84%
Natural Casing	2 oz	18	178	91%
(Hormel)				
12 oz pkg	1	10	100	90%
1 lb pkg	1	13	140	84%
(Oscar Meyer)	~ 1.5 oz	13	145	81%
Bun Length	2 oz	17	185	83%
Jumbo	2 oz	17	185	83%
(Wranglers)-smoked	1	15	170	79%

FRENCH FRIES (See POTATO, or FAST FOOD)
FRENCH ONION SOUP (See SOUP)
FRENCH TOAST

Food and Description	Amount	Fat Grams	Total Calories	% Fat Calories
Frozen				
Aunt Jemima				
Cinnamon	2 slices	4	170	21%
Cinnamon swirl	2 slices	7	210	30%
Original	2 slices	7	230	27%
plain	2 slices	4	170	21%
Raisin	2 slices	4	170	21%
Downyflake				
Cinnamon	2 slices	7	210	30%
plain	2 slices	14	270	36%
Great Starts				
Cinnamon swirl	6½ oz	28	480	53%
Cinnamon swirl w/sausages	6½ oz	26	470	50%
Oatmeal Cinnamon Swirl w/lite links	6.66 oz	13	310	38%
plain w/sausages	6½ oz	25	450	50%
Krusteaz				
Cinnamon swirl	2 slices	5	270	17%
Classic style	2 slices	6	260	21%
Oat bran	2 slices	3	210	13%
(Weight Watchers) w/links	4¾ oz	12	260	42%

Food and Description	Amount	Fat Grams	Total Calories	% Fat Calories
Standard Home Recipe (USDA)	1 slice	7	155	41%
FRITTER				
apple/frozen (Pepperidge Farm)	2	13	270	43%
homemade	1	7.5	132	51%
FROG LEGS				
fried-floured	1 oz	5	70	64%
	3 oz	17	250	61%
raw	3 oz	< 1	63	7%
FROSTING (*See* CAKE ICING)				
FROZEN DAIRY DESSERT (*See also* ICE CREAM)				
(Diet Count)-Dietetic				
chocolate	½ cup	6	120	45%
strawberry	½ cup	5	140	32%
vanilla	½ cup	7	120	53%
(Dreyer's)				
American Dream Frozen Dairy Desert				
chocolate chip	3 oz	1	100	9%
mocha almond fudge	3 oz	1	110	8%
rocky road	3 oz	1	110	9%
vanilla	3 oz	< 1	80	6%
vanilla, chocolate, strawberry	3 oz	1	80	11%
Frozen Dietary Dessert				
chocolate	4 oz	7	140	45%
chocolate fudge	4 oz	9	160	51%
strawberry	4 oz	6	120	45%
vanilla	4 oz	7	130	49%
Light Dairy Desert				
bananapolitan	½ cup	4	110	33%
candy bar	½ cup	5	140	32%
chocolate fudge mousse	½ cup	5	130	35%
malt ball'n fudge	½ cup	5	140	32%
rocky road	½ cup	5	130	35%
(Edy's)				
chocolate	½ cup	7	140	45%
marble fudge	½ cup	9	160	51%
strawberry	½ cup	6	120	45%
vanilla	½ cup	7	130	49%
(Knudsen) Free Frozen Dessert				
chocolate	½ cup	–	100	–
vanilla	½ cup	–	100	–
vanilla flavored				
strawberry royal	½ cup	–	100	–
(Knudsen) Free Frozen Dessert Bars				
chocolate fudge	1 bar	–	90	–

Food and Description	Amount	Fat Grams	Total Calories	% Fat Calories
vanilla fudge	1 bar	–	80	–
vanilla strawberry	1 bar	–	80	–
Simple Pleasures (Simplesse)-Frozen Dairy Dessert				
chocolate	½ cup	< 1	140	4%
coffee	½ cup	–	120	–
peach	½ cup	< 1	120	4%
rum raisin	½ cup	< 1	130	4%
strawberry	½ cup	–	120	–
toffee crunch	½ cup	< 1	130	4%
Simple Pleasures Light				
chocolate	4 oz	< 1	80	5%
chocolate caramel sundae	4 oz	< 1	90	5%
vanilla	4 oz	< 1	80	6%
vanilla fudge	4 oz	< 1	90	5%
(Slimmery) Skinny Dip Bars	1 Bar	7	110	57%
(Sweet'N Low)				
butter pecan	4 oz	6	120	45%
chocolate	4 oz	2	90	20%
strawberry	4 oz	1	80	11%
vanilla	4 oz	2	80	23%
(Thrifty)-Light Frozen Dairy Dessert				
chocolate chocolate chip	4 oz	6	130	42%
swiss mocha	4 oz	5	120	38%
vanilla	4 oz	5	120	38%
wild berry	4 oz	4	110	33%
FROZEN NON-DAIRY DESSERT				
(Carnation)-Lite Wonder				
chocolate	½ cup	3	110	25%
mocha fudge	½ cup	3	120	23%
neapolitan	½ cup	3	110	25%
strawberry	½ cup	3	110	25%
vanilla	½ cup	3	100	27%
vanilla praline	½ cup	5	130	35%
Mellorine (Costello's)				
fudge revel	½ cup	6	130	42%
vanilla	½ cup	7	130	49%
(Mocha Mix)-(lower in saturated fat)				
chocolate chip	4 oz	9	180	45%
dutch chocolate	4 oz	8	130	55%
mocha almond fudge	4 oz	8	150	48%
neopolitan	4 oz	7	130	49%
strawberry swirl	4 oz	7	140	45%
toasted almond	4 oz	9	150	54%
vanilla	4 oz	7	140	45%

Food and Description	Amount	Fat Grams	Total Calories	% Fat Calories
vanilla, chocolate chocolate almond	4 oz	9	150	54%
vanilla-chocolate covered bars	1 bar	21	300	63%
FROZEN ENTREE/DINNER				
(Armour Classics)/Frozen Dinners				
Dining Light				
Cheese Cannelloni	9 oz	9	310	23%
Cheese Lasagna	9 oz	6	260	21%
Chicken Ala King	9 oz	7	240	26%
Chicken Chow Mein	9 oz	2	180	10%
Chickken w/noodles	9 oz	7	240	26%
Fettucini	9 oz	12	290	37%
Lasagna w/meat sauce	9 oz	5	240	19%
Salisbury Steak	9 oz	8	200	36%
Sauce & Sweedish meatballs	9 oz	10	280	32%
Spaghetti	9 oz	8	220	33%
Dinner Classics				
BBQ Chicken	10 oz	8	280	26%
Beef Stroganoff	10 oz	12	320	34%
Boneless Beef Short Ribs	10.5 oz	19	390	44%
Chicken & Noodles	12 oz	13	340	34%
Chicken Fricasse	11.75 oz	11	340	29%
Chicken Hawaiian	10.5 oz	5	280	16%
Chicken Milan	11.5 oz	10	320	28%
Chicken Parmesan	10.75 oz	20	370	49%
Chicken w/wine and mushroom sauce	10.75 oz	18	350	46%
Ham Steak	11 oz	13	350	33%
Salisbury Steak	11 oz	25	460	49%
Salisbury Steak w/red sauce	9.75 oz	18	310	52%
Seafood Newburg	11.5 oz	12	300	36%
Sirloin Roast	11 oz	8	250	29%
Sirloin Tips	11 oz	10	290	31%
Swedish Meatballs	12.5 oz	27	480	51%
Turkey and Dressing	11.25 oz	14	330	38%
Veal Parmigiana	10.75 oz	22	400	50%
Yankee Pot Roast	12 oz	17	390	39%
Dinner Classics-Light				
Baby Bay Shrimp	10.5 oz	6	260	21%
Beef Pepper Steak	10 oz	5	240	19%
Beef Stroganoff	10 oz	7	250	25%
Chicken Ala King	9 oz	5	240	19%
Chicken & Noodles	10.5 oz	9	250	32%
Chicken w/wine and mushroomsauce	10 oz	11	300	33%

Food and Description	Amount	Fat Grams	Total Calories	% Fat Calories
Chicken Breast w/mushroom and tomato sauce	10 oz	5	240	19%
Chicken Burgundy	10 oz	2	190	10%
Chicken Cacciatore	11 oz	4	250	14%
Chicken Fettuccini	10 oz	11	300	33%
Chicken Mesquite	9.5 oz	15	370	37%
Chicken Oriental	10 oz	2	230	8%
Chicken Parmigiana	10.75 oz	20	370	49%
Glazed Chicken	10.25 oz	16	320	45%
Meat Loaf	9.75 oz	14	340	37%
Salisbury Steak w/mushroom gravy, broccoli, carrots, and red peppers	10.5 oz	11	250	40%
Salisbury Steak w/mushroom gravy, peas, carrots, and potatoes	11.25 oz	20	430	42%
Seafood w/natural herbs	10.5 oz	4	220	16%
Shrimp Creole	10 oz	4	180	20%
Steak Diane	10 oz	9	270	30%
Sweedish Meatballs	10 oz	15	300	45%
Sweet and Sour Chicken	10.5 oz	2	240	8%
Tortellini w/meat	10 oz	10	250	36%
Turkey w/dressing and gravy	11.25 oz	5	250	18%
Veal Parmigiana	10 oz	18	340	48%
(Banquet)/Frozen				
Beef Meat Pie	7 oz	32	500	58%
Supreme-microwave	7 oz	29	439	60%
Casseroles				
Macaroni & Cheese	8 oz	17	344	45%
Spaghetti w/meat sauce	8 oz	8	270	27%
Cookin' Bags				
Beef w/gravy	4 oz	5	100	45%
Barbecue Sauce and Sliced Beef	4 oz	2	100	18%
Breaded Veal Parmigiana	4 oz	11	230	43%
Chicken & Vegetables Primavera	4 oz	2	100	18%
Chicken Ala King	4 oz	5	110	41%
Creamed Chipped Beef	4 oz	4	100	36%
Gravy & Salisbury Steak	5 oz	14	190	66%
Gravy & Sliced Beef	4 oz	5	100	45%
Gravy & Sliced Turkey	5 oz	6	100	54%
Meat Loaf	4 oz	14	200	63%
Mostaccioli	7 oz	3	170	16%

Food and Description	Amount	Fat Grams	Total Calories	% Fat Calories
Mushroom Gravy and Charbroiled Beef Patty	5 oz	15	210	64%
Salisbury Steak	5 oz	14	190	66%
Sweet & Sour Chicken	4 oz	2	130	14%
Dinners				
Beans & Frankfurters Dinner	10 oz	25	510	44%
Chopped Beef Dinner	11 oz	31	420	66%
Fried Chicken Dinner	10 oz	21	400	47%
Meat Loaf Dinner	11 oz	27	440	55%
Salisbury Steak Dinner	11 oz	34	495	62%
Turkey Dinner	10.5 oz	20	385	47%
Western Dinner	11 oz	40	630	57%
Extra Helping Dinners				
Beef Dinner	16 oz	61	865	64%
Chicken Nuggets Dinner w/BBQ sauce	10 oz	36	640	51%
Chicken Nuggets Dinner w/sweet & sour sauce	10 oz	33	650	46%
Fried Chicken Dinner	16 oz	28	560	45%
Fried Chicken Dinner, All White Meat	16 oz	28	560	45%
Lasagna Dinner	16.5 oz	23	645	32%
Salisbury Steak Dinner	18 oz	60	910	59%
Salisbury Steak Dinner w/mushroom gravy	18 oz	58	890	59%
Turkey Dinner	19 oz	41	750	49%
Family Entrees				
Beef Stew	7 oz	5	140	32%
Chicken & Dumplings	7 oz	14	280	45%
Chicken & Vegetables Primavera	7 oz	3	140	9%
Gravy & Salisbury Steak	8 oz	22	300	66%
Gravy & Sliced Beef	8 oz	5	160	28%
Gravy & Sliced Turkey	8 oz	8	150	48%
Lasagna w/meat sauce	7 oz	10	270	33%
Macaroni & Cheese	8 oz	13	290	40%
Mostaccioli & Meat Sauce	7 oz	3	170	16%
Mushroom Gravy & Charbroiled Beef Patties	8 oz	21	270	70%
Noodles & Beef w/gravy	8 oz	7	200	32%
Noodles & Julienne Beef w/sauce	7 oz	3	170	16%
Onion Gravy & Beef Patties	8 oz	21	300	63%
Stroganoff Sauce w/Beef and Noodles	7 oz	6	190	28%

Food and Description	Amount	Fat Grams	Total Calories	% Fat Calories
Veal Parmagian Patties	8 oz	18	370	44%
Family Favorites Dinners				
Chicken & Dumplings Dinner	10 oz	24	420	51%
Macaroni & Cheese Dinner	10 oz	20	415	43%
Noodles & Chicken Dinner	10 oz	15	340	40%
Spaghetti & Meatballs Dinner	10 oz	9	290	28%
Platters				
All White Meat Fried Chicken	9 oz	21	430	44%
All White Meat Hot'n Spicy Fried Chicken	9 oz	21	430	44%
Beef Platter	10 oz	33	460	65%
Boneless Chicken Drumsnacker	7 oz	18	430	38%
Boneless Chicken Nuggets	6.4 oz	21	425	45%
Boneless Chicken Pattie Platter	7.5 oz	20	370	49%
Fish Platter	8.75 oz	22	445	45%
Ham Platter	10 oz	16	400	36%
Supreme Entrees				
Beef Stew	8 oz	5	180	25%
Chicken Ala King	8 oz	11	260	38%
Chicken & Dumplings	8 oz	11	260	38%
Lasagna w/meat sauce	8 oz	5	190	24%
Macaroni & Beef	8 oz	6	210	26%
Macaroni & Cheese	9 oz	8	300	24%
Macaroni & Cheese w/frankfurters	7.5 oz	13	280	42%
Mini Ravioli	8 oz	3	200	14%
Spaghetti & Meat Sauce	8 oz	6	210	26%
(Budget Gourmet)/Frozen				
Light & Healthy Dinners				
Chicken Breast Parmigiana	11 oz	8	260	28%
Herbed Chicken Breast w/Fettucine	11 oz	7	240	26%
Italian Style Meat Loaf	11 oz	10	270	33%
Sirloin Salisbury Steak	11 oz	9	260	31%
Special Recipe Sirloin Beef	11 oz	10	250	36%
Stuffed Turkey Breast	11 oz	6	230	23%
Teriyaki Chicken Breast	11 oz	9	310	26%
Light Entrees				
Beef Stroganoff	8.75 oz	12	290	37%
Cheese Ravioli	9.5 oz	10	290	31%
Chicken Au Gratin	9.1 oz	11	250	40%
Chicken Enchilada Suiza	8.75 oz	12	290	37
French Recipe Chicken and Vegetables	10 oz	9	240	38%
Glazed Turkey	9 oz	5	270	17%
Lasagna w/meat sauce	9.4 oz	13	300	39%

Food and Description	Amount	Fat Grams	Total Calories	% Fat Calories
Mandarin Chicken	10 oz	7	300	21%
Oriental Beef	10 oz	9	290	28%
Sirloin Beef in Herb Sauce	9.5 oz	10	270	33%
Sirloin Salisbury Steak	8.5 oz	13	260	45%
Light & Healthy Dinners				
Beef Pot Roast	10.5 oz	8	210	34%
Chicken Breast Parmigiana	11 oz	8	260	28%
Herbed Chicken	11 oz	7	240	26%
Italian Style Meatloaf	11 oz	10	270	30%
Sirloin Salisbury Steak	11 oz	9	260	31%
Sliced Sirloin in Wine	11 oz	8	270	26%
Special Recipe Sirloin Beef	11 oz	10	250	36%
Stuffed Turkey Breast	11 oz	6	230	23%
Teriyaki Chicken Breast	11 oz	6	270	13%
Regular Entrees				
Cheese Manicotti w/meat Sauce	10 oz	25	450	50%
Chicken & Egg Noodles w/broccoli	10 oz	26	450	52%
Chicken Marsala	10 oz	5	500	9%
Chicken w/Fettucini	10 oz	21	400	47%
Italian Sausage Lasagna	10 oz	20	420	43%
Italian Style Meatballs				
w/noodles and peppers	10 oz	12	310	35%
Linguini w/shrimp	10 oz	15	330	41%
Pasta Shells & Beef	10 oz	14	340	37%
Pepper Steak w/rice	10 oz	9	300	27%
Roast Sirloin	9.5 oz	14	560	23%
Seafood Newberg	10 oz	12	350	31%
Shrimp Fettucini	9.5 oz	20	630	29%
Sirloin Tips w/countrystyle vegetables	10 oz	18	310	52%
Spaghetti w/Italian sausage	10 oz	19	400	43%
Swedish Meatballs w/Noodles	10 oz	39	600	59%
Sweet & Sour Chicken w/rice	10 oz	7	350	18%
Three Cheese Lasagna	10 oz	17	400	38%
Turkey A La King w/rice	10 oz	18	390	42%
Side Dishes				
Cauliflower in cheddar cheese sauce	5 oz	5	110	41%
Cheddared Potatoes	5.5 oz	13	230	51%
Cheddared Potatoes & Broccoli	5 oz	4	130	28%
Cheese Tortellini	5.5 oz	6	180	30%
Country Style Corn	5.75 oz	5	140	32%
Glazed Apples in Raspberry Sauce	5 oz	3	110	25%
Macaroni & Cheese	5.3 oz	8	210	34%
Nacho Potatoes	5 oz	10	180	50%
New England Recipe Vegetables	5.5 oz	10	210	43%

Food and Description	Amount	Fat Grams	Total Calories	% Fat Calories
New Potatoes in Sour Cream Sauce	5 oz	6	120	45%
Oriental Rice & Vegetables	5.75 oz	10	210	43%
Pasta Alfredo w/broccoli	5.5 oz	8	200	36%
Peas & Cauliflower in Cream Sauce	5.75 oz	7	170	37%
Peas & Water Chestnuts Oriental	5 oz	3	120	23%
Rice Pilaf w/green beans	5.5 oz	9	240	34%
Spinach Au Gratin	6 oz	5	120	38%
Spring Vegetables in cheese sauce	5 oz	3	90	30%
Sweet Corn in butter sauce	5.5 oz	6	190	28%
Three Cheese Potatoes	5.75 oz	11	230	43%
Ziti in Marinara Sauce	6.25 oz	9	220	37%
Slim Selects				
Beef Stroganoff	8.75 oz	12	290	37%
Cheese Ravioli	10 oz	10	290	31%
Chicken Au Gratin	9.1 oz	11	250	40%
Chicken Enchilada Suiza	8.8 oz	12	290	37%
Fettucini w/meat sauce	10 oz	10	290	31%
French Recipe Chicken	10 oz	10	260	35%
Glazed Turkey	9 oz	5	270	17%
Ham & Asparagus Au Gratin	9 oz	12	290	37%
Lasagna w/meat sauce	10 oz	10	290	31%
Linguini w/scallops & clams	9.5 oz	11	290	34%
Mandarin Chicken	10 oz	6	300	18%
Oriental Beef	10 oz	9	290	28%
Sirloin of Beef in herb sauce	9.5 oz	10	270	33%
Sirloin EnchiladaRanchero	8.75 oz	9	270	30%
Sirloin Salisbury Steak	9 oz	13	260	45%
Three Dish Dinners				
Beef Mexicana	12.8 oz	15	510	27%
Chicken Cacciatore	11 oz	13	300	39%
Chicken Mexicana	12.8 oz	15	510	27%
Roast Chicken	11.2 oz	7	280	23%
Scallops & Shrimp Mariner	11.5 oz	9	320	25%
Sirloin Salisbury Steak	11.5 oz	22	410	48%
Sirloin Tips in burgundy sauce	11 oz	11	310	32%
Sliced Turkey Breast	11.1 oz	9	290	28%
Swiss Steak	11.2 oz	22	450	44%
Teriyaki Chicken	12 oz	12	360	30%
Turkey Breast Dijon	11.2 oz	12	340	32%
Veal Parmigiana	12 oz	20	440	41%
Yankee Pot Roast	11 oz	21	380	50%
(Campbell's)/Frozen Souper-Combo				
Chicken & Stars Soup and				
Breaded Chicken Nuggets	1 Serving	15	320	42%

Food and Description	Amount	Fat Grams	Total Calories	% Fat Calories
Chicken Noodle Soup and Grilled Ham and Cheese	1 Serving	19	460	37%
Chicken NoodleO's Soup and Hot Dog On a Bun	1 Serving	15	310	44%
Chicken Rice Soup and Vegetable Egg Rolls	1 Serving	12	290	37%
Chili With Beans and Hot Dog on a Bun	1 Serving	22	510	39%
Cream of Broccoli and Ham & Cheese Croissant	1 Serving	26	450	52%
Cream of Mushroom Soup and Breaded Chicken	1 Serving	29	520	50%
Minnestrone Soup and Breaded Mozzarella Breaded Sticks	1 Serving	18	400	41%
New England Clam Chowder and Breaded Fish Sandwich	1 Serving	19	460	37%
Vegetable Soup and Cheeseburger	1 Serving	22	410	48%
Tomato Soup and Grilled Cheese Sandwich	1 Serving	22	400	50%
(Celentano)/Frozen Entrees				
Baked Pasta & Cheese	12 oz	21	530	36%
Broccoli Stuffed Shells	11.5 oz	17	400	38%
Cannelloni Florentine	12 oz	17	380	40%
Cavatelli	3.2 oz	1	270	3%
Chicken Cutlets Parmigiana	9 oz	5	310	15%
Chicken Primavera	11.5 oz	9	270	30%
Eggplant Parmigiana	8 oz	22	320	62%
Eggplant Rollettes	11 oz	30	420	64%
Lasagne (16 oz)	8 oz	16	320	45%
Lasagne Primavera	11 oz	9	300	27%
Manicotti				
w/sauce	8 oz	15	300	45%
w/o sauce	7 oz	18	380	43%
Mini Ravioli	4 oz	6	250	22%
Ravioli	6.5 oz	12	410	26%
Stuffed Shells w/sauce	8 oz	11	330	30%
(Freezer Queen)/Frozen Family Supper				
Gravy & 6 Salisbury Steaks	7 oz	13	200	59%
Gravy & Sliced Turkey	7 oz	5	110	41%
Mushroom Gravy & 6 Charbroiled Beef Patties	7 oz	11	180	55%
Onion Gravy & Beef Patties	7 oz	12	200	54%
Salisbury Steak	7 oz	13	200	59%

Food and Description	Amount	Fat Grams	Total Calories	% Fat Calories
Tomato Sauce & Meatloaf	7 oz	13	230	51%
(Golden)/Frozen Entrees				
Apple Blintz	1 serving	1.8	92	18%
Apple-Raisin Blintz	1 serving	2.5	105	21%
Blueberry Blintz	1 serving	1.9	92	19%
Blueberry-Cheese Blintz	1 serving	2.5	92	25%
Cheese Blintz	1 serving	3	102	26%
Cherry Blintz	1 serving	1.9	105	16%
Potato Blintz	1 serving	6	125	43%
Potato Cheese Pierogie	1 serving	4	108	33%
Potato Onion Pierogie	1 serving	4	80	45%
Potato Pancakes	1 serving	5.6	70	72%
Stawberry-Rhubarb Blintz	1 serving	1.8	92	18%
(Healthy Choice)/Frozen				
Dinners				
Beef Pepper Steak	11 oz	6	290	19%
Breast of Turkey	10.5 oz	5	290	16%
Chicken & Pasta Divan	11.5 oz	4	310	12%
Chicken Oriental	11.25 oz	2	220	8%
Chicken Parmigiana	11.5 oz	3	280	10%
Herb Roasted Chicken	11 oz	3	260	10%
Mesquite Chicken	10.5 oz	2	310	6%
Oriental Pepper Steak	11 oz	6	290	19%
Salisbury Steak	11.5 oz	7	300	21%
Shrimp Creole	11.25 oz	1	210	4%
Shrimp Marinara	10.5 oz	1	220	4%
Sirloin Tips	11.75 oz	6	290	19%
Sole Au Gratin	11 oz	5	270	17%
Sweet & Sour Chicken	11.5 oz	2	280	6%
Yankee Pot Roast	11 oz	4	260	14%
Entrees				
Baked Cheese Ravioli	9 oz	2	240	8%
Beef Pepper Steak	7.5 oz	3	200	14%
Cheese Manicotti	9.25 oz	4	230	16%
Chicken A L 'Orange	9 oz	2	260	7%
Chicken Chow Mein	8.5 oz	3	220	12%
Fettucini Alfredo	8 oz	7	240	26%
Glazed Chicken	8.5 oz	3	220	12%
Lasagna w/meat sauce	9 oz	5	260	17%
Linguini w/Shrimp	9.5 oz	2	230	8%
Roasted Turkey & Mushroom				
Gravy	8.5 oz	3	200	14%
Seafood Newburg	8 oz	3	200	14%
Sole w/Lemon Butter Sauce	8.25 oz	4	230	16%

Food and Description	Amount	Fat Grams	Total Calories	% Fat Calories
Spaghetti w/meat sauce	10 oz	6	310	17%
Zucchini Lasagna	11.5 oz	3	240	11%
(Hormel)/Microwave Entrees				
Microcup				
Chili Mac	7.5 oz	10	200	45%
Chili No Beans	7-3/8 oz	28	380	66%
Chili With Beans	7-3/8 oz	11	250	40%
Dinty Moore Beef Stew	7.5 oz	9	190	43%
Hot Chili W/Beans	7-3/8 oz	11	250	40%
Lasagna	7.5 oz	13	250	47%
Macaroni & Cheese	7.5 oz	6	190	28%
Noodles & Chicken	7.5 oz	8	180	40%
Pork & Beans	7.5 oz	5	250	18%
Ravioli in Tomato Sauce	7.5 oz	11	250	40%
Scalloped Potatoes & Ham	7.5 oz	16	260	55%
Spaghetti & Meatballs	7.4 oz	7	204	31%
Top Shelf				
Beef Oriental	10.3 oz	10	290	31%
Beef Stroganoff	10 oz	11	300	33%
Boneless Beef Ribs	10 oz	19	400	43%
Breast of Chicken Acapulco	10 oz	16	410	35%
Cheese Tortellini in Marinara Sauce	10 oz	4	210	17%
Cheese Tortellini w/Shrimp & Seafood	10 oz	8	280	26%
Chicken Ala King	10 oz	12	340	32%
Chicken Cacciatore	10 oz	2	190	9%
Chili Con Carne Suprema	10 oz	11	310	32%
Glazed Breast Chicken	10 oz	2	190	9%
Italian Style Lasagna	10 oz	16	350	41%
Linguini	10 oz	19	350	49%
Salisbury Steak	10 oz	19	340	50%
Spaghettini	10 oz	6	260	21%
Sukiyaki	10.3 oz	8	320	23%
Sweet & Sour Chicken	10 oz	2	260	7%
Tender Roast Beef	10 oz	7	250	25%
Vegetable Lasagna	10 oz	9	280	26%
(Kibun Gold)/Frozen Entrees				
Chicken Oriental	8 oz	3	230	12%
Ellen's Homestyle Chicken	10 oz	4	300	12%
Honey Garlic Chicken	10 oz	4	290	12%
Lemon Ginger Beef	8 oz	4	230	16%
Pasta & Chicken				

Food and Description	Amount	Fat Grams	Total Calories	% Fat Calories
w/dressing	½ package	9	220	37%
w/o dressing	½ package	2	150	12%
Pasta & Turkey Ham				
w/dressing	½ package	12	250	43%
w/o dressing	½ package	2	140	13%
Sweet & Sour Chicken	10 oz	1	310	3%
(Kid's Cuisine)/Frozen				
Entrees				
Cheese Beef Patty Sandwich	6.25 oz	19	400	43%
Cheese Nuggets	6.25 oz	19	400	43%
Cheese Pizza	6.50 oz	4	240	15%
Chunky Chicken Supreme	10 oz	23	430	48%
Fish Nuggets	7 oz	15	320	42%
Fried Chicken	7.5 oz	23	425	49%
Macaroni & Cheese				
w/mini franks	9 oz	14	380	33%
Mini Cheese Ravioli	8.75 oz	2	250	7%
Spaghetti w/meatsauce	9.25 oz	12	310	35%
(Kraft)/Frozen				
Eating Right Entrees				
Beef Pepper Steak	10 oz	10	290	31%
Beef Sirloin Tips				
& Noodles	9 oz	8	250	29%
Chicken Breast & Vegetables	9 oz	4	200	18%
Fettucini Alfredo	10 oz	7	220	29%
Glazed Chicken Breast	9 oz	4	220	16%
Lasagna w/meat sauce	10 oz	7	270	23%
Macaroni & Cheese	9 oz	8	270	27%
Shrimp Vegetable STir Fry	9 oz	4	220	16%
Sirloin Salisbury Steak	9.5 oz	8	230	31%
Sliced Turkey Breast	10 oz	7	250	25%
Sweedish Meatballs				
& Noodles	10 oz	7	290	22%
Regular Entrees				
Barbecue Beef w/corn	9 oz	12	340	32%
Beef Stew	10 oz	12	250	43%
Cheese Enchilada	9.8 oz	20	390	46%
Chicken A La King	10 oz	14	350	36%
Chicken And Egg Noodles	10 oz	20	420	43%
Chili w/Beef & Beans	9.7 oz	22	380	52%
Creamed Chipped Beef	9 oz	27	380	64%
Fettucini Alfredo	10 oz	30	465	58%
Lasagna w/meat sauce	10 oz	16	390	37%
Macaroni & Beef	11.5 oz	16	370	39%

Food and Description	Amount	Fat Grams	Total Calories	% Fat Calories
Macaroni & Cheese	12 oz	30	610	44%
Ravioli	10 oz	11	320	31%
Salisbury Steak & Fries	9 oz	20	360	50%
Sirloin Chili w/Steak Fries	9 oz	23	390	53%
Spaghetti & Meatballs	9.7 oz	15	340	40%
Tuna Noodle Casserole	10.2 oz	20	370	47%
Turkey & Dressing	9 oz	10	300	30%
Microwave				
Beef Stew	10 oz	4	230	16%
Beef Stroganoff	9 oz	13	330	35%
Cheese Tortellini	10 oz	8	320	23%
Chicken Cacciatore	10 oz	6	260	21%
Chicken Fettuccine	9 oz	12	270	40%
Lasagna	10.2 oz	14	370	34%
Salisbury Steak	9 oz	13	300	39%
Spaghetti & Meatballs	10 oz	12	360	25%
Sweet & Sour Chicken	9 oz	1	290	3%
(Le Menu)/Frozen Dinners				
Beef Sirloin Tips	11.5 oz	19	400	43%
Beef Stroganoff	10 oz	25	450	50%
Chicken a la King	10.25 oz	14	330	38%
Chicken Cordon Bleu	11 oz	20	470	38%
Chicken Florentine	10.75 oz	10	340	27%
Chicken Parmigiana	11.5 oz	19	390	44%
Chopped Sirloin Beef	12.25 oz	25	440	51%
Ham Steak	10 oz	10	300	30%
Pepper Steak	11.5 oz	13	370	32%
Salisbury Steak	10.5 oz	24	400	61%
Sliced Breast of Turkey w/Mushroom Gravy	10.5 oz	6	270	13%
Sweet & Sour Chicken	11.25 oz	22	450	44%
Veal Parmigiana	11.5 oz	18	400	41%
Yankee Pot Roast	11 oz	15	370	37%
Entrees				
Beef Burgandy	7.5 oz	23	330	63%
Chicken Kiev	8 oz	39	530	66%
Manicotti, Cheese Filled	8.5 oz	20	410	44%
Oriental Chicken	10.5 oz	9	330	25%
Healthy				
Chicken Cacciatore	10 oz	8	270	27%
Chicken Cannelloni	10.25 oz	5	270	17%
Chicken Chow Mein	10 oz	4	260	14%
Glazed Chicken Breast	10 oz	6	270	20%
Herb Roasted Chicken	9.25 oz	6	220	25%

Food and Description	Amount	Fat Grams	Total Calories	% Fat Calories
Salisbury Steak	10.5 oz	7	220	29%
3-Cheese Stuffed Shells	10 oz	8	280	26%
Turkey Divan	10 oz	9	280	29%
Veal Marsala	10 oz	6	260	21%
Light Style Entrees				
Cheese Tortellini	8 oz	8	250	29%
Chicken Dijon	8 oz	7	240	26%
Chicken Enchiladas	8 oz	8	280	26%
Chicken A 'La King	8 oz	5	240	19%
Empress Chicken	8 oz	5	210	21%
Glazed Turkey	8 oz	6	260	21%
Herb Roasted Chicken	8 oz	6	260	14%
Lasagna w/meat sauce	10 oz	8	290	25%
Spaghetti w/meat sauce	8 oz	6	280	19%
Sweedish Meatballs	8 oz	8	260	28%
Traditional Turkey	8 oz	5	200	23%
Vegetable Lasagna	10 oz	8	260	28%
Lean Cuisine (Stouffer's)/Frozen Entrees				
Beef & Pork Cannelloni w/Mornay Sauce	9⅝ oz	10	260	35%
Beefsteak Ranchero	9¼ oz	9	270	30%
Breast of Chcicken in Herb Cream Sauce	9½ oz	10	260	35%
Breast of Chicken Marsala w/Vegetables	8⅛ oz	5	190	24%
Breast of Chicken Parmesan	10 oz	8	250	29%
Cheese Cannelloni w/tomato sauce	9⅛ oz	10	260	35%
Chicken al'Orange w/almond rice	8 oz	5	260	17%
Chicken & Vegetables w/vermicelli	11¾ oz	8	270	27%
Chicken Cacciatore w/vermicelli	10⅞ oz	9	270	30%
Chicken Chow Mein w/rice	11¼ oz	5	250	18%
Chicken Oriental	9⅜ oz	6	240	23%
Filet of Fish Divan	12⅜ oz	8	260	28%
Filet of Fish Florentine	9 oz	9	240	34%
Filet of Fish Jardiniere w/Souffléd Potatoes	11¼ oz	10	280	32%
French Bread Pizza Mexican Style	6⅛ oz	10	330	27%
Glazed Chicken w/vegetable rice	8½ oz	8	270	27%
Lasagna w/Meat & Sauce	10¼ oz	8	270	27%
Linguini w/Clam Sauce	9⅝ oz	7	260	24%
Meatball Stew	10 oz	10	250	36%
Oriental Beef w/Vegetables & Rice	8⅝ oz	7	250	25%
Rigatoni Bake w/Meat Sauce & Cheese	9¾ oz	10	260	35%

Food and Description	Amount	Fat Grams	Total Calories	% Fat Calories
Salisbury Steak	9.5 oz	9	260	31%
Salisbury Steak w/Italian Style Sauce & Vegetables	9½ oz	15	280	48%
Shrimp & Chicken Cantonese w/Noodles	10⅛ oz	9	260	17%
Sliced Turkey Breast in Mushroom Sauce	8 oz	7	240	26%
Spaghetti w/Beef & Mushroom Sauce	11½ oz	7	280	23%
Stuffed Cabbage w/Meat in Tomato Sauce	10¾ oz	10	220	41%
Szechwan Beef w/Noodles & Vegetables	9.25 oz	10	260	35%
Tuna Lasagna w/Spinach Noodles & Vegetables	9¾ oz	10	270	33%
Turkey Dijon	9.5 oz	10	270	33%
Veal Primavera	9⅛ oz	9	250	32%
Vegetable & Pasta Mornay w/Ham	9⅜ oz	11	280	35%
Zucchini Lasagna	11 oz	7	260	24%
Lean Pockets (Chef America)/Frozen				
Beef & Broccoli	1 pocket	8	250	29%
Chicken Parmesan	1 pocket	6	250	22%
Chicken Supreme	1 pocket	4	210	17%
Pizza Deluxe	1 pocket	10	280	32%
(Lunch Bucket)/Light Balance Microwavable Meals				
Beef Americana	8.25 oz	3	190	14%
Beef & Pasta Bordeaux	8.25 oz	1	180	5%
Chicken Cacciatre	8.25 oz	1	210	4%
Chicken Fiesta	8.25 oz	4	210	17%
Pasta & Garden Vegetables	8.25 oz	1	170	5%
Mushroom Stroganoff	8.25 oz	6	190	28%
(Micro Magic)/Frozen Sandwiches				
Cheeseburger	4.75 oz	25	450	50%
Chicken	4.5 oz	16	390	37%
Hamburger	4 oz	18	350	46%
(Morton)/Frozen Dinners				
Beans & Frankfurters Dinner	10 oz	13	343	34%
Beef Meat Pie	7 oz	31	430	65%
Fish Dinner	10 oz	12	367	29%
Ham Dinner	10 oz	3	286	9%
Meatloaf Dinner	10 oz	17	306	50%
Salisbury Steak Dinner	10 oz	17	294	52%
Sliced Beef Dinner	10 oz	4	215	17%

Food and Description	Amount	Fat Grams	Total Calories	% Fat Calories
Spaghetti & Meatball Dinner	10 oz	2	198	9%
Turkey Dinner	10 oz	6	226	24%
Veal Parmigian Dinner	10 oz	8	252	29%
Western Dinner	10 oz	13	289	41%
New Traditions (Hormel)/Frozen Microwavable Sandwiches				
Bacon Cheeseburger	4.5 oz	20	390	46%
Cheeseburger	4.5 oz	19	380	45%
Chicken	4 oz	11	300	33%
Fish Fillet	4.9 oz	21	430	44%
(Pitaria) Pita Stuffs/Frozen				
Gyros	6 oz	29	520	50%
Ham'N Swiss	6 oz	17	420	36%
Pizza	6 oz	18	430	38%
Taco	6 oz	16	390	37%
(Prego)				
Beef Marsala w/noodles	11.3 oz	15	384	35%
(Schwan's)-Home Delivery - frozen				
BBQ Beef	3.5 oz	8	180	40%
BBQ Beef Brisket				
Chopped	3.5 oz	12	210	51%
Sliced	3.5 oz	5	150	30%
BBQ Ribs	3.5 oz	15	260	52%
Ball Tip Steaks	6 oz	10	240	38%
Beef Patties	4 oz	24	300	72%
Beef Patty Melt	4 oz	28	330	76%
Big Sam Steaks	6 oz	18	300	54%
Breaded Beef Steak Fingers	3.5 oz	7	220	29%
Chopped Beef Steak	5.33 oz	31	390	72%
Cross cut Tenderloin Steak	6 oz	41	500	74%
Floured Cubed Beef Steak	4 oz	20	290	62%
Haugin's Pride Dinner Steaks	7 oz	45	560	72%
Pizza Patties	3.5 oz	22	270	73%
Ribeye Steak	8 oz	64	730	79%
Sirloin Fillet of Beef Steak	4 oz	12	200	54%
Strip Steak				
Lean & fat	10 oz	65	790	74%
Lean only	10 oz	20	430	42%
(Schwan's), Home Delivery/Frozen Entrees & Sandwiches				
Bagel Dogs	4.5 oz	21	410	46%
Beef Casserole	3.5 oz	9	160	51%
Beef Lasagna	3.5 oz	6	150	34%
Beef Teriyaki	11 oz	14	430	29%
Beef Tortellini	3.5 oz	8	270	27%
Chese Tortellini	3.5 oz	5	220	21%

Food and Description	Amount	Fat Grams	Total Calories	% Fat Calories
Chicken 'ala Orange	9.5 oz	8	300	24%
Chicken Casserole	3.5 oz	8	150	48%
Chicken Oriental	10.25 oz	7	270	23%
Club Croissant Sandwich	1	22	400	50%
Grandma's Chicken Casserole	3.5 oz	9	160	51%
Jumbo Beef Ravioli	3.5 oz	4	180	20%
Macaroni & Cheese	3.5 oz	10	160	56%
Ranchero Sandwich	1	19	450	38%
Roast Beef & Swiss Croissant	1	20	370	49%
Round Cheese Ravioli	3.5 oz	8	200	36%
Shrimp Oriental	10 oz	3	190	14%
Sweet & Sour Chicken-bag	11 oz	15	530	26%
Sweet & Sour Chicken-plate	11 oz	15	420	32%
Vegetable Lasagna	3.5 oz	3	130	21%

(Stouffer's)/Frozen Entrees

Regular

Food and Description	Amount	Fat Grams	Total Calories	% Fat Calories
Bar B Que Style Chicken	10.5 oz	23	390	53%
Beef Chop Suey w/rice	12 oz	11	340	29%
Beef Fajitas	6⅞ oz	12	330	32%
Beef Pie	10 oz	32	500	58%
Beef Short Rib in Gravy	9 oz	20	350	51%
Beef Stroganoff w/Parsley Noodles	9.75 oz	20	390	46%
Beef Teriyaki in Sauce w/rice & vegetables	9.75 oz	8	290	25%
Cashew Chicken in Sauce w/rice	9.5 oz	16	380	38%
Chicken a la King w/rice	9.5 oz	9	290	28%
Chicken Chow Mein w/o noodles	8 oz	4	130	28%
Chicken Divan	8.5 oz	20	320	56%
Chicken Fajitas	7 oz	10	330	27%
Creamed Chicken	6.5 oz	21	300	63%
Creamed Chipped Beef	5.5 oz	16	230	63%
Escalloped Chicken & Noodles	10 oz	25	420	54%
Green Pepper Steak w/rice	10.5 oz	11	330	30%
Ham & Asparagus Bake	9.5 oz	35	510	62%
Homestyle Chicken & Noodles	10 oz	15	310	44%
Lasagna-21 oz	10.5 oz	13	360	33%
Lasagna, Single Serving	10.5 oz	13	360	33%
Lobster Newburg	6.5 oz	32	380	76%
Macaroni & Beef w/tomatoes-11.5 oz	5.75 oz	7	170	37%
Macaroni & Cheese-12 oz	6 oz	13	250	47%
Roast Beef Hash	10 oz	22	380	52%
Salisbury Steak in Gravy	9⅞ oz	14	250	50%
Southern Fried Chicken	10⅝ oz	23	450	46%
Spaghetti w/meatballs	12⅝ oz	15	380	36%

Food and Description	Amount	Fat Grams	Total Calories	% Fat Calories
Spaghetti w/meat sauce	12⅞ oz	11	370	27%
Stuffed Green Peppers w/beef in tomato sauce-15.5 oz	7.75 oz	9	200	41%
Sweedish Meatballs in Gravy w/parsley noodles	11 oz	26	480	49%
Tortellini				
Cheese in Alfredo Sauce	8⅞ oz	40	600	60%
Cheese w/tomato sauce	9⅝ oz	16	360	40%
Cheese w/vinaigrette dressing	6⅞ oz	27	400	61%
Veal in Alfredo Sauce	8⅝ oz	30	500	54%
Tuna Noodle Casserole	10 oz	13	310	38%
Turkey Casserole w/gravy & Dressing	9¾ oz	17	360	43%
Turkey Tetrazzini	10 oz	20	380	47%
Vegetable Lasagna	10.5 oz	24	420	51%
Welsh Rarebit-10 oz	5 oz	30	350	77%
Right Course				
Barbecue Chicken	7.5 oz	6	270	20%
Beef Dijon w/Pasta & Vegetables	9.5 oz	9	290	28%
Beef Ragout w/Rice Pilaf	10 oz	8	300	24%
Broiled Chicken Tenderloins w/vegetables & rice	9¼ oz	8	300	57%
Chicken Italiano	9⅝ oz	8	280	26%
Chicken Tenderloins in BBQ Sauce w/rice pilaf	8.75 oz	6	270	20%
Chicken Tenderloins in Peanut Sauce w/linguini & vegetables	9.25 oz	10	330	27%
Chicken Italiano w/Fettucini & Vegetables	9⅝ oz	8	280	26%
Fiesta Beef w/corn pasta	8⅞ oz	7	270	23%
Homestyle Pot Roast	9.25 oz	7	220	29%
Sesame Chicken	10 oz	9	320	25%
Sliced Turkey in a Mild Curry Sauce w/rice pilaf	8.75 oz	8	320	23%
Shrimp Primavera	9⅝ oz	7	240	26%
Vegetarian Chili	1 serving	7	240	26%
Side Dishes				
Corn Souffle-12 oz	4 oz	7	160	39%
Creamed Spinach-9 oz	4.5 oz	14	170	74%
Escalloped Apples-12 oz	4 oz	2	130	14%
Fettucini Alfredo-10 oz	5 oz	19	270	63%
Green Bean Mushroom Casserole-9.5 oz	4.75 oz	11	160	62%

Food and Description	Amount	Fat Grams	Total Calories	% Fat Calories
Noodles Romanoff-12 oz	4 oz	9	170	48%
Pasta Carbonara	9¾ oz	45	620	65%
Pasta Casino	9¼ oz	10	300	30%
Pasta Oriental	9⅞ oz	14	300	42%
Pasta Primavera-10-5/8 oz	~ 5.25 oz	21	270	70%
Potatoes au Gratin-11.5 oz	~ 4 oz	6	110	49%
Scalloped Potatoes-11.5 oz	~ 4 oz	4	90	40%
Spinach Soufle-12 oz	4 oz	9	140	58%
(Swanson)/Frozen				
Chicken Duet Gourmet Nuggets				
Ham & Cheese	2.70 oz	12	190	57%
Mexican Style	2.70 oz	12	200	54%
Pizza Style	2.70 oz	11	190	52%
Salisbury Steak	10.75 oz	18	410	40%
Spinach & Herb	2.70 oz	12	200	54%
Budget Dinners				
Beans & Franks	10.5 oz	19	440	39%
Fried Chicken	7.25 oz	24	470	46%
Macaroni & Beef	12 oz	15	380	36%
Macaroni & Cheese	12.25 oz	15	370	36%
Spaghetti & Meatballs	12.5 oz	15	370	36%
Dinners-3 Compartment				
Beans & Franks	10.5 oz	20	440	41%
Fried Chicken Platter edible portion	7.75 oz	16	340	42%
Macaroni & Beef	12 oz	15	370	37%
Macaroni and Cheese	12.25 oz	15	380	36%
Noodles and Chicken	10.5 oz	9	260	31%
Spaghetti & Meatballs	12.5 oz	16	370	39%
Dinners-4 Compartment				
Beef	11.25 oz	8	340	21%
Beef in Barbecue Sauce	11 oz	15	460	29%
Chicken in Barbecue Sauce	11.75 oz	13	460	25%
Chicken Nuggets	8.75 oz	25	460	49%
Chopped Sirloin Beef	11 oz	19	370	46%
Fish'n'Chips	10 oz	20	500	36%
Fish Nuggest	9.5 oz	19	410	42%
Fried Chicken, BBQ flavored edible portion	10 oz	21	520	36%
Fried Chicken, White Meat edible portion	10.25 oz	25	560	40%
Fried Chicken, Dark Meat edible portion	9.75 oz	28	560	45%
Loin of Pork	10.75 oz	12	310	35%
Meatloaf	10.75 oz	22	430	46%

Food and Description	Amount	Fat Grams	Total Calories	% Fat Calories
Salisbury Steak	10.75 oz	18	410	40%
Sweet'n Sour Chicken	12 oz	11	380	26%
Swiss Steak	10 oz	11	340	29%
Turkey	11.5 oz	11	350	28%
Veal Parmigiana	12.25 oz	22	450	44%
Western Style	11.5 oz	21	450	42%
Entrees				
Chicken Duet Entrees				
Creamy Broccoli	6 oz	19	320	53%
Creamy Green Bean	6 oz	19	330	52%
Saucy Tomato	6 oz	18	340	48%
Savory Wild Rice	6 oz	20	330	55%
Homestyle Recipe				
Cheese Ravioli	8.75 oz	9	250	32%
Chicken & Noodles	9 oz	16	400	36%
Chicken Cacciatore	11 oz	8	260	28%
Chicken Nibbles edible portion	4.25 oz	24	340	64%
Fish N Chips	6.5 oz	18	370	44%
Fish'n'Fries	6.5 oz	17	350	44%
Fried Chicken edible portion	7 oz	21	380	50%
Lasagna w/meat sauce	10.5 oz	16	400	36%
Macaroni & Cheese	10 oz	21	400	47%
Salisbury Steak	10 oz	34	480	64%
Scalloped Potatoes & Ham	9 oz	16	340	42%
Sirloin Tips in Burgandy Sauce	7 oz	10	270	33%
Spaghetti w/Italian Style Meatballs	13 oz	19	460	37%
Sweedish Meatballs	8.5 oz	22	350	57%
Tuna Noodle Casserole	9 oz	11	250	40%
Turkey w/Dressing & Potatoes	9 oz	13	290	40%
Veal Parmigiana	10 oz	13	330	36%
Hungry Man Dinners				
Boneless Chicken	17.75 oz	28	700	36%
Chopped Beef Steak	16.75 oz	37	640	52%
Fried Chicken, White Meat edible portion	14.25 oz	46	870	48%
Fried Chicken-Dark Meat edible portion	14.25 oz	45	860	47%
Salisbury Steak	18.25 oz	41	680	54%
Sliced Beef	15.25 oz	12	450	24%
Turkey	17 oz	18	550	30%
Veal Parmigiana	18.25 oz	23	560	37%
(Tyson)/Frozen				
Gourmet Entrees				
Beef Champignon	10.5 oz	15	370	37%

Food and Description	Amount	Fat Grams	Total Calories	% Fat Calories
Chicken & Beef Luau	10.5 oz	10	330	27%
Lasagna	11.5 oz	14	380	33%
Pasta Trio	11 oz	16	420	34%
Pepper Steak	11 oz	11	330	30%
Salisbury Supreme	10 oz	26	430	54%
Short Ribs	11 oz	24	470	46%
Looney Tunes				
Bugs Bunny Chicken Chunks	1 serving	14	340	37%
Daffy Duck Spaghetti & Meatballs	1 serving	10	320	28%
Road Runner Chicken Sandwich	1 serving	11	320	31%
Speedy Gonzales Beef Enchilada	1 serving	16	400	36%
Sylvester Fish Sandwich	1 serving	11	270	37%
Tweety Macaroni & Cheese	1 serving	8	280	26%
Yosemite Sam BBQ Glazed Chicken	1 serving	21	420	45%
Wile E Coyote Hamburger Pizza	1 serving	12	300	36%
(Ultra Slim Fast)/Frozen Entrees				
Chicken & Vegetables	12 oz	3	310	9%
Chicken Fettuccine	12 oz	10	400	23%
Mesquite Chicken	12 oz	1	360	3%
Pasta Primavera	12 oz	9	340	24%
Roasted Chicken w/mushrooms	12 oz	5	300	15%
Shrimp Marinara	12 oz	3	290	9%
Shrimp Creole	12 oz	4	240	15%
Spaghetti w/beef & mushrooms	12 oz	9	370	22%
Sweet & Sour Chicken	12 oz	2	330	5%
Turkey Medallions	12 oz	5	320	14%
(Weight Watchers)/Frozen Entrees				
Baked Cheese Ravioli	9 oz	12	290	37%
Beef Salisbury Steak Romana	8.75 oz	13	310	38%
Beef Sirloin Tips & Mushrooms in Wine Sauce	7.5 oz	8	250	29%
Beef Steak Chopped	9 oz	17	280	55%
Breaded Chicken Cordon Bleu	8 oz	11	230	43%
Broccoli & Cheese Baked Potato	10.5 oz	7	250	25%
Cheese Manicotti	9.25 oz	13	300	39%
Chicken Divan Baked Potato	11 oz	4	270	13%
Chicken Patty Parmigiana	8.06 oz	16	280	51%
Fillet of Fish Au Gratin	9.25 oz	6	200	27%
Garden Lasagna	11 oz	12	330	33%
Imperial Chicken	9.25 oz	4	230	16%
Italian Cheese Lasagna	12 oz	14	380	33%
Lasagna w/Meat Sauce	11 oz	11	330	30%
London Broil in Mushroom Sauce	7.37 oz	3	140	19%
Oven-Fried Fish	6.81 oz	13	300	39%

Food and Description	Amount	Fat Grams	Total Calories	% Fat Calories
Pasta Primavera	8.5 oz	11	260	38%
Pasta Rigati	11 oz	9	290	28%
Seafood Linguini	9 oz	7	210	30%
Southern Fried Chicken Patty	6.5 oz	16	340	42%
Spaghetti w/meat sauce	10.5 oz	7	280	23%
Stuffed Sole w/Newburg Sauce	10.5 oz	9	310	26%
Sweet'N Sour Chicken Tenders	10.19 oz	1	240	4%
FRUIT (*See* individual listings)				
FRUIT BITS/dried				
(Sun Maid)	2 oz	.5	160	3%
FRUIT COCKTAIL				
canned				
in water	½ cup	–	40	–
in juice	½ cup	–	56	–
in heavy syrup	½ cup	–	93	–
in extra hvy syrup	½ cup	–	115	–
(Del Monte)	½ cup	–	80	–
Lite	½ cup	–	50	–
(Nutradiet)	½ cup	–	40	–
(S&W)				
Heavy syrup	½ cup	–	90	–
Natural style	½ cup	–	90	
FRUIT CUP				
(Hunt's) Snack Pack	5 oz	< 1	120	4%
FRUIT DRINK				
Caribbean Cooler				
Crystal Light Powder	8 oz	–	3	–
Citrus Blend (Crystal Light)mix-diet	8 oz	–	4	–
Citrus Fruit Juice Drink	8 oz	–	113	–
Fruit Juicy Red (Hawaiian Punch)	8 oz	–	90	–
Lite	8 oz	–	60	–
Fruit Medley (Libby's)	8 oz	–	80	–
Island Fruit Cocktail				
(Hawaiian Punch)	6 oz	–	90	–
Juice Medley	6 oz	–	80	–
Kool-Aid Flavored Drinks				
all flavors	8 oz	–	2	–
with sugar added	8 oz	–	100	–
pre-sweetened	8 oz	–	80	–
sugar-free	8 oz	–	4	–
FRUIT ICES				
Berry Blend Pops-(Crystal Light)	1	–	14	–
Chilly Things-Light/all flavors	1	–	12	–
(Eskimo) Rainbow Twin Pops	1	–	60	–

Food and Description	Amount	Fat Grams	Total Calories	% Fat Calories
Fresh Lites (Dole)				
Cherry	1	–	25	–
Lemon	1	–	25	–
Pineapple Orange	1	–	25	–
Raspberry	1	–	25	–
Frozfruit-On A Stick-all flavors	1	–	70	–
Fruit And Cream Bars (Dole)				
Blueberry	1 bar	1	90	10%
Chocolate/Banana	1 bar	9	175	46%
Chocolate/Strawberry	1 bar	8	140	51%
Peach	1 bar	1	90	10%
Raspberry	1 bar	1	90	10%
Strawberry	1 bar	1	90	10%
Fruit And Yogurt Bars (Dole)				
Cherry	1 bar	.5	80	6%
Raspberry	1 bar	.5	70	6%
Strawberry	1 bar	.5	70	6%
Fruit Bars-(Jell-O)				
all flavors-averaged data	1 bar	–	45	–
Fruit Ice-(Haagan Dazs)				
Boysenberry	½ cup	–	90	–
Lemon	½ cup	–	140	–
Lime	½ cup	–	123	–
Orange	½ cup	–	140	–
Raspberry	½ cup	–	100	–
Fruit Juice Bars (Minute Maid)				
cherry	1 bar	–	60	–
fruit punch	1 bar	–	60	–
grape	1 bar	–	60	–
orange	1 bar	–	60	–
strawberry	1 bar	–	60	–
Fruit Juice Bars (Welch's)				
Grape	1 bar	–	45	–
Raspberry	1 bar	–	45	–
Strawberry	1 bar	–	45	–
no sugar added				
Grape	1 bar	–	25	–
Raspberry	1 bar	–	25	–
Strawberry	1 bar	–	25	–
Fruit'N Juice Bars (Dole)				
Pina Colada	1 bar	3	90	30%
Pineapple	1 bar	< 1	70	6%
Raspberry	1 bar	< 1	70	6%
Strawberry	1 bar	< 1	70	6%

Food and Description	Amount	Fat Grams	Total Calories	% Fat Calories
Fruit Punch Pops-(Crystal Light)	1 bar	–	14	–
Fruit Slush (Wyler's)-Freeze & Eat				
Cherry	4 oz	–	157	–
Fruit Punch	4 oz	–	157	–
Grape	4 oz	–	157	–
Orange	4 oz	–	157	–
Pink Lemonade	4 oz	–	157	–
Strawberry	4 oz	–	157	–
Tropical Punch Fruit	4 oz	–	157	–
Fruit Sorbet (Dole)				
Peach	4 oz	< 1	110	4%
Pineapple	4 oz	< 1	100	5%
Strawberry	4 oz	< 1	120	4%
Gelatin Pops-(Jell-O)				
all flavors-averaged data	1 bar	–	35	–
(Good Humor)				
Calippo				
Cherry	1 bar	–	140	–
Lemon	1 bar	–	112	–
Orange	1 bar	–	110	–
Cherry Italian Ice	1 bar	–	138	–
Cool Shark Bar	1 bar	–	70	–
Ice Stripes				
Cherry/orange	1 bar	–	35	–
Grape/Lemon	1 bar	–	35	–
Jumbo Jet Star	1 bar	–	85	5%
Strawberry Finger	1 bar	–	50	–
Stripes	1 bar	–	35	–
(Koolaid) Kool-pops/all flavors	1 bar	–	40	–
Life Saver Pops-(Nabisco)				
all flavors	1 bar	–	40	–
(Natural Nectar)-Tropical Delight	1 bar	–	63	–
Wildberry Fruit'N Cream	1 bar	–	93	5%
Pink Lemonade Pops-(Crystal Light)	1 bar	–	13	–
(Popsicle) Ice Pops				
sugar-free/all flavors	1 bar	–	18	–
regular/all flavors	1 bar	–	50	–
Snowburst (Jell-O)				
Lemon	1 bar	–	45	–
Sorbet-(Dole)				
Mandarin Orange	4 oz	–	110	–
Peach	4 oz	–	120	–
Pineapple	4 oz	–	120	–
Raspberry	4 oz	–	110	–

Food and Description	Amount	Fat Grams	Total Calories	% Fat Calories
Strawberry	4 oz	–	110	–
Spot Pops				
Diet 7-up	1 pop	–	15	–
Diet Cherry 7-up	1 pop	–	15	–
(Sunkist)				
Coconut Bar	4 oz	8	138	52%
Lemonade Bar	4 oz	–	68	–
Orange Juice Bar	4 oz	–	72	–
Orange & Cream	4 oz	.5	84	16%
Wild Berry Fruit & Juice	4 oz	.5	103	4%
SunTops-(Dole)				
Fruit Punch	1 bar	–	40	–
Grape	1 bar	–	40	–
Lemonade	1 bar	–	40	–
Tropical Orange	1 bar	–	40	–
(Trix) Pops/all flavors	1 bar	–	40	–
FRUIT JUICE				
Juicy Juice (Libby's)	6 oz	–	100	–
Paradise Punch/from frozen conc.	8 oz	1	100	9%
Tropical-Juicy Juice (Libby's)	6 oz	–	100	–
Tropical Nectar (Kern's)	6 oz	–	112	–
Tropical Squeeze (Chiquita)	6 oz	< 1	90	5%
FRUIT MEDLEY				
(Mariani)				
dried	¼ cup	1	150	5%
dried Tropical	1 oz	1	90	10%
FRUIT, MIXED				
canned heavy syrup	1 cup	–	184	–
(Del Monte)				
chunky	½ cup	–	80	–
chunky lite	½ cup	–	50	–
cup	5 oz	–	100	–
(Nutradiet) natural in water	½ cup	–	40	–
(S&W) natural style juice	½ cup	–	90	–
dried	4 oz	.6	278	2%
(Del Monte)	2 oz	–	130	–
(Mariani) Fancy	¼ cup	–	140	–
frozen				
sweetened	1 cup	.5	245	2%
unsweetened	3.5 oz	< 1	45	10%
frozen syrup (Birds Eye)	5 oz	–	120	–
FRUIT'N NUT MIX (Planters)	1 oz	9	150	54%
FRUIT PECTIN				
Certo	1 Tbs	–	2	–

Food and Description	Amount	Fat Grams	Total Calories	% Fat Calories
Sure Jell				
light	¼ pkg	–	36	–
sweetened	¼ pkg	–	40	–
FRUIT PUNCH				
canned	6 oz	–	87	–
(Bama)	8.45 oz	–	130	–
(Crystal Light)-mix-diet	8 oz	–	4	–
(Kern's) Islander Punch	8 oz	–	120	–
(Mott's)	10 oz	–	170	–
	9.5 oz	–	150	–
concentrate (Hawaiian Punch)	6 oz	–	90	–
drink powder				
(Crystal Light) Paradise Punch	8 oz	–	3	–
(Tropicana)				
2 round tsp	8 oz	–	97	–
single serve	10 oz	–	148	–
frozen concentrate	8 oz	–	113	–
fruit punch juice drink	6 oz	–	123	–
gelatin drinking powder				
1 packet +water	4 oz	–	67	–
(Knox)-with Nutrasweet	1 env.	–	39	–
mix (Wyler's)				
all flavors w/sugar	8 oz	–	90	–
w/o sugar	8 oz	–	2	–
Mountain Berry Punch	8.45 oz	–	140	
Rainbow Punch (Mountain Berry)	8.45 oz	–	130	–
Tropical Punch(Mountain Berry)	8.45 oz	–	130	–
Red-Squeezit (Betty Crocker)	6.75 oz	–	110	–
FRUIT SALAD				
canned				
in water	½ cup	< 1	37	12%
in juice	½ cup	< 1	62	7%
in heavy syrup	½ cup	< 1	94	15%
in xtra hvy syrup	½ cup	< 1	114	4%
canned				
(Del Monte)	½ cup	–	90	–
(Kraft)	½ cup	–	50	–
tropical				
canned hvy syrup	½ cup	–	110	–
(Del Monte)	½ cup	–	90	–
FRUIT SNACKS				
Candied Fruit (*See* individual fruit listings)				
(Estee)-Tropi Mix-assorted				
sugar-free	2 pieces	–	25	–

Food and Description	Amount	Fat Grams	Total Calories	% Fat Calories
(Featherweight)-Sweet Pretenders				
Berry Patch Blend	1 piece	–	12	–
Orange Blend	1 piece	–	12	–
Tropical Blend	1 piece	–	12	–
Flippits (Sunkist)-chocolate covered fruit				
snacks/all flavors	1 pouch	4	110	33%
Fruit & Nut Mix (Estee)	4 pieces	2	35	51%
Fruit Bears (Flavor Tree)				
assorted	1.05 oz	1.6	117	12%
Fruit Circus (Flavor Tree)				
assorted	1.05 oz	1.6	117	12%
(Fruit Corners)				
Berry Bears				
Assorted Fruit	1 pouch	.5	100	5%
Fruit Punch	1 pouch	.5	100	5%
Shark Bites				
Assorted Fruit	1 pouch	.5	100	5%
Fruit Punch	1 pouch	.5	100	5%
Fruit Nibbles				
Assorted	1.05 oz	2	120	15%
Cherry & Yogurt	1.05 oz	4	130	28%
Orange	1.05 oz	4	130	28%
Strawberry	1.05 oz	5	140	32%
Fruit Roll (Flavor Tree)				
Apple	1 roll	–	80	–
Apricot	1 roll	.5	80	6%
Cherry	1 roll	–	80	–
Fruit Punch	1 roll	–	70	–
Grape	1 roll	–	80	–
Raspberry	1 roll	–	80	–
Strawberry	1 roll	–	80	–
(Fruit Roll-Ups)-all flavors	1 roll	.5	50	9%
Peel-Outs-all flavors	1 roll	.5	50	9%
(Fruit Wrinkles)-all flavors	1 pouch	1	100	9%
Fun Fruits-(Sunkist)				
all shapes/all flavors	1 pouch	1	100	9%
Fun Fruits-(Sunkist)-Creme Supremes-				
Strawberry/yogurt covered	.9 oz	3.6	114	28%
(Nintendo)				
Link	1 pouch	–	100	–
Super Mario Bros	1 pouch	–	100	–
(Squeezit)				
apple, orange,				
red punch, wild berry	6.75 oz	.5	110	4%

Food and Description	Amount	Fat Grams	Total Calories	% Fat Calories
cherry, grape (higher sodium)	6.75 oz	.5	110	4%
Sierra Trail Mix (Del Monte)	.9	7	130	49%
2-T Fruit (Sunkist)/all flavors	1 pouch	1	90	10%
Tropical Fruit Punch (Del Monte)	.9 oz	1	90	10%
(Weight Watchers)-fruit snacks				
apple	½ oz	.5	50	9%
cinnamon	.5	.5	50	9%
peach	.5	.5	50	9%
strawberry	.5	.5	50	9%
Yogurt Raisins (Del Monte)	.9 oz	5	120	38%
FRUIT SQUARES				
frozen (Pepperidge Farm)				
Apple	1	12	220	49%
Blueberry	1	11	220	45%
Cherry	1	12	230	47%

G

Food and Description	Amount	Fat Grams	Total Calories	% Fat Calories
GARBANZO BEAN (*See* CHICKPEA)				
GARLIC/raw, minced	1 clove	–	4	–
GARLIC CLOVE/raw	1 clove	–	5	–
GARLIC POWDER	1 tsp	–	9	–
GAZPACHO (*See* SOUP)				
GEFILTE FISH				
commercial				
sweet	1 piece			
	~ 1.5 oz	.7	35	18%
(Manischewitz)				
homestyle	3.5 oz	3.89	111	32%
sweet	3.5 oz	4	132	27%
(Mother's) Old Fashioned				
sweetened	1 fishball	1	70	13%
w/o sugar	1 fishball	1	54	17%
(Rokeach)				
with Natural Broth	2 oz	1	46	20%
Old Vienna	2.6 oz	2	68	27%
GELATIN				
Dry	1 pkt	–	23	–

Food and Description	Amount	Fat Grams	Total Calories	% Fat Calories
Mix				
(D-Zerta) Low-Calorie/all flavors				
averaged data	½ cup	–	8	–
(Estee) Low-Cal Gelatin Desserts	½ cup	–	8	–
(Jell-O)/1-2-3				
Cherry	⅔ cup	2	130	14%
Orange	⅔ cup	2	130	14%
Strawberry	⅔ cup	2	130	14%
Triple Fruit Rainbow	⅔ cup	2	130	14%
(Jell-O)/regular				
Apricot	½ cup	–	80	–
Black Cherry	½ cup	–	80	–
Black Raspberry	½ cup	–	80	–
Blackberry	½ cup	–	80	–
Cherry	½ cup	–	80	–
Concord Grape	½ cup	–	80	–
Lemon	½ cup	–	80	–
Lime	½ cup	–	80	–
Mixed Fruit	½ cup	–	80	–
Orange	½ cup	–	80	–
Orange Pineapple	½ cup	–	80	–
Peach	½ cup	–	80	–
Raspberry	½ cup	–	80	–
Strawberry	½ cup	–	80	–
Strawberry Banana	½ cup	–	80	–
Wild Strawberry	½ cup	–	80	–
(Jell-O)/sugar-free				
Hawaiian Pineapple	½ cup	–	8	–
Lemon	½ cup	–	8	–
Lime	½ cup	–	8	–
Mixed Fruit	½ cup	–	8	–
Orange	½ cup	–	8	–
Peach	½ cup	–	8	–
Raspberry	½ cup	–	8	–
Strawberry	½ cup	–	8	–
Strawberry Banana	½ cup	–	8	–
Triple Berry	½ cup	–	8	–
(Jell-O)/unflavored	½ cup	–	6	–
(Jell-Well)/regular				
Cherry	½ cup	–	80	–
Lemon	½ cup	–	80	–
Lime	½ cup	–	80	–
Mixed Fruit	½ cup	–	80	–
Orange	½ cup	–	80	–

Food and Description	Amount	Fat Grams	Total Calories	% Fat Calories
Raspberry	½ cup	–	80	–
Strawberry	½ cup	–	80	–
Strawberry Banana	½ cup	–	80	–
(Jell-Well)/sugar-free				
Orange	½ cup	–	8	–
Raspberry	½ cup	–	8	–
Strawberry	½ cup	–	8	–
Strawberry Banana	½ cup	–	8	–
(Royal)/regular				
Apple	½ cup	–	80	–
Blackberry	½ cup	–	80	–
Cherry	½ cup	–	80	–
Concord Grape	½ cup	–	80	–
Lemon	½ cup	–	80	–
Lemon-Lime	½ cup	–	80	–
Lime	½ cup	–	80	–
Mixed Berry	½ cup	–	80	–
Orange	½ cup	–	80	–
Peach	½ cup	–	80	–
Pineapple	½ cup	–	80	–
Raspberry	½ cup	–	80	–
Strawberry	½ cup	–	80	–
Strawberry Banana	½ cup	–	80	–
Tropical Fruit	½ cup	–	80	–
(Royal)/sugar-free				
Cherry	½ cup	–	6	–
Lime	½ cup	–	6	–
Orange	½ cup	–	6	–
Raspberry	½ cup	–	6	–
Strawberry	½ cup	–	6	–
GIN (See DISTILLED LIQUOR)				
GINGER/ground	1 tsp	–	6	–
GINGER ROOT/raw	¼ cup	–	17	–
	5 Slices	–	8	–
GINKGO				
canned	1 oz	.5	32	14%
dried	1 oz	.57	99	5%
raw	1 oz	–	52	–
GOAT/raw-boneless	1 oz	6.6	177	34%
GOOSE/domestic				
meat & skin-roasted	~ 2 lb	69.69	2362	65%
meat only-roasted	1¼ lb	74.86	1406	48%
Goose Gizzard/raw	3 o	4.5	119	34%

Food and Description	Amount	Fat Grams	Total Calories	% Fat Calories
Goose Liver				
pate-smoked, canned	1 oz	12	131	82%
raw	3 oz	3.6	114	28%
GOOSEBERRY				
canned in light syrup	½ cup	–	93	–
raw	1 cup	.87	67	12%
GRANDILLA (*See* PASSION FRUIT)				
GRANOLA (*See also* CEREAL)				
GRANOLA BARS				
Health Valley				
apple bake	2 bars	4	150	24%
date bake	2 bars	4	160	23%
raisin bake	2 bars	4	150	24%
Jack LaLane-Chewey Fruit & Nut				
apple nut	1 bar	2	90	20%
banana nut	1 bar	2	90	20%
date nut	1 bar	2	90	20%
orange nut	1 bar	3	100	27%
Kudos				
butter almond	1 bar	10	180	50%
chocolate chip	1 bar	10	180	50%
cookies & creme	1 bar	10	180	50%
crunchy nut	1 bar	11	180	55%
nutty fudge	1 bar	12	200	54%
peanut butter	1 bar	12	190	57%
raisin	1 bar	9	170	48%
Nature Valley				
almond	1 bar	5	120	38%
chocolate chip	1 bar	4	110	33%
cinnamon	1 bar	5	120	38%
oat bran	1 bar	4	110	33%
oats & honey	1 bar	5	120	38%
peanut	1 bar	5	120	38%
peanut butter	1 bar	6	120	45%
Nature's Choice				
carob chip	1 bar	3	90	30%
cinnamon & raisin	1 bar	3	90	30%
oats & honey	1 bar	3	90	30%
peanut butter	1 bar	4	90	40%
New Trail-Chocolate Covered				
chocolate chip	1 bar	11	200	50%
cocoa creme	1 bar	9	190	43%
cookies & creme	1 bar	11	200	50%
peanut butter	1 bar	11	200	50%

Food and Description	Amount	Fat Grams	Total Calories	% Fat Calories
Quaker				
Chewy				
apple	1 bar	3	120	23%
chocolate chip	1 bar	5	130	35%
choc graham marshmallow	1 bar	4	126	29%
chunky nut	1 bar	6	130	42%
honey & oats	1 bar	4	125	29%
nut & raisin	1 bar	6	130	42%
peanut butter	1 bar	4	120	30%
peanut butter choc chip	1 bar	6	130	42%
raisin cinnamon	1 bar	5	128	35%
s'mores	1 bar	4	130	28%
strawberry	1 bar	3	120	23%
Dipps				
caramel nut	1 bar	6	150	36%
chocolate chip	1 bar	6	140	39%
chocolate fudge	1 bar	8	160	45%
peanut butter	1 bar	9	170	48%
peanut butter choc chip	1 bar	10	170	53%
Fudge Dipped Chewy				
chocolate chip	1.63 oz bar	11	220	45%
oats & honey	1.38 oz bar	10	190	47%
w/peanuts	1.38 oz bar	12	200	54%
	2.25 oz bar	18	300	54%
w/raisins	1.5 oz bar	12	200	54%
Sunbelt/Chewy				
chocolate chip	1.25 oz bar	7	150	42%
	1.75 oz bar	9	220	37%
oats & honey	1 oz bar	5	130	35%
w/almonds	1 oz bar	6	120	45%
w/raisins	1.25 oz bar	6	150	36%
GRAPE				
Concord				
fresh	½ cup	.75	33	21%
(S&W)				
heavy syrup	½ cup	–	100	–
Thompson				
seedless-fresh	½ cup	–	48	–
canned in heavy syrup	½ cup	–	94	–
GRAPE-APPLE DRINK (Mott's)	10 oz	–	167	–
	9.5 oz	–	158	–
GRAPE-CRANBERRY JUICE COCKTAIL				
(Seneca)	6 oz	–	110	–

Food and Description	Amount	Fat Grams	Total Calories	% Fat Calories
GRAPE DRINK				
Grape Drink				
(Bama)	8.45 oz	–	120	–
(Hawaiian Punch)	6 oz	–	90	–
(Juice Works)	6 oz	–	98	–
(Kool-Aid Kooler)	8.45 oz	–	140	–
(Tang) Fruit Box	8.45 oz	–	130	–
Grape Juice Drink/canned	6 oz	–	94	–
Grape Medley (Libby's)	6 oz	–	90	–
Grape-Squeezit (Betty Crocker)	6.75 oz	–	110	–
GRAPE JUICE				
Grape, Concord (S&W)-unsweetened	6 oz	–	100	–
Grape/from frozen concentrate	8 oz	–	128	–
frozen-undiluted	6 oz	–	385	–
Grape-Juicy Juice (Libby's)	6 oz	–	100	–
Grape, Purple				
bottled	6 oz	–	120	–
frozen				
(Birds Eye)	6 oz	–	90	–
(Seneca)	6 oz	–	115	–
(Welch's)	6 oz	–	100	–
Juice Bowl-Grape (Campbell's)	6 oz	–	110	–
(Kraft) Pure 100%	6 oz	–	104	–
(Seneca)-Natural	6 oz	–	100	–
(Sippin' Pak) from concentrate	8.45 oz	–	130	–
(Sunglo)	8.45 oz	–	169	–
(Tree Top)	6 oz	–	120	–
(Welch's)	6 oz	–	120	–
Grape, Red (Welch's)-sparkling	6 oz	–	128	–
Grape, White/bottled	6 oz	–	110	–
(Welch's)	6 oz	–	120	–
sparkling	6 oz	–	120	–
GRAPEFRUIT				
Pink, White, & Red	½ fruit	–	38	–
canned				
in water	½ cup	–	44	–
in juice	½ cup	–	46	–
in light syrup	½ cup	–	76	–
sections				
(Kraft)	½ cup	–	50	–
(Nutradiet)	½ cup	–	40	–
(S&W)				
light syrup	½ cup	–	80	–
natural	½ cup	–	40	–

Food and Description	Amount	Fat Grams	Total Calories	% Fat Calories
GRAPEFRUIT DRINK				
Pink Grapefruit Drink				
(Tropicana) Twister	8 oz	–	112	–
GRAPEFRUIT JUICE				
canned	8 oz	–	93	–
canned-sweetened	8 oz	–	116	–
canned-unsweetened	8 oz	–	95	–
(Del Monte)	6 oz	–	70	–
(S&W)	6 oz	–	80	–
from frozen concentrate	8 oz	–	102	–
frozen (Birds Eye)	6 oz	–	70	–
Juice Bowl (Campbell's)	6 oz	–	80	–
(Kraft) Pure 100%	6 oz	–	70	–
(Libby's)	6 oz	–	70	–
(Mott's) unsweetened	10 oz	–	124	–
(Sunglo)	8.45 oz	–	94	–
(Sunkist)-fresh squeezed	8 oz	–	96	–
	6 oz	–	56	–
(Tropicana)	8 oz	–	101	–
fresh	8 oz	–	96	–
white grapefruit (Ocean Spray)	6 oz	–	70	–
GRAPEFRUIT JUICE COCKTAIL				
Pink Grapefruit Juice Cocktail				
(Minute Maid)	6 oz	–	80	–
(Ocean Spray)	6 oz	–	80	–
GRAPEFRUIT-ORANGE JUICE				
canned				
sweetened	8 oz	–	125	–
unsweetened	8 oz	–	108	–
frozen	8 oz	–	110	–
GRAPEFRUIT PEEL				
candied	1 oz	–	90	–
GRAVY (*See also* SAUCE)				
canned & jars				
Au jus	1 cup	.5	38	12%
	1 can	.6	201	3%
(Franco-American)	2 oz	–	10	–
(Heinz)	2 oz	–	10	–
Beef	1 cup	5.5	124	40%
	1 can	6.8	156	39%
Brown	4 oz	6	94	57%
(Franco-American)	2 oz	1	25	36%
with onions				
(Franco-American)	4 oz	1	25	36%

Food and Description	Amount	Fat Grams	Total Calories	% Fat Calories
(Heinz)	2 oz	1	25	36%
Chicken	1 cup	13.6	189	65%
	1 can	17	236	65%
(Franco-American)	2 oz	4	45	80%
(Heinz)	2 oz	1	25	36%
Chicken Giblet				
(Franco-American)	2 oz	2	30	60%
Mushroom	1 cup	6.5	120	49%
	1 can	8	150	48%
(Franco-American)	2 oz	1	25	36%
(Heinz)	2 oz	–	16	–
Pork	4 oz	5	76	59%
(Franco American)	2 oz	3	40	68%
(Heinz)	2 oz	–	18	–
Turkey	1 cup	5	122	37%
	1 can	6	152	36%
(Franco American)	2 oz	2	30	60%
(Heinz)	2 oz	1	25	36%
homestyle	4 oz	4	58	62%
GRAVY/DEHYDRATED: Prepared as directed.				
Au jus	1 cup	.8	19	38%
(Durkee)	2 cups	–	62	–
Roastin' Bag w/gravy	1 pkg	1	64	14%
(French's)	¼ cup	–	10	–
(Knorr)	1 oz	< 1	4	75%
Beef	1 cup	–	9	–
Brown	1 cup	–	9	–
(Durkee)	1 cup	–	59	–
(Estee)	¼ cup	–	14	–
(French's)	¼ cup	1	20	45%
(McCormick/Schilling)	¼ cup	.8	23	31%
(Pillsbury)	¼ cup	–	15	–
Brown w/Mushrooms				
(Durkee)	1 cup	.5	59	8%
Brown w/Onions				
(Durkee)	1 cup	.5	66	7%
Chicken	1 cup	1.9	83	21%
(Durkee)	1 cup	1	92	10%
Roastin' Bag w/gravy	1 pkg	1	122	7%
(French's)	¼ cup	1	25	36%
(McCormick/Schilling)	¼ cup	< 1	22	20%
(Pillsbury)	¼ cup	1	25	36%
Chicken & Herb				
(Estee)	¼ cup	–	20	–

Food and Description	Amount	Fat Grams	Total Calories	% Fat Calories
Chicken, Creamy				
(Durkee)	1 cup	9	156	52%
Roastin' Bag w/gravy	1 pkg	12	242	45%
Chicken-Italian Style				
(Durkee)				
Roastin'Bag w/gravy	1 pkg	1	144	6%
Homestyle				
(Durkee)	1 cup	2	70	26%
(French's)	¼ cup	1	20	45%
(Pillsbury)	¼ cup	–	15	–
(La Loma)				
Quik-Brown	1 pkt	2	88	21%
Chicken	1 pkt	2	88	21%
Country	1 pkt	2	88	21%
Mushroom	1 pkt	2	88	21%
Onion	1 pkt	2	90	29%
Mushroom	1 cup	.9	70	12%
(Durkee)	1 cup	1	60	15%
(French's)	¼ cup	1	20	45%
(McCormick/Schilling)	¼ cup	.5	19	24%
Onion/(contains beef fat and coconut oil)	1 cup	.7	80	8%
(Durkee)	1 cup	.5	84	5%
(French's)	¼ cup	1	25	36%
(McCormick/Schilling)	¼ cup	.6	22	25%
Onion Pot Roast				
(Durkee)				
Roastin' Bag w/gravy	1 pkg	–	124	–
Pork	1 cup	1.9	76	23%
(Durkee)	1 cup	.5	70	6%
Roastin' Bag w/gravy	1 pkg	1	130	7%
(French's)	¼ cup	1	20	45%
Pot Roast& Stew				
(Durkee)				
Roastin'Bag w/gravy	1 pkg	1	125	7%
Swiss Steak				
(Durkee)	1½ cups	–	68	–
Roastin' Bag w/gravy	1 pkg	.9	115	7%
Turkey	1 cup	1.9	87	20%
(Durkee)	1 cup	–	87	–
(French's)	¼ cup	1	25	36%
(McCormick/Schilling	¼ cup	.5	22	21%
GREAT NORTHERN BEANS				
boiled	½ cup	–	104	–
canned	½ cup	.5	150	3%

Food and Description	Amount	Fat Grams	Total Calories	% Fat Calories
(Joan of Arc/Green Giant)	½ cup	1	80	11%
w/liquid	8 oz	1	300	3%
canned-Seasoned w/Pork				
(Luck's)	7.25 oz	5	220	21%
	7.5 oz	6	230	24%
dry-cooked	½ cup	.5	105	4%
GREEK SOUP (See SOUP)				
GREEN (SNAP) BEAN				
boiled	½ cup	–	22	–
canned	½ cup	–	13	–
(Del Monte)				
cut	½ cup	–	20	–
French style	½cup	–	20	–
Italian Cut	½ cup	–	25	–
whole	½ cup	–	20	–
(Festal)				
cut	½ cup	–	20	–
French Style	½ cup	–	20	–
(Green Giant)				
50% Less Salt	½ cup	–	20	–
1-½" cut	½ cup	< 1	20	23%
French style	½ cup	–	20	–
Kitchen Cut	½ cup	–	20	–
(Joan of Arc)	½ cup	–	25	18%
(Libby)-cut	½ cup	–	20	–
(Nutradiet)-cut	½ cup	–	20	–
(S&W)				
cut	½ cup	–	20	–
dilled	½ cup	–	60	–
Fancy stringless whole	½ cup	–	20	–
Premium Blue Lake-cut	½ cup	–	20	–
Premium Blue Lake-French style	½ cup	–	20	–
Vertical Pack whole	½ cup	–	20	–
(Luck's)-cut & shelled				
Seasoned w/Pork	8 oz	8	200	36%
frozen	½ cup	–	25	–
french style	½ cup	–	26	–
(Freshlike)	3 oz	–	25	–
(Health Valley)	4.5 oz	–	36	–
(Green Giant)	½ cup	–	14	–
(Freshlike)				
cut	3 oz	–	25	–
(Harvest Frest)	½ cup	–	16	–

Food and Description	Amount	Fat Grams	Total Calories	% Fat Calories
Italian				
(Birds Eye)	3.3 oz	–	30	–
(Freshlike)	3 oz	–	30	–
whole				
(Freshlike)	3 oz	–	25	–
microwaveable				
(Green Giant) Pantry Express	½ cup	–	12	–
raw	½ cup	–	17	–
seasoned/canned				
(Del Monte)	½ cup	–	20	–
GREEN BEAN DISHES				
Bavarian Style Recipe (Birds Eye)	3.3 oz	6	110	49%
Blue Lake Green Beans, Potatoes,				
& Julienne Carrots in Grey Poupon Dijon Mustard Sauce				
Vegetable Classics (Del Monte)				
microwave	3⅓ oz	4	70	51%
Cut Green Beans in Butter Sauce				
frozen				
(Green Giant)	½ cup	1	30	30%
Cut Green Beans & Cut Wax Beans				
canned				
(S&W)	½ cup	–	20	–
French Style W/Almonds				
frozen				
(Birds Eye)	½ cup	1.6	52	28%
French Style Green Beans in Butter Sauce				
(Green Giant)	½ cup	1	35	26%
German Style Green Bean Salad				
canned				
(Read)	1 cup	7	180	35%
Green Beans With Mushrooms Casserole				
frozen				
(Birds Eye)	5 oz	5	90	50%
GRITS (*See* CORN GRITS)				
GROUNDCHERRY				
raw	½ cup	.5	37	12%
GROUPER				
cooked-dry heat	3 oz	1	100	9%
raw	3 oz	.9	78	10%
GUAVA				
fresh	1 med	.5	45	10%
GUAVA BUTTER	1 Tbs	–	39	–
GUAVA JUICE				
Guava Juice/canned	1 cup	–	172	

Food and Description	Amount	Fat Grams	Total Calories	% Fat Calories
Guava Nectar				
bottled (Kern's)	6 oz	–	110	–
from frozen conc.	6 oz	–	90	–
Guava, Ripe Nectar (Libby's)	8 oz	–	140	–
GUAVA SAUCE				
cooked	½ cup	–	43	–
GUAVA STRAWBERRY/raw	1 cup	1.5	169	8%
	1 med	–	4	–
GUAVA PUNCH				
Mauna Lai Hawaiian Guava				
(Ocean Spray)	6 oz	–	100	–
Mauna Lai Hawaiian Guava Passion				
(Ocean Spray)	6 oz	–	100	–
GUINEA HEN/meat & skin				
raw-meat only	3.5 oz	2.5	110	20%
raw-ready to cook	1 lb	23	568	36%
GUINEA PIG/raw	3 oz	1.7	82	19%
GUM				
Big Red	1 stick	–	10	–
Bubble Yum				
regular	1 piece	–	25	–
sugar-free	1 piece	–	20	–
Candy-Coated Pieces	12 pieces	–	63	–
Diet				
(Carefree)	1 stick	–	8	–
(Carefree)-bubble gum	1 stick	–	10	–
(Extra)-sugarfree				
bubble gum	1 piece	–	7	–
cinnamon	1 piece	–	8	–
peppermint	1 piece	–	8	–
spearmint	1 piece	–	8	–
winter fresh	1 piece	–	8	–
Doublemint (Wrigley's)	1 stick	–	10	–
(Freedent)				
Cinnamon	1 stick	–	10	–
Peppermint	1 stick	–	10	–
Spearmint	1 stick	–	10	–
Fruit Stripes-all flavors	1 stick	–	10	–
(Hubba Bubba)				
Blueberry	1 piece	–	23	–
Cola	1 piece	–	23	–
Grape	1 piece	–	23	–
Original	1 piece	–	23	–
Raspberry	1 piece	–	23	–

Food and Description	Amount	Fat Grams	Total Calories	% Fat Calories
Strawberry (Hubba Bubba)-sugar free	1 piece	–	23	–
Grape	1 piece	–	13	–
Original	1 piece	–	14	–
(Juicy Fruit)	1 stick	–	10	–
Spearmint (Wrigley's)	1 stick	–	10	–

H

Food and Description	Amount	Fat Grams	Total Calories	% Fat Calories
HADDOCK (*See also* SEAFOOD DINNER/ENTREE)				
breaded & fried	3 oz	9.7	194	45%
cooked-dry heat	3 oz	.79	95	8%
raw	3 oz	.6	74	7%
smoked	3 oz	.8	99	7%
HALIBUT (*See also* SEAFOOD DINNER/ENTREE)				
Atlantic & Pacific				
batter-fried	3 oz	6	153	35%
broiled w/butter	3 oz	6	140	39%
cooked-dry heat	3 oz	2.49	119	19%
raw	3 oz	1.95	93	19%
smoked	3 oz	12.7	190	60%
Greenland				
raw	3 oz	12	160	68%
HAM (*See also* LUNCHEON MEAT)				
Bits (Hormel)	2 Tbs	5	103	44%
Bone-In (Hormel)	4 oz	15	210	64%
Boneless				
Canned-Black Label (Hormel)				
1½ lb	4 oz	7	150	42%
3 lb	4 oz	7	140	45%
5 lb	4 oz	7	140	45%
Chopped	1 oz	4.89	65	68%
canned (Hormel)	1 oz	5	68	66%
12 oz	2 oz	9	120	68%
8 lb	3 oz	21	240	79%
Chunk (Hormel)	6¾ oz	20	310	58%

Food and Description	Amount	Fat Grams	Total Calories	% Fat Calories
Country Style-Center Slice-Lean				
& fat-cold	1 oz	3.66	57	58%
Cured				
regular	3 oz	11	163	61%
roasted	3 oz	13	194	60%
Cured-lean	3 oz	4	103	35%
Curemaster (Hormel)	4 oz	5	140	32%
Deviled-canned	1 Tbs	4	46	78%
	1 oz	9	100	81%
	1 cup	72.7	790	83%
Extra Lean (5%fat)				
cold	1 oz	1	37	24%
roasted	3 oz	4.7	123	34%
(Wilson) Masterpiece				
95% fat-free	3 oz	4	110	33%
Extra Lean (4% fat)				
cold	1 oz	1	34	27%
roasted	3 oz	4	116	31%
(Wilson)-96% fat-free	1 oz	1	30	30%
Extra Lean Deli-10 lb	4 oz	6	130	42%
Holiday Glaze Ham 3 lb	4 oz	4	130	28%
(Hormel)-Extra Lean	4 oz	6	120	45%
Light & Lean (Hormel)-BBQ	2 slices	2	50	36%
boneless	2 oz	2	60	30%
chopped	2slices	4	70	51%
cooked	2 slices	2	50	36%
glazed	2 slices	2	50	36%
red peppered	2 slices	2	50	36%
smoked cooked	2 slices	2	50	36%
Minced	1 oz	5.86	75	70%
(Oscar Meyer)-Boneless-Jubilee	1 oz	3	45	60%
Breakfast, Honey	1 slice	2	50	36%
Canned-Jubilee w/natural				
juices	1 oz	1	30	30%
Slice-Jubilee-95% fat-free	1 oz	1	30	30%
Steaks-Jubilee-95% fat-free	2 oz	2	60	30%
Patties-grilled	1 pattie	18	203	80%
unheated	1 pattie	18	206	79%
(Hormel)-canned	1 pattie	16	180	80%
(Swift)-Premium brown'n				
serve ham patties	1 pattie	13	130	90%
Premium sugarplum	1 oz	1	30	30%
Regular/cooked				
cold	1 oz	2	46	39%

Food and Description	Amount	Fat Grams	Total Calories	% Fat Calories
roasted	3 oz	6.5	140	42%
Regular (11% fat)				
cold	1 oz	3	52	52%
roasted	3 oz	7.66	151	46%
Roasted	3 oz	4	117	31%
Sliced/frozen (Schwan's)	3.5 oz	5	130	35%
Spread/canned (Underwood)	½ can	16	190	76%
Steak, Extra Lean(Boneless)-cold	2 oz	2	69	26%
(Swift)-Premium Hostess	1 oz	1	30	30%
(Underwood)	½ can/			
	2.25 oz	20	220	82%
Whole				
cold-lean only	1 oz	1.6	42	34%
roasted-lean & fat	3 oz	14	207	61%
roasted-lean only	3 oz	4.67	133	32%
HAM AND CHEESE				
Loaf or Roll	1 oz	5.7	73	70%
Roll (Hormel)	4 oz	10	170	53%
Spread	1 Tbs	2.78	37	68%
HAM SALAD	1 Tbs	2	32	56%
	1 oz	4	61	59%
HAMBURGER (*See* BEEF)				
HAMBURGER HELPER				
(Betty Crocker) Box Mix				
Beef Noodle	1 Serving	15	320	42%
Beef Romanoff	1 Serving	16	350	41%
Cheeseburger Macaroni	1 Serving	18	360	45%
Cheesy Italian	1 Serving	17	360	43%
Chili Tomato	1 Serving	14	330	38%
Chili With Beans	1 Serving	17	350	44%
Hamburger Hash	1 Serving	15	320	42%
Hamburger Pizza Dish	1 Serving	14	360	35%
Hamburger Stew	1 Serving	14	300	42%
Lasagna	1 Serving	14	340	37%
Meat Loaf	1 Serving	22	350	57%
Pizzabake	1 Serving	14	320	39%
Potatoes Au Gratin	1 Serving	15	320	42%
Potato Stroganoff	1 Serving	15	320	42%
Rice Oriental	1 Serving	14	340	37%
Sloppy Joe Bake	1 Serving	15	340	40%
Spagetti	1 Serving	15	340	40%
Stroganoff	1 Serving	20	390	46%
Tacobake	1 Serving	15	320	42%
Tamale Pie	1 Serving	16	380	38%

Food and Description	Amount	Fat Grams	Total Calories	% Fat Calories
Zesty Italian	1 Serving	14	330	38%
12 Minute Microwave (Betty Crocker)-Box mix				
Beefy Noodle	1 Serving	20	370	49%
Cheeseburger Spiral	1 Serving	19	380	45%
Lasagna	1 Serving	19	400	32%
Mushroom w/Wild Rice	1 Serving	20	400	45%
HAMBURGER PATTIES				
Frozen				
(Banquet)				
Charbroiled w/mushroom gravy	8 oz	21	270	70%
(Freezer Queen)	7 oz	11	180	55%
w/onion gravy	8 oz	16	240	60%
HAMBURGER VEAL PATTIES				
Broiled (4 oz raw)	2.4 oz	8.9	156	51%
HAMBURGERS-MINI				
Refrigerated-microwavable				
(Jimmy Dean)	1 Burger	5	120	38%
With cheese-mini				
Refrigerated-microwavable				
(Jimmy Dean)	1	6	140	39%
HASH (See CORNED BEEF HASH and ROAST BEEF HASH)				
HERRING				
Atlantic				
breaded & fried	3 oz	18	279	58%
canned-tomato sauce	2 oz	6	100	54%
cooked-dry heat	3 oz	9.85	172	52%
dried	1 oz	5	72	63%
kippered	1 piece/ ~ 1.5 oz	4.95	87	51%
pickled	1 piece/ ~ 1/2 oz	2.7	39	62%
	3 oz	13	190	62%
raw	3 oz	7.68	134	52%
roe-raw	3 oz	1.7	111	14%
Pacific				
raw	3 oz	11.8	166	64%
HICKORY NUT				
dried	1 oz	18	187	87%
HOKI				
raw	3.5 oz	.8	74	10%
HOLLANDAISE SAUCE (See SAUCE)				
HOMINY				
white/canned (Van Camp's)	1 cup	.7	138	5%
yellow/canned (Van Camp's)	1 cup	.6	128	4%

Food and Description	Amount	Fat Grams	Total Calories	% Fat Calories
HOMINY GRITS (*See* CORN GRITS)				
HONEY	1 Tbs	–	64	–
	½ cup	–	512	–
HONEYDEW				
~ 4.5 oz	1/10 fruit	< 1	47	10%
	1 cup	< 1	50	9%
HORSERADISH (*See also* SAUCE)				
prepared	1 oz	–	11	–
(Kraft)				
cream style	1 Tbs	1	10	90%
regular	1 Tbs	1	14	64%
raw	1 oz	–	18	–
HOT DOGS (*See* FRANKFURTERS)				
HUMMUS				
homemade	1 cup	21	420	45%
mix (Casbah)	1 oz	5	110	41%
mix-bean dip w/sesame tahini (Casbah)	2 oz	10	220	41%
HUNTER'S SOUP (*See* SOUP)				
HYACINTH BEAN				
boiled	½ cup	.56	114	4%
raw	½ cup	2	350	5%

Food and Description	Amount	Fat Grams	Total Calories	% Fat Calories
ICE CREAM (*See also* FROZEN DAIRY DESSERT, FROZEN NON-DAIRY DESSERT)				
(Baskin Robbins)				
chocolate	4 oz	13	264	44%
chocolate mousse royale	4 oz	14	293	43%
chocolate raspberry truffle	4 oz	17	310	49%
french vanilla	4 oz	19	290	59%
pralines'n cream	4 oz	13	283	41%
rocky road	4 oz	11	291	34%
strawberry	4 oz	10	226	40%
vanilla	4 oz	13	235	50%
very berry strawberry	4 oz	10	220	41%
world class chocolate	4 oz	14	280	45%
(Baskin Robbins) fat free				
chocolate vanilla twist	4 oz	–	100	–

Food and Description	Amount	Fat Grams	Total Calories	% Fat Calories
just peachy	4 oz	–	100	–
(Baskin Robbins) light				
praline dream	4 oz	6	130	42%
strawberry royal	4 oz	3	110	25%
(Baskin Robbins) sugar free				
jamoca swiss almond	4 oz	2	90	20%
strawberry	4 oz	1	80	11%
(Borden)				
chocolate swirl	½ cup	6	130	42%
strawberry	½ cup	6	130	42%
Olde Fashioned Recipe				
dutch chocolate	½ cup	6	130	42%
strawberries'n cream	½ cup	5	130	35%
vanilla flavored	½ cup	7	130	49%
(Breyers) Original				
butter almond	½ cup	10	170	53%
butter pecan	½ cup	12	180	60%
cherry	½ cup	7	140	45%
cherry-vanilla	½ cup	7	140	45%
chocolate	½ cup	8	160	45%
chocolate chocolate chip	½ cup	10	180	50%
mint chocolate chip	½ cup	10	170	53%
peach	½ cup	6	140	39%
strawberry	½ cup	6	130	42%
vanilla	½ cup	8	150	48%
vanilla w/chocolate almonds	½ cup	10	170	53%
vanilla fudge swirl	½ cup	8	160	45%
(Breyers) Light				
chocolate	½ cup	4	120	30%
chocolate fudge swirl	½ cup	4	130	28%
praline almond crunch	½ cup	5	130	35%
strawberry	½ cup	3	110	25%
vanilla raspberry parfait	½ cup	3	130	21%
(Dreyer's) Grand				
chocolate chip	½ cup	9	150	54%
cookies 'n'cream	½ cup	9	160	51%
marble fudge	½ cup	8	150	48%
rocky road	½ cup	10	170	53%
vanilla	½ cup	10	160	56%
Other Flavors (listed below)	½ cup	7-10	130-180	49%-50%
almond praline				
Butter Pecan				
chocolate				
chocolate chocolate chip				

Food and Description	Amount	Fat Grams	Total Calories	% Fat Calories
chocolate fudge mousse				
coffee				
creamy caramel nut				
dark dutch chocolate				
french vanilla				
international stripes				
mocha almond fudge				
mocha mania				
mom's lemon cream pie				
new york blueberry cheesecake				
strawberry				
toasted almond				
vanilla-chocolate-strawberry				
very vanilla				
(Dreyer's) Grand Light				
almond roca crunch	4 oz	5	120	38%
almond praline	4 oz	4	110	33%
ameretto fudge	4 oz	4	120	30%
banana politan	½ cup	4	110	33%
berry wonderful	½ cup	4	110	33%
cafe au lait	½ cup	4	110	33%
chocolate chip	½ cup	5	120	38%
chocolate fudge mousse	½ cup	5	130	35%
cookies'n'cream	½ cup	5	120	38%
dreamy caramel cream	½ cup	5	120	38%
fudgescotch swirls	4 oz	4	110	33%
malt ball'n fudge	4 oz	5	110	41%
marble fudge	½ cup	4	120	30%
mocha fudge	½ cup	4	110	33%
raspberry truffle	½ cup	4	110	33%
rocky road	½ cup	5	130	35%
strawberries 'n'cream	½ cup	4	110	33%
strawberry cheesecake	½ cup	4	110	33%
vanilla	½ cup	4	100	36%
vanilla/chocolate/strawberry	½ cup	4	110	33%
very vanilla	½ cup	4	100	36%
(Dreyer's & Edy's) Limited Editions				
candy bar	½ cup	5	120	38%
chocolate chocolate chip	½ cup	5	120	38%
english toffee	½ cup	5	110	41%
malted milk ball	½ cup	5	110	41%
mandarin orange chip	½ cup	5	110	41%
(Eagle Brand)				
homestyle vanilla-all natural	½ cup	9	150	54%

Food and Description	Amount	Fat Grams	Total Calories	% Fat Calories
(Haagen-Dazs)				
butter pecan	½ cup	1	290	53%
carob	½ cup	17	260	59%
cherry-vanilla	½ cup	17	260	59%
chocolate	½ cup	17	270	57%
chocolate chip	½ cup	18	290	56%
chocolate swiss almond	½ cup	17	250	61%
coffee	½ cup	15	260	52%
cookies & cream	½ cup	17	270	57%
elberta peach	½ cup	16	250	58%
honey vanilla	½ cup	16	250	58%
macadamia nut	½ cup	24	330	66%
maple walnut	½ cup	19	290	59%
mocha chip	½ cup	18	270	60%
pralines 'n cream	½ cup	16	260	55%
rum raisin	½ cup	17	260	59%
strawberry	½ cup	15	250	54%
vanilla	½ cup	17	260	59%
vanilla chip	½ cup	17	280	55%
vanilla swiss almond	½ cup	19	290	59%
(Haagen-Dazs)-Special Additions				
chocolate chocolate mint	½ cup	20	300	60%
deep chocolate fudge	½ cup	15	300	45%
deep chocolate peanut butter	½ cup	19	330	52%
macadamia brittle	½ cup	18	280	58%
mocha double nut	½ cup	20	290	62%
(Lady Borden)				
buttered pecan	½ cup	12	180	60%
(Kemps)-all flavors	½ cup	6	140	39%
(Lucerne)				
chocolate chip	½ cup	8	150	48%
coffee ice cream	½ cup	7	140	45%
french vanilla	½ cup	8	150	48%
Light-Dairy				
chocolate	½ cup	4	115	31%
cookie cream	½ cup	5	130	35%
mocha almond	½ cup	4	125	29%
rocky road	½ cup	4	130	28%
strawberry cream	½ cup	3	105	26%
mint chocolate chip	½ cup	8	150	48%
neapolitan	½ cup	7	140	45%
ranch pecan	½ cup	9	160	51%
rocky road	½ cup	8	150	48%
strawberry cheesecake	½ cup	6	140	39%

Food and Description	Amount	Fat Grams	Total Calories	% Fat Calories
vanilla	½ cup	8	140	39%
(Pet)				
black sweet cherry	½ cup	6	120	45%
butter pecan	½ cup	9	140	58%
chocolate	½ cup	7	130	49%
chocolate chip	½ cup	7	120	53%
cookies n'cream	½ cup	7	140	45%
heavenly hash	½ cup	7	140	45%
neapolitan	½ cup	6	130	42%
strawberry cheesecake	½ cup	5	130	35%
vanilla	½ cup	7	130	49%
vanilla fudge swirl	½ cup	6	130	42%
(Schwan's) Ice Cream & Ice Milk Home Delivery				
black raspberry	½ cup	7	140	45%
butter brickle	½ cup	7	150	42%
butter pecan	½ cup	9	150	54%
buttersctoch ripple	½ cup	7	140	45%
cherry nut	½ cup	7	140	45%
cherry vanilla	½ cup	7	140	45%
chip & mint	½ cup	8	150	48%
chocolate (Schwan's)	½ cup	7	140	45%
chocolate almond	½ cup	8	150	48%
chocolate chip	½ cup	8	150	48%
chocolate french silk	½ cup	7	150	42%
chocolate fudge ripple	½ cup	7	140	45%
chocolate marshmallow ripple	½ cup	6	140	39%
coffee	½ cup	7	140	45%
cookies & cream	½ cup	8	160	45%
dark sweet cherry	½ cup	6	140	39%
french vanilla	½ cup	8	150	48%
holiday special	½ cup	6	140	39%
maple nut	½ cup	9	150	54%
neapolitan	½ cup	7	140	45%
peach (Schwan's)	½ cup	6	130	42%
peanut butter fudge ripple	½ cup	7	150	42%
pecan praline	½ cup	7	150	42%
pink divinity	½ cup	7	150	42%
raspberry delight	½ cup	5	130	35%
raspberry ripple	½ cup	7	140	45%
rocky road	½ cup	6	150	36%
strawberry	½ cup	7	140	45%
strawberry ripple	½ cup	7	140	45%
summer's dream	½ cup	5	130	35%
tin roof sundae	½ cup	7	150	42%

Food and Description	Amount	Fat Grams	Total Calories	% Fat Calories
vanilla	½ cup	7	140	45%
(Sealtest)				
butter pecan	½ cup	10	160	56%
chocolate	½ cup	6	140	39%
cubic scoops	½ cup	4	130	28%
french vanilla	½ cup	7	140	45%
fudge royale	½ cup	7	140	45%
heavenly hash	½ cup	7	150	42%
strawberry	½ cup	5	130	35%
strawberry, chocolate, vanilla	½ cup	6	140	39%
(Thrifty)				
apple cinnamon	½ cup	7	150	42%
black cherry	½ cup	6	130	42%
butter pecan	½ cup	9	150	54%
chocolate	½ cup	7	140	45%
chocolate almond amaretto	½ cup	9	160	51%
chocolate brownie	½ cup	9	170	48%
chocolate chip	½ cup	8	150	48%
chocolate malted krunch	½ cup	8	160	45%
coconut pineapple	½ cup	6	130	42%
cookies'n cream	½ cup	7	150	42%
french vanilla	½ cup	8	150	48%
½ & ½ (vanilla ice cream & orange sherbet)	½ cup	4	130	28%
marble fudge	½ cup	6	140	39%
mint'n chip	½ cup	8	150	48%
pecan praline	½ cup	8	160	45%
pistachio nut	½ cup	8	150	48%
raspberry fudge torte	½ cup	7	160	39%
rocky road	½ cup	8	160	45%
strawberry	½ cup	6	130	42%
vanilla	½ cup	7	140	45%
(Weight Watchers)-Grand Collection				
chocolate swirl, pralines & cream	½ cup	3	120	23%
neopolitan	½ cup	3	110	25%
strawberries'n creme	½ cup	3	120	23%
vanilla	½ cup	3	100	27%
Ice Cream & Frozen Custard				
chocolate	1 cup	16	295	49%
french vanilla-soft serve	1 cup	22.5	377	54%
strawberry	1 cup	12	250	43%
vanilla (10% fat)	1 cup	14.3	269	48%
vanilla (16% fat)	1 cup	24	350	62%

Food and Description	Amount	Fat Grams	Total Calories	% Fat Calories
Ice Cream mixed w/Sorbet-(Haagen-Dazs)				
key lime sorbet & vanilla ice cream	½ cup	7	190	33%
orange sorbet & vanilla ice cream	½ cup	8	190	38%
raspberry sorbet & vanilla ice cream	½ cup	7	180	35%
ICE CREAM BAR				
(A & P)/vanilla w/chocolate coating	1 bar	10	151	60%
(Baskin Robbins)/vanilla-dark choc. coat.	10	21	310	61%
(Baskin Robbins) sundae bar				
light/chocolate with caramel ribbon	1	5	150	30%
pralines 'n cream	1	13	310	38%
Brownie Sundaes (Betty Crocker)				
vanilla fudge swirl	1	10	240	38%
(Creamsicle)	1	3	103	26%
sugar-free cream pops	1	1	25	36%
(Dolly Madison)/vanilla-chocolate coating	1 Bar	12	197	55%
(Dove Bar)				
almond bar	1	23	350	59%
choc.-dark chocolate coating	1	22	350	57%
choc.-milk chocolate coating	1	21	340	56%
Crunchy Cookies	1	20	330	55%
vanilla-milk chocolate coating	1	21	340	56%
vanilla-dark chocolate coating	1	22	340	58%
(Dove Light)				
vanilla w/milk choc coating	1	12	230	47%
vanilla w/dark chocolate coating	1	12	230	47%
(Dreyer's)/vanilla-dark chocolate coating	1	20	295	61%
(Drumstick) Sundae Cone				
caramel surprise	1	19	352	49%
vanilla	1	19	332	52%
(Freezer Pleezer)/vanilla-choc. coating	1	10	147	61%
(Fudgesicle) fudge pop	1	1	70	13%
(Fudgetastics)-sundaes on a stick				
plain	1	15	220	61%
crunchy	1	14	230	55%
Gold Rush Bar (Betty Crocker)				
peanut butter	1	16	233	62%
vanilla	1	13	208	56%
(Good Humor)				
almond supreme	1	23	350	59%
bubble o bill	1	8	149	48%
chip candy crunch	1	17.9	255	63%
chocolate eclair	1	10	188	48%
chocolate fudge cake	1	15	214	63%
fat frog	1	9	154	53%

Food and Description	Amount	Fat Grams	Total Calories	% Fat Calories
fudge bar	1		127	4%
fudge cake	1	15	214	63%
halo bar	1	13.7	230	54%
king cone	5.5 oz	12	290	37%
boysenberry	5 oz	13	340	34%
laser blazer	1	3	131	21%
milk supreme	1	16.8	278	54%
chocolate chip cookie				
chocolate	1	8	204	35%
vanilla	1	10.5	246	38%
vanilla ice cream sdw.	2.5 oz	4.9	165	27%
	3 oz	5.7	191	27%
milky pop	3 oz	.8	47	15%
strawberries & cream	4 oz	1	94	10%
strawberry shortcake	3 oz	8	176	41%
supreme	1	25	375	60%
toasted almond	3 oz	11.8	212	50%
vanilla cup	3 oz	5	98	46%
vanilla-chocolate combo cup	6 oz	9	201	40%
vanilla w/chocolate coating	1 Bar	13.7	198	62%
whammy	1 Bar	7	95	66%
(Haagen-Dazs)				
choc.-dark chocolate coating	1 Bar	27	390	62%
vanilla-dark chocolate coating	1 Bar	27	360	68%
vanilla-milk chocoalte coating	1 Bar	27	360	68%
vanilla-milk choc coating w/almonds	1 Bar	27	370	66%
(Klondike)				
choc.-milk chocolate coating	1 Bar	20	287	63%
vanilla-milk choccolate coating	1 Bar	20	294	61%
(Klondike)-Frozen Dessert Bar-Lite	1 Bar	10	140	64%
sensation w/almnds	1 Bar	13	190	61%
(Natural Nectar)-cocoa fudge'n cream	1 Bar	< 1	110	4%
(Nestle)				
vanilla-milk chocolate coating	1 Bar	18.5	286	58%
alpine white premium	1 Bar	25	350	64%
(Nestle) Crunch/vanilla-milk choc. coating	1 Bar	13	180	65%
light	1 Bar	10	150	60%
(Nestle) Quik/choc.-milk chocolate				
coating	1 Bar	14	210	60%
(Nestle) milk chocolate premium	1 Bar	20	300	60%
(Nestle) milk chocolate w/almonds				
premium	1 Bar	23	350	59%
(Nestle) semi-sweet premium	1 Bar	21	310	61%
(Oreo)/cookies cream on a stick	1 Bar	15	220	61%

Food and Description	Amount	Fat Grams	Total Calories	% Fat Calories
(Pathmark)/vanilla-chocolate coating	1 Bar	10	151	60%
(Polar Bar)/vanila-milk chocolate coating	1 Bar	17.5	234	67%
(Rondos)				
chicago cherry	.75 oz	4	60	60%
classic vanilla	1 Bar	4	60	60%
french vanilla	1 Bar	4	60	60%
original chocolate	1 Bar	4	60	60%
(Schwan's)-home delivery				
chocolate scooter crunch	1 Bar	9	170	48%
english toffee	1 Bar	12	190	57%
gold'n nugit	1 Bar	16	260	55%
peaches & cream bar	1 Bar	1	80	11%
pecan sundae cone	1 cone	12	270	40%
peanut stick bars	1 Bar	13	190	62%
raspberry cordial Bar	1 Bar	13	210	56%
rootbeer float	1 Bar	2	90	21%
schwan bar	1 Bar	12	190	57%
silver mint bar	1 Bar	10	160	56%
strawberries & cream	1 Bar	2	80	23%
sundae cones	1 Bar	11	210	47%
swiss chocolate almond sundae cone	1 Bar	13	260	45%
tin roof sundae bar	1 Bar	16	250	58%
(Snickers)	1 Bar	14	220	57%
(Steve's)/vanilla-milk chocolate coating	1 Bar	29	439	60%
(3 Musketeers)				
chocolate	1 Bar	10	170	53%
vanilla	1 Bar	10	170	53%
sugar free vanilla	1 Bar	4	50	72%
(Weight Watchers)				
chocolate mint treat	1 Bar	1	60	15%
chocolate mousse	1 Bar	.8	35	21%
chocolate treat	1 Bar	1	100	9%
cookies & cream	1 Bar	1	120	8%
double fudge	1 Bar	1	60	15%
dutch chocolate	1 Bar	1	100	9%
golden vanilla	1 Bar	1	100	9%
neopolitan	1 Bar	1	100	9%
orange-vanilla treat	1 Bar	1	60	15%
peanut butter fudge	1 Bar	.8	60	12%
vanilla sandwich bar	1 Bar	3	150	18%

ICE CREAM CONE

Cones only

  (Baskin-Robbins)

| Cake | 1 cone | – | 19 | – |

Food and Description	Amount	Fat Grams	Total Calories	% Fat Calories
Sugar	1 cone	1	57	16%
(Comet)				
Cones	1 cone	–	40	–
Cups	1 cup	–	40	–
(Country Inn)	1 cone	–	18	–
(Disney) Cakes	1 cone	–	17	–
(Disney) Sugar Cones	1 cone	–	53	–
(Disney) Waffle Cones	1 cone	–	59	8%
(Keebler) Ice Cream Cups	1 cup	–	15	30%
Little Debbie) Ice Cream Cups	1 cup	–	15	–
Ice Cream Nuggets-Bon Bon				
(Carnation)				
Vanilla				
w/dark chocolate coating	5 nuggets	11	170	58%
w/milk chocolate coating	5 nuggets	11	165	60%
ICE CREAM SANDWICH				
(Eskimo Pie)				
original dark choc. coating	1	12	140	71%
dark chocolate coating	1	15	209	65%
Fudge Bars-sugar free	1	1	60	15%
Light-sugar free	1	9	140	58%
Sandwich-sugar free	1	6	170	32%
w/crispy rice-sugar free	1	11	150	66%
Good Humor Sandwich	1	5	162	28%
Oreo sandwich	1 Bar	11	240	41%
Schwan's Sandwiches	1 Bar	6	160	34%
ICE CREAM TOPPING				
Butterscotch				
(Kraft)	1 Tbs	1	60	15%
(Smucker's)	2 Tbs	–	140	–
Caramel				
(Kraft)	1 Tbs	–	60	–
(Smucker's)	2 Tbs	–	140	–
Cherry-(Smucker's)	1 Tbs	–	53	–
Chocolate				
(Kraft)	1 Tbs	–	60	–
(Smucker's)	2 Tbs	2	130	14%
Chocolate Fudge				
(Hershey)	2 Tbs	4	100	36%
(Smucker's)	2 Tbs	1	130	7%
Chocolate Fudge Magic Shell				
(Smucker's)	2 Tbs	15	190	71%
Chocolate Sauce/homemade	1 Tbs	2	55	33%

Food and Description	Amount	Fat Grams	Total Calories	% Fat Calories
Chocolate Syrup				
(Estee)	1 Tbs	–	6	–
(Hershy)	1 Tbs	–	36	–
(Nestle)	1.22 oz	1	100	9%
Chocolate Nut-Magic Shell				
(Smucker's)	1.22 oz	16	200	72%
Hard Sauce-homemade	1.22 oz	6	95	57%
Hot Caramel-(Smucker's)	1.22 oz	4	150	24%
Hot Fudge				
(Kraft)	1 Tbs	3	70	39%
(Mrs. Richardson's)-Lite	2 Tbs	1	90	10%
(Smucker's)	2 Tbs	4	110	33%
Lemon Sauce/homemade	2 Tbs	1.5	60	23%
Marshmallow-(Baker's)	2 Tbs	–	120	–
Peanut Butter Caramel-(Smucker's)	2 Tbs	2	150	12%
Pecans in Syrup-(Smucker's)	2 Tbs	1	130	7%
Pineapple	1 Tbs	–	50	–
(Smucker's)	2 Tbs	–	130	–
(Planter's) Nut Topping	1 oz	16	180	80%
Special Recipe Butterscotch Caramel-Flavored				
(Smucker's)	2 Tbs	3	160	17%
Special Recipe Dark Chocolate				
(Smucker's)	2 Tbs	1	130	7%
Special Recipe Hot Fudge				
(Smucker's)	2 Tbs	5	150	30%
Strawberry				
(Kraft)	1 Tbs	–	50	–
(Smucker's)	2 Tbs	–	120	–
Swiss Milk Chocolate Fudge				
(Smucker's)	2 Tbs	1	140	6%
Walnuts in Syrup (Smucker's)	2 Tbs	1	130	7%
Whipped Toppings (*See also* CREAM)				
Frozen				
(Birds Eye)				
Cool Whip Extra Creamy	1 Tbs	1	16	56%
Cool Whip Non-Dairy	1 Tbs	1	12	75%
Lite	1 Tbs	< 1	8	56%
(Rich Whip)	1 Tbs	1	12	75%
(Kraft)	¼ cup	3	35	77%
Real Cream Topping	¼ cup	2	30	60%
Mix				
(Dream Whip)-prepared w/ whole milk	2 Tbs	1	10	90%
(D-Zerta) reduced calorie	1 Tbs	< 1	8	90%

Food and Description	Amount	Fat Grams	Total Calories	% Fat Calories
(Estee)	1 Tbs	< 1	4	90%
(Featherweight)	1 Tbs	–	4	–
Pressurized				
cream	1 Tbs	< 1	8	90%
	½ cup	7	75	84%
non dairy	1 Tbs	1	10	90%
	½ cup	8	95	76%
ICE MILK				
(Carnation)-Smooth'N Lite-96% Fat Free				
cherry vanilla	½ cup	3	100	27%
chocolate	½ cup	2	90	20%
chocolate chip	½ cup	4	110	33%
cookies 'n cream	½ cup	3	120	23%
double dutch fudge	½ cup	3	150	18%
marble fudge	½ cup	4	150	24%
neapolitan	½ cup	3	100	27%
praline pecan	½ cup	6	180	30%
rocky road	½ cup	4	120	30%
strawberry	½ cup	2	90	20%
vanilla	½ cup	2	90	20%
vanilla bean	½ cup	4	140	26%
(Light N'Lively)				
caramel nut	½ cup	4	120	30%
chocolate chip	½ cup	4	120	30%
cookies'n cream	½ cup	3	120	23%
heavenly hash	½ cup	3	120	23%
vanilla	½ cup	3	100	27%
vanilla, chocolate, strawberry	½ cup	3	110	25%
vanilla flavored & chocolate covered				
almonds	½ cup	4	120	30%
vanilla, fudge twirl	½ cup	3	110	25%
(Schwan's)-See ICE CREAM				
(Steve's)-Light Ice Milk				
butter pecan	4 oz	8	190	38%
cherry chocolate chunk	4 oz	8	190	38%
deep chocolate peanut butter	4 oz	8	200	36%
fudge nut fantasy	4 oz	8	200	36%
heath bar crunch	4 oz	8	210	34%
vanilla	4 oz	8	190	38%
Strawberry (Borden)	½ cup	2	90	20%
Vanilla	1 cup	5.6	184	27%
(Borden)	½ cup	2	90	20%
soft serve (3%)	1 cup	5	225	20%
(Weight Watchers)	½ cup	3	100	27%

Food and Description	Amount	Fat Grams	Total Calories	% Fat Calories
(Weight Watchers)-Grand Collection				
chocolate	½ cup	3	150	18%
fudge marble	4 oz	3	120	23%
neopolitan	½ cup	3	100	27%
strawberry'n creme	4 oz	3	120	23%
swiss vanilla	4 oz	3	120	23%
(Weight Watchers) One-Ders				
chocolate chip	4 oz	4	120	30%
heavenly hash	4 oz	3	120	23%
pecan pralines 'n creme	4 oz	4	120	30%
strawberry	4 oz	3	110	25%
ICE MILK BAR				
(Crystal Light) Cool'N Creamy				
bavarian bar	1 Bar	2	50	36%
chocolate amaretto	1 Bar	2	60	30%
double chocolate fudge	1 Bar	2	50	36%
orange	1 Bar	1	50	18%
(Sweet'N Low) vanilla				
w/chocolate coating	1 Bar	6	90	60%
(3 Musketeers)	1 Bar	4	50	72%
(Weight Watchers)				
english toffee crunch bar	1 Bar	8	120	60%
vanilla-choc coating	1 Bar	6.8	111	55%
ICES (See FRUIT ICES)				
INDIAN PUDDING (See PUDDING)				

J

Food and Description	Amount	Fat Grams	Total Calories	% Fat Calories
JACKFRUIT/raw	1 medium	–	107	–
JAM/JELLY/PRESERVES				
(Bama)				
Apple jelly	2 tsp	–	30	–
Grape jelly	2 tsp	–	30	–
Peach preserves	2 tsp	–	30	–
Red Plum Jam	2 tsp	–	30	–
Strawberry preserves	2 tsp	–	30	–
(Country Pure)-Jam				
Apricot	2 tsp	–	35	–

Food and Description	Amount	Fat Grams	Total Calories	% Fat Calories
Blackberry	2 tsp	–	35	–
Red Cherry	2 tsp	–	35	–
Red Raspberry	2 tsp	–	35	–
Strawberry	2 tsp	–	35	–
(Empress)				
Apple Jelly	2 tsp	–	35	–
Apricot Pineapple Preserves	2 tsp	–	35	–
Apricot Preserves	2 tsp	–	35	–
Black Cherry Preserves	2 tsp	–	35	–
Black Raspberry Preserves	2 tsp	–	35	–
Blackberry Jelly	2 tsp	–	35	–
Boysenberry Preserves	2 tsp	–	35	–
California Orange Marmalade	2 tsp	–	35	–
Concord Grape Jam	2 tsp	–	35	–
Grape Jam	2 tsp	–	35	–
Mixed Fruit Jelly	2 tsp	–	35	–
Peach Pineapple Preserves	2 tsp	–	35	–
Peach Preserves	2 tsp	–	35	–
Plum Preserves	2 tsp	–	35	–
Red Cherry Preserves	2 tsp	–	35	–
Red Currant Jelly	2 tsp	–	35	–
Red Raspberry Preserves	2 tsp	–	35	–
Seedless Blackberry Preserves	2 tsp	–	35	–
Strawberry Preserves	2 tsp	–	35	–
(Estee)-Preserves & Jelly-all flavors	1 tsp	–	2	–
(Featherweight) Fruit Spreads-all flavors	1 tsp	–	4	–
(Kraft)				
Jam-all flavors	1 tsp	–	17	–
Jelly-all flavors	1 tsp	–	17	–
reduced calorie-grape	1 tsp	–	8	–
Preserves-all flavors	1 tsp	–	17	–
reduced calorie-strawberry	1 tsp	–	8	–
(Mary Ellen)				
Apricot Jam	2 tsp	–	35	–
Grape Jam	2 tsp	–	35	–
Grape Jelly	2 tsp	–	35	–
Red Raspberry Jam	2 tsp	–	35	–
Seedless Blackberry Jam	2 tsp	–	35	–
Strawberry Jam	2 tsp	–	35	–
Strawberry Jelly	2 tsp	–	35	–
(Nutradiet)/sugar-free				
Jam				
Blackberry	1 tsp	–	4	–
Red Raspberry	1 tsp	–	4	–

Food and Description	Amount	Fat Grams	Total Calories	% Fat Calories
Strawberry	1 tsp	–	4	–
Jelly				
Concord Grape	1 tsp	–	4	–
Marmalade				
orange	1 tsp	–	4	–
Preserves				
Apricot-Pineapple	1 tsp	–	4	–
Boysenberry	1 tsp	–	4	–
Red Tart Cherry	1 tsp	–	4	–
(Poiret)-100% Pure Fruit Spreads				
Apple spread	½ tsp	–	17	–
Pear,apricot,apple spread	½ tsp	–	17	–
Pear, black cherry spread	½ oz	–	35	–
Pear, strawberry spread	½ oz	–	35	–
Pear,strawberry,apple spread	½ tsp	–	17	–
(Polaner)-All Fruit Spread				
Apricot	1 tsp	–	14	–
Black cherry	1 tsp	–	14	–
Blackberry	1 tsp	–	14	–
Blueberry	1 tsp	–	14	–
Raspberry	1 tsp	–	14	–
Strawberry	1 tsp	–	14	–
(Pritikin)-Fruit Spread-all flavors	1 tsp	–	14	–
(R W Knudsen)-All Fruit Spread				
Blackberry	2 tsp	–	35	–
Red Raspberry	2 tsp	–	35	–
Strawberry	2 tsp	–	35	–
(Smucker's)				
Imitation Grape Jelly & Strawberry				
Jam (artificially sweetened)	1 tsp	–	2	–
Jam-all flavors	1 tsp	–	18	–
Low-Sugar Spreads-all flavors	1 tsp	–	8	–
Mint Apple Jelly	1 tsp	–	18	–
Natural, Cider, Simply Fruit &				
Autumn Harvest	1 tsp	–	12	–
Orange Marmalade	1 tsp	–	18	–
Preserves-all flavors	1 tsp	–	18	–
Simply Fruit Spread-all flavors	1 tsp	–	16	–
Slenderella-low-cal imitation				
jams and jellies	1 tsp	–	8	–
(Weight Watchers)-spreads				
all flavors	2 tsp	–	16	–
(Welch's)-Jams-all flavors	2 tsp	–	35	–
Jelly-all flavors	2 tsp	–	35	–

Food and Description	Amount	Fat Grams	Total Calories	% Fat Calories
Preserves	2 tsp	–	35	–
Squeezables	2 tsp	–	35	–
JAPANESE FOOD (See ORIENTAL FOOD)				
JELLO (See GELATIN)				
JELLY (See JAM/JELLY/PRESERVES)				
JICAMA				
cooked	½ cup	< 1	46	10%
raw-sliced	1 cup	< 1	50	9%
JUICE (See individual flavors)				
JUJUBE				
dried	3 oz	.9	246	3%
raw	3 oz	–	68	–

K

Food and Description	Amount	Fat Grams	Total Calories	% Fat Calories
KALE				
fresh-cooked	½ cup	–	21	–
frozen-cooked	½ cup	–	20	–
raw	½ cup	–	17	–
KANPYO/(Dried Gourd Strips)	3 strips	–	49	–
KETCHUP (See CATSUP)				
KIDNEY BEAN				
boiled	½ cup	< 1	112	4%
canned	½ cup	< 1	104	4%
(Nutradiet)	½ cup	1	90	10%
dried	½ cup	.5	130	4%
raw	½ cup	1	300	3%
Dark Red				
canned (Van Camp's)	1 cup	1	180	5%
canned dry (Joan of Arc)				
(Green Giant)	½ cup	< 1	90	5%
(Ranch Style)	7.5 oz	1	170	5%
(S&W) 50% Less Salt	½ cup	1	120	8%
Light Red				
canned dry				
(Joan of Arc/Green Giant)	½ cup	< 1	90	5%
(Van Camp's)	1 cup	1	180	5%

Food and Description	Amount	Fat Grams	Total Calories	% Fat Calories
Red				
boiled	½ cup	< 1	112	4%
canned	½ cup	< 1	108	4%
baked (B&M)	~ 1 cup	7	290	22%
(Progresso)	8 oz	1	190	5%
New Orleans Style (Van Camp's)	1 cup	1	180	5%
Seasoned w/Pork (Luck's)	7.5 oz	6	220	25%
Special Cook/canned (Luck's)	7.5 oz	4	190	19%
White				
canned (Progresso)	8 oz	1	180	5%
KIELBASA (*See* LUNCHEON MEAT)				
KINGFISH				
cooked-dry heat	3 oz	11	219	45%
raw	3 oz	2.57	90	26%
KIWI-BANANA DRINK	3 oz	–	98	–
KIWI DRINK				
Kiwi Juice Drink	6 oz	–	98	–
KIWIFRUIT/raw	1 medium	< 1	46	10%
	1 large	< 1	55	8%
KIWI-PEACH DRINK	6 oz	–	98	–
KIWI-STRAWBERRY DRINK	6 oz	–	98	–
KNOCKWURST (*See* LUNCHEON MEATS)				
KOHLRABI				
fresh-cooked	½ cup	–	24	–
raw	½ cup	–	19	–
KUMQUAT/raw	1	–	12	–

L

Food and Description	Amount	Fat Grams	Total Calories	% Fat Calories
LAMB				
(NOTE: All portions are cooked, unless otherwise stated.				
Lean = all separable fat has been trimmed.				
Lean & fat = untrimmed and cooked as purchased.)				
Chop, arm/lean & fat-braised	2.2 oz	15	220	61%
Chop, arm/lean-braised	3 oz	14	270	47%
Chop, loin				
lean & fat-broiled	4 oz	23	336	62%
lean-broiled	3 oz	8	182	40%

Food and Description	Amount	Fat Grams	Total Calories	% Fat Calories
Chop, rib				
lean & fat-broiled	2.5 oz	25	289	79%
lean-broiled	2 oz	7	130	49%
Chop, shoulder/lean	7 oz (raw wt)	9	185	39%
Chop, shoulder/lean & fat	7 oz (raw wt)	34	427	72%
Ground-cooked-1.7 oz meat	4 oz (raw wt)	22.5	275	74%
Heart-braised	½ cup	10	189	48%
Hocks	4 oz	16	236	61%
Leg, roast/lean & fat-roasted	3 oz	16	237	61%
Leg, roast/lean-roasted	3 oz	7	162	39%
Liver/broiled	1.6 oz slice	5.6	117	43%
Ribs/cooked-3 oz meat	6 oz (raw wt)	8.9	178	45%
Shoulder				
lean & fat-roasted	3 oz	23	287	72%
lean-roasted	3 oz	8.5	174	44%
Sweetbreads-cooked	3 oz	5	149	30%
Tongue/braised	2 oz	10	144	63%
lamb/sheep	2 oz	14	183	69%
LAMB DISHES				
Lamb Curry/homemade	1 cup	23	460	45%
Lamb Stew/homemade	1 cup	7	165	38%
LAMB'S-QUARTERS				
fresh-cooked	1 cup	.6	29	19%
LARD	1 Tbs	12.8	115	100%
	1 cup	205	1850	100%
	8 oz	227	2046	100%
LASAGNE				
Frozen-w/meat sauce				
(Banquet)	7 oz	10	270	33%
(Swanson's)	10.5 oz	16	400	36%
Homemade	~7.5 oz	18	320	51%
w/mushrooms (Van de Kamp's)	11 oz	25	430	52%
w/meat sauce (Weight Watchers)	11 oz	13	330	36%
Standard Home Recipe (USDA)				
~2-½"x4" piece	~7 oz	12	325	33%
Vegetable Lasagna				
(Impromptu Lite)	10.6 oz	11	270	37%
(Weight Watchers)				
Italian Cheese Lasagna-frozen	11 oz	14	380	33%
Whole Wheat				
(Westbrae Natural)-dry	2 oz	2	210	9%
LEEK				
cooked	¼ cup	–	8	–

Food and Description	Amount	Fat Grams	Total Calories	% Fat Calories
freeze-dried	¼ cup	–	3	–
raw	¼ cup	–	16	–
	1 leek	–	17	–
LEMON	1 medium	–	17	–
	1 large	–	25	–
LEMON JUICE				
bottled	⅓ cup	–	17	–
	1 Tbs	–	5	–
fresh	⅓ cup	–	20	–
	1 Tbs	–	4	–
frozen	1 Tbs	–	3	–
(Sunkist)	1 oz	–	7	–
(Realemon)	1 oz	–	6	–
refrigerated	1 oz	–	6	–
LEMON-LIME DRINK				
(Country Time)				
mix	6 oz	–	80	–
sugar-free	6 oz	–	4	–
(Crystal Light)				
diet soft drink mix	6 oz	–	4	–
LEMON PEEL				
candied	1 oz	–	90	–
grated	1 Tbs	–	–	–
LEMONADE				
(Country Time)-mix	8 oz	–	80	–
sugar free	8 oz	–	4	–
(Crystal Light) Mix-sugar free	8 oz	–	4	–
(Tropicana)-single serve	8 oz	–	120	–
Lemonade Flavor Drink Mix	2 Tbs mix + 8 oz water	–	113	–
from frozen concentrate	8 oz	–	100	–
(Birds Eye)-frozen	6 oz	–	70	–
Lemonade Powder Mix	1 Tbs powder + 4 oz water	–	102	–
Pink Lemonade				
(Country Time)-mix	8 oz	–	80	–
(Country Time)-sugar-free	8 oz	–	4	–
LENTIL				
boiled	½ cup	–	115	–
canned	½ cup	–	130	–
cooked	½ cup	–	103	–
dry	½ cup	1	374	2%
green (Arrowhead Mills)	2 oz	1	190	5%
red (Arrowhead Mills)	2 oz	1	190	5%

Food and Description	Amount	Fat Grams	Total Calories	% Fat Calories
split/dry	½ cup	1	379	2%
sprouts	½ cup	–	40	–
LENTIL PILAF-Zesty (Health Valley)	4 oz	2.75	110	23%
LENTIL SOUP (*See* SOUP)				
LETTUCE				
Butterhead	1 head	–	21	–
Iceburg	1 head	1	70	13%
Looseleaf or Simpson	½ cup	–	5	–
Romaine/shredded	½ cup	–	4	–
LICHEE (LYCHEE) NUTS				
dried/shelled	3 oz	.9	237	3%
raw	~6 nuts	–	45	–
raw/shelled	4 oz	1	314	3%
	1 cup	.8	125	6%
LIMA BEAN				
canned				
(Dennison's) w/ham	7.5 oz	7	250	25%
(Libby)	½ cup	–	80	–
frozen				
(Green Giant)	½ cup	–	100	–
(Harvest Fresh)	½ cup	–	60	–
Baby				
boiled	½ cup	–	115	–
frozen	½ cup	–	94	–
(Birds Eye)	3.3 oz	–	130	–
(Freshlike)	3.3 oz	–	130	–
raw	½ cup	1	330	3%
Giant				
canned-Seasoned w/Pork (Luck's)	7.5 oz	7	230	27%
Green				
canned (Del Monte)	½ cup	–	70	–
Large				
boiled	½ cup	–	108	–
canned	½ cup	–	95	–
frozen	½ cup	–	85	–
raw	½ cup	.5	300	2%
Small green				
canned-Seasoned w/Pork (Luck's)	7.5 oz	7	220	29%
fancy (S&W)	12 cup	–	80	–
Thin/frozen (Health Valley)	6 oz	.5	188	2%
LIMA BEAN DISHES				
In butter sauce				
frozen				
(Green Giant)	½ cup	2	100	18%

Food and Description	Amount	Fat Grams	Total Calories	% Fat Calories
With ham				
canned (Dennison's)	7.5 oz	7	250	25%
LIME	1	–	20	–
LIME JUICE				
fresh	⅓ cup	–	22	–
bottled	⅓ cup	–	17	–
	1 Tbs	–	3	–
(Realime)	1 oz	–	6	–
LIMEADE/from frozen concentrate	8 oz	–	102	–
LINGCOD/raw	3 oz	1	70	13%
LIQUEUR:				
Anisette	¾ fl oz	–	74	–
B & B	1 fl oz	–	94	–
Benedictine	¾ fl oz	–	69	–
Brandy-fruit flavored	1.5 fl oz	–	129	–
Brandy-coffee	1.5 fl oz	–	132	–
Cherry Hering	1.5 fl oz	–	120	–
Coffee	1.5 fl oz	–	174	–
Coffee/with cream	1.5 fl oz	7	154	41%
Creme de Almonde	1.5 fl oz	–	151	–
Creme de Banane	1.5 fl oz	–	144	–
Creme de Cacao	1.5 fl oz	–	150	–
Creme de Cassis	1.5 fl oz	–	122	–
Creme deMenthe	1.5 fl oz	–	186	–
Curacao	3/4 fl oz	–	54	–
Drambuie	1.5 fl oz	–	165	–
Gin-Citrus	1.5 fl oz	–	114	–
Kirsch	1.5 fl oz	–	124	–
Maraschino	1.5 fl oz	–	112	–
Peppermint Schnapps	1.5 fl oz	–	124	–
Pernod	1.5 fl oz	–	117	–
Rock & Rye	1.5 fl oz	–	140	–
Sloe Gin	1.5 fl oz	–	124	–
Southern Comfort	1.5 fl oz	–	180	–
Tia Maria	1.5 fl oz	–	138	–
Triple Sec	1.5 fl oz	–	121	–
Vodka-Citrus	1.5 fl oz	–	150	–
LIVER LOAF (*See* LUNCHEON MEAT)				
LIVERWURST (*See* LUNCHEON MEAT)				
LOAF, LUNCHEON (*See* LUNCHEON MEAT)				
LOBSTER (*See also* SEAFOOD ENTREE/DINNER)				
Northern				
boiled	3 oz	.5	83	5%
	1 cup	.86	142	6%

Food and Description	Amount	Fat Grams	Total Calories	% Fat Calories
raw -1 lobster	~ 5 oz	1	140	6%
Spiny-raw	3 oz	1	95	10%
LOBSTER BISQUE (*See* SOUP)				
LOBSTER PASTE	1 Tbs	2	39	46%
LOBSTER SALAD				
homemade-includes mayonnaise, tomato				
celery, carrots, onion, & egg	3 oz	5.5	94	53%
LOGANBERRY				
canned				
in water	½ cup	–	40	–
in heavy syrup	½ cup	–	89	–
frozen	1 cup	.5	80	56%
raw	½ lb	–	45	–
LOGANBERRY JUICE	8 oz	–	100	–
LOQUAT	1	–	5	–
	½ lb	–	84	–
LOTUS ROOT				
cooked	1 root	–	50	–
raw	1 root	–	64	–
LOTUS SEED				
dried	1 oz	.6	94	6%
	1 cup	.6	106	5%
raw	1 oz	–	25	–
LUNCHEON MEAT (*See also* BACON, HAM, SAUSAGE)				
(Armour/Armour Star)				
Canned-Deviled Ham	1.5 oz	9	110	74%
Deviled Treet	1.5 oz	10	120	75%
Potted Meat	1.5 oz	6	80	68%
Sliced Dried Beef	1 oz	2	60	30%
Vienna Sausage-in beef broth	2 oz	17	180	85%
smoked	2 oz	17	180	85%
Cold Cuts-barbecue loaf	1 oz	3	50	54%
bologna-beef	1 oz	9	100	81%
lower salt	1 oz	8	90	80%
liverwurst	1 oz	8	90	80%
Old Fashioned Loaf	1 oz	7	80	90%
Pepperoni				
Italian	1 oz	11	130	76%
Sliced	1 oz	11	130	76%
Salami				
Genoa	1 oz	10	110	82%
Hard	1 oz	10	120	75%
Italian Hard	1 oz	10	120	75%
Lower salt	1 oz	7	80	79%

Food and Description	Amount	Fat Grams	Total Calories	% Fat Calories
Sliced	1 oz	10	120	75%
Spiced Luncheon Meat				
w/chicken	3 oz	24	280	77%
regular	3 oz	25	280	80%
Summer Sausage Cheese	1 oz	8	100	72%
Turkey Bologna	2 oz	8	110	66%
Turkey Cotto Salami	2 oz	5.5	90	55%
Turkey Ham	2 oz	2	70	26%
Sausages				
links/raw	1 oz	11	110	90%
lower salt	1 oz	11	110	90%
patties/raw	1.5 oz	16	160	90%
lower salt	1.5 oz	16	160	90%
rolls/raw	1 oz	11	110	90%
lower salt	1 oz	11	110	90%
Barbeque Loaf-pork and beef	~1 oz	2.5	49	46%
(Eckrich)	1 slice/1 oz	2	35	51%
Beef				
Slender sliced (Eckrich)	1 oz	1	35	26%
Thin sliced (Carl Buddig)	1 oz	2	40	45%
Beef Loaf-jellied/(Hormel)	2 slices	4	90	40%
Beef Sausage Sticks/(Red Baron)				
smoked	1 oz	10	120	75%
Beerwurst, Beer Salami/Beef	1 slice/1 oz	6.76	75	81%
Beef & Pork (Eckrich)	1 oz	6	70	77%
(Beer Salami)	1 slice/			
	2¾" dia	1	14	64%
	1 oz	4	55	66%
Pork	1 oz	4	55	66%
Berliner/Beef, Pork	1 oz	4.88	65	68%
Blood Sausage	1 oz	9.78	107	82%
Bockwurst	1 link/~2 oz	18	200	81%
Bologna/Beef	1 oz	8	89	81%
(Eckrich)				
plain	1 slice/1 oz	8	90	80%
thick sliced	1.5 oz	12	130	83%
	1.8 oz	15	170	79%
(Health Valley)	3.5 oz	30	310	87%
(Hebrew National)-Original				
Deli style	1 oz	3	90	30%
(Hormel)	2 slices	16	170	85%
coarse ground	2 oz	14	160	79%
(Oscar Meyer)	1 oz	8	90	80%
Garlic Beef	1 oz	8	90	80%

Food and Description	Amount	Fat Grams	Total Calories	% Fat Calories
Lebanon	1 oz	3	50	54%
Bologna/Beef and Pork	1 oz	8	89	81%
(Eckrich)-w/cheese	1 slice/1 oz	9	90	90%
garlic	1 oz	9	90	90%
German Brand	1 oz	7	80	79%
Lite	1 oz	6	70	77%
plain	1 oz	9	100	81%
Sandwich	1 oz	9	100	81%
thick sliced	1 slice/ 1.7 oz	15	160	84%
(Hormel)-coarse ground	2 oz	14	160	79%
fine ground	2 oz	16	170	85%
plain	2 slices	16	180	80%
(Oscar Meyer)	1 oz	8	90	80%
w/cheese	1 oz	7	75	84%
Wisconsin Made Ring	1 oz	8	85	85%
Bologna/Chicken				
(Health Valley)	3.5 oz	30	310	87%
(Weaver)	1 slice	3.7	44	76%
Bologna/Pork	1 oz	4.6	57	73%
	1 oz	5.6	70	72%
Bologna/Turkey	2 slices/2 oz	8.6	113	69%
(Butterball)	1 slice/1 oz	6	70	77%
Deli	1 oz	6	70	77%
Slice'N Serve	1 oz	6	70	77%
variety pak	¾ oz	4	50	72%
Bratwurst/cooked-Pork	1 link/3 oz	22	256	77%
	1 oz	7	85	74%
(Eckrich)	1 link	30	310	87%
fresh (Schwan's)	1 link/4 oz	34	370	83%
Braunschweiger (Liverwurst)/Pork	1 oz	9	102	79%
(Hormel)	1 oz	7	80	79%
(Oscar Meyer)				
German Brand-tube	1 oz	8	95	76%
Liver Sausage	1 oz	9	95	85%
Brotwurst/Pork, Beef				
(w/nonfat dry milk)	1 oz	7.88	92	77%
	1 link/ ~2.5 oz	19.5	226	78%
(Butterball) Fresh Deli				
Honey Roasted Turkey Breast	1 slice	< 1	20	23%
Oven Roasted Turkey Breast	1 slice	< 1	20	23%
Smoked Chicken Breast	1 slice	< 1	20	23%
Smoked Turkey Breast	1 slice	< 1	20	23%

Food and Description	Amount	Fat Grams	Total Calories	% Fat Calories
Turkey Ham	1 slice	< 1	20	23%
Capocollo/(Hormel)-dry	1 oz	6	80	68%
Cervalat-Viking/dry (Hormel)-chub	1 oz	8	90	80%
Cheesefurter	1/1.5 oz	12.5	141	80%
Chicken/Thin sliced (Carl Buddig)	1 oz	4	60	60%
Chicken Hickory Breast/(Weaver)	1 slice	.8	26	28%
Chicken Oven Roasted Breast/ (Weaver)	1 slice	.8	25	29%
Chicken Roll-Light Meat	3 oz	6	135	40%
(Weaver)	1 slice	1.4	26	49%
Chicken Sandwich Makin's/(Hormel) canned	½ oz	2	25	72%
Chorizo Sausage	1 link/~2 oz	23	273	76%
Corned Beef				
Slender sliced (Eckrich)	1 oz	1	40	23%
Thin sliced (Carl Buddig)	1 oz	2	40	45%
Corned Beef Loaf/canned (Libby's)	2.3 oz	9	160	51%
Cotto Salami				
(Eckrich)	1 slice/1 oz	6	70	77%
Beef	1 slice/1 oz	8	100	72%
(Hormel)	2 slices	7	105	60%
dried chub	1 oz	9	100	81%
Dutch Brand Loaf	1 oz	5	68	66%
(Gallo Salame) 96% fat free				
Deli Style				
Ham/Smoked	1 slice	< 1	10	45%
Italian Dry Salame	1 slice	1	14	64%
Pastrami	1 slice	< 1	12	38%
Turkey Breast	1 slice	< 1	10	45%
Genoa Salami-dry/(Hormel)	1 oz	10	110	82%
Di Lusso	1 oz	8	100	72%
Gran Valore	1 oz	10	110	82%
San Remo Brand	1 oz	10	118	76%
Gourmet Loaf/(Eckrich)	1 slice/1 oz	1	30	30%
Ham-Pork				
Boiled	3/4 oz	1	25	36%
Boneless-Prosciutto (Hormel)-dry	1 oz	7	90	70%
Chopped				
(Eckrich)	1 slice/1 oz	2	45	40%
(Hormel)	2 slices	5	88	51%
Chopped-canned	1.5 oz	5	68	66%
(Hormel)-12 oz can	2 oz	9	120	68%
Chopped-spiced/canned	1.5 oz	5	68	66%
Cooked-Lite (Eckrich)	1 oz	1	25	36%

Food and Description	Amount	Fat Grams	Total Calories	% Fat Calories
Danish (Danola)				
sliced 98% fat free	2 slices	.5	45	10%
Deviled/canned	3.5 oz	32	348	83%
(Libby's)	1.5 oz	11	130	76%
(Hormel)	1 Tbs	3	35	77%
(Underwood)	2.25 oz	20	220	82%
Hostess (Swift Premiium)	1 oz	1	30	30%
Loaf (Eckrich)	1 slice/1 oz	4	50	72%
Minced	1 oz	5.86	75	70%
Patties (Hormel)	1 patty	16	180	80%
Slender sliced (Eckrich)	1 oz	2	40	45%
Sliced (extra lean 5% fat)	1 oz	1.5	37	37%
Sliced (regular 11% fat)	1 oz	3	52	52%
Sliced w/black cracked pepper/pkg	¾ oz	.9	24	34%
Smoked (97% fat free)	2 slices/			
	~.5 oz	1.5	20	68%
Spiced/(Hormel)	3 oz	21	240	79%
Thin sliced (Carl Buddig)	1 oz	3	50	54%
Ham and Cheese Loaf or Roll	1 oz	5.7	73	70%
(Eckrich)	1 oz	4	50	72%
(Hormel)	3 oz	22	260	76%
	2 slices	7	110	57%
Ham and Cheese Patties/(Hormel)	1 patty	18	190	85%
Ham and Cheese Spread	1 Tbs	2.78	37	68%
Ham Salad Spread	1 oz	4	61	59%
	1 Tbs	2	32	56%
Headcheese/Pork	1 oz	4	60	60%
(Hillshire Farm)				
Bologna				
large	1 oz	8	90	80%
ring	1 oz	8	89	81%
Deli Select				
Cajun Ham	1 oz	< 1	31	15%
Corned Beef	1 oz	< 1	31	15%
Honey Ham	1 oz	< 1	31	15%
Oven Roasted Cured Beef	1 oz	< 1	31	15%
Oven Roasted Turkey Breast	1 oz	< 1	31	15%
Pastrami	1 oz	< 1	30	15%
Smoked Chicken Breast	1 oz	< 1	31	15%
Smoked Beef	1 oz	< 1	31	15%
Smoked Ham	1 oz	< 1	31	15%
Smoked Turkey Breast	1 oz	< 1	31	15%
Flavorseal				
Beef & Cheddar	2 oz	15	190	71%

Food and Description	Amount	Fat Grams	Total Calories	% Fat Calories
Beef Polska Kielbasa	2 oz	17	190	81%
Beef Smoked Sausage	2 oz	16	180	80%
Country Recipe	2 oz	16	180	80%
Hot Smoked Sausage	2 oz	16	180	80%
Lite Polska Kielbasa	2 oz	13	160	73%
Lite Smoked Sausage	2 oz	13	160	73%
Mild Polska Kielbasa	2 oz	17	190	81%
Polska Kielbasa	2 oz	17	190	81%
Smoked Sausage	2 oz	17	190	81%
Smoked Sausage-Italian	2 oz	18	200	81%
Links				
Beef Hot Links	2 oz	17	190	81%
Bun Size Beef Wieners	2 oz	16	180	80%
Bun Size Beef Smoked Sausage	2 oz	16	180	80%
Bun Size Cheddarwurst	2 oz	18	200	81%
Bun Size Cheese Wieners	2 oz	16	180	80%
Bun Size Kielbasa	2 oz	16	180	80%
Bun Size Smoked Sausage	2 oz	16	180	80%
Bun Size Wieners	2 oz	16	180	80%
Cheddarwurst	2 oz	17	190	81%
Fresh Bratwurst	2 oz	17	190	81%
Fully Cooked Brats	2 oz	16	170	85%
Hot Italian Sausage	2 oz	17	180	85%
Hot Links	2 oz	16	190	76%
Knockwurst	2 oz	16	180	80%
Mild Italian Sausage	2 oz	17	190	81%
Natural Casing Wieners	2 oz	17	180	85%
Polish Sausage Links	2 oz	17	190	81%
Polska Kielbasa Links	2 oz	17	190	81%
Smoked Bratwurst	2 oz	17	190	81%
Smoked Sausage Links	2 oz	18	190	85%
Spicy Bratwurst	2 oz	17	180	85%
Semi-Dry Sausage				
Beef Summer Sausage	2 oz	17	190	81%
Summer Sausage	2 oz	16	180	80%
Summer Sausage w/ Cheese	2 oz	18	200	81%
Thuringer	2 oz	15	180	75%
Honey Loaf/Pork, Beef	1 oz	1	36	25%
(Eckrich)	1 oz	1	35	26%
(Hormel)	2 slices	5	90	50%
Honey Roll Sausage/Beef	1 oz	2.98	52	52%
Iowa Brand Loaf/(Hormel)	2 slices	6	90	60%
Italian Sausage/Pork-raw	3 oz	28.5	315	81%
/Pork-cooked	3 oz	21	268	71%

Food and Description	Amount	Fat Grams	Total Calories	% Fat Calories
(Kahn's)				
Family Pack				
Beef Bologna	1 slice	6	70	77%
Beef Pickle	1 slice	5	60	75%
Beef Salami	1 slice	5	60	75%
Beef Spice	1 slice	5	60	75%
Cotto Salami	1 slice	3	45	60%
Deluxe Club Bologna	1 slice	6	70	77%
Pickle Loaf	1 slice	6	70	77%
Spice Loaf	1 slice	6	70	77%
Links				
Beef Frank	1	13	140	84%
Beef n'Cheddar Frank	1	16	180	80%
Big Red Smokey	1	14	170	74%
Bratwurst	1	17	190	81%
Bun Size Beef Frank	1	17	190	81%
Bun Size Beef Smokey	1	17	190	81%
Bun Size Frank	1	17	190	81%
Bun Size Polska	1	17	190	81%
Cheese Wiener	1	13	150	78%
Jumbo Beef Frank	1	18	190	85%
Jumbo Frank	1	17	190	81%
Wieners	1	13	140	84%
Sliced Pack Luncheon Meats				
Beef Bologna-8 oz	1 slice	8	90	80%
Beef n'Cheddar Bologna-8 oz	1 slice	8	90	80%
Beef Pounder	1 slice	8	90	80%
Beef Salami-8 oz	1 slice	6	70	77%
Chopped Ham-8 oz	1 slice	3	50	54%
Cooked Ham-5 oz	1 slice	1	30	30%
Cooked Salami-8 oz	1 slice	4	60	60%
Deluxe Club Bologna-8 oz	1 slice	8	90	80%
Deluxe Club Pounder	1 slice	8	90	80%
Dutch Loaf-8 oz	1 slice	7	80	79%
Garlic Bologna-8 oz	1 slice	8	90	80%
Giant Beef Bologna-12 oz	1 slice	8	90	80%
Giant Deluxe-12 oz	1 slice	8	90	80%
Giant Thick Deluxe-12 oz	1 slice	10	110	82%
Ham & Cheese Loaf	1 slice	6	70	77%
Ham Bologna-12 oz	1 slice	8	90	80%
Honey Loaf-8 oz	1 slice	2	40	45%
Jalapeno Loaf-8 oz	1 slice	6	70	77%
Liver Loaf	1 slice	15	170	79%
Low Salt Ham-5 oz	1 slice	1	30	30%

Food and Description	Amount	Fat Grams	Total Calories	% Fat Calories
P & B Loaf-8 oz	1 slice	2	40	45%
Pepper Loaf-8 oz	1 slice	2	40	45%
Pickle Loaf-8 oz	1 slice	7	80	79%
Souse Loaf-8 oz	1 slice	7	90	70%
Spiced Luncheon Loaf-8 oz	1 slice	7	80	79%
Thick Deluxe-8 oz	1 slice	13	140	84%
Thin Sliced Deluxe-8 oz	1 slice	5	60	75%
Kielbasa, Kalbassy Sausage/				
Pork or Beef	1 oz	7.7	88	79%
(Hormel)-skinless	½ link	14	180	70%
Polska (Eckrich)-Lite	1 oz	6	70	77%
Skinless	1 oz	16	180	80%
Polska (Louis Rich)-turkey	1 oz	3	50	54%
Knackwurst, Knockwurst-Pork, Beef	1 oz	7.87	87	81%
(Best's)-Beef Lower Fat	3 oz	16	210	69%
(Hebrew National)-Beef	3 oz	25	260	87%
Kolbase Polish Sausage/(Hormel)	3 oz	19	220	78%
Lebanon Bologna/Beef	1 oz	4	64	56%
Light & Lean (Hormel) Lunch Meats				
BBQ Ham	2 slices	2	50	36%
Black Peppered Ham	2 slices	2	50	36%
Bologna	2 slices	12	140	77%
Bologna-thin sliced	2 slices	6	70	77%
Breast of Turkey	2 slices	2	60	30%
Canadian Style Bacon	2 slices	1	35	26%
Chopped Ham	2 slices	4	70	51%
Cooked Ham	2 slices	2	50	36%
Cotto Salami	2 slices	6	80	68%
Glazed Ham	2 slices	2	50	36%
Ham & Cheese Loaf	2 slices	6	90	60%
New England Brand Luncheon Meat	2 slices	6	90	60%
Pickle Loaf	2 slices	6	100	54%
Red Peppered Ham	2 slices	2	50	36%
Smoked Cooked Ham	2 slices	2	50	36%
Spiced Luncheon Meat	2 slices	9	120	68%
Summer Sausage	2 slices	8	100	72%
Liver Cheese/Pork	1 oz	7	86	73%
Liver Loaf/(Hormel)	2 slices	13	160	73%
Liver Sausage, Liverwurst/Pork	1 oz	8	93	77%
(Oscar Meyer)				
sliced	1 oz	9	95	85%
tube	1 oz	9	95	85%
(Louis Rich)-Cold Cuts				
Chopped Turkey Ham	1 slice	2	40	45%

Food and Description	Amount	Fat Grams	Total Calories	% Fat Calories
Deluxe Oven Roasted				
Chicken Breast	1 slice	1	30	30%
Hickory Smoked Chicken Breast	1 slice	1	30	30%
Hickory Smoked Turkey Breast-				
92% fat free	1 slice	< 1	20	23%
Honey Cured Turkey Ham	1 slice	.5	25	18%
Honey Roasted Turkey Breast	1 slice	1	30	30%
Mild Turkey Bologna	1 slice	5	60	75%
Oven Roasted Turkey Breast	1 slice	1	30	30%
Oven Roasted White Chicken	1 slice	2	40	45%
Smoked Turkey	1 slice	1	30	30%
Smoked Turkey Breast	1 slice	.5	20	23%
Turkey Bologna	1 slice	5	60	75%
82% fat free	1 slice	4	45	80%
Turkey Cotto Salami	1 slice	4	50	72%
86% fat free	1 slice	3	40	68%
Turkey Ham-round	1 slice	1	35	26%
square 96% fat free	1 slice	< 1	25	18%
Turkey Luncheon Loaf	1 slice	3	45	60%
Turkey Pastrami-round	1 slice	1	35	26%
Turkey Pastrami-square	1 slice	.5	25	18%
Turkey Salami	1 slice	4	55	66%
Turkey Summer Sausage	1 slice	4	55	66%
Lumberjack Beef Roll-dry/(Hormel)	1 oz	9	101	80%
Luncheon meat, beef-sliced thin	1 oz	.9	35	23%
smoked beef (97% fat free)	2 slices			
	~.5 oz	1.5	20	68%
spiced (Hormel)				
canned	3 oz	26	280	84%
pkg	2 slices	9	118	69%
Luncheon Loaf/chicken (Hormel)-				
canned	2 oz	10	130	69%
Luxury Loaf	1 oz	1	40	23%
Macaroni-Cheese Loaf/(Eckrich)	1 oz/			
	1 slice	6	75	72%
Minced Roll Sausage/(Eckrich)	1 oz/			
	1 slice	7	80	79%
Mortadella/Beef, Pork	1 oz	7	88	72%
Mother's Loaf	1 oz	6	80	68%
New England Brand Sausage	1 oz	2	46	39%
Old Fashioned Loaf/Pork and Beef	1 oz	5	68	66%
(Eckrich)	1 oz	6	70	77%
Olive Loaf/Beef & Pork-(Eckrich)	1 oz	6	80	68%

Food and Description	Amount	Fat Grams	Total Calories	% Fat Calories
Pork	1 oz	4.68	67	63%
(Hormel)	2 slices	7	110	57%
(Oscar Meyer) Cold Cuts				
Bar-B-Que Loaf-93% fat free	1 slice	2	50	36%
Beef-smoked-97% fat-free	1 slice	.5	15	30%
Chicken Breast-oven roasted-97% fat-free	1 slice	.5	30	15%
Chicken Breast-smoked-97% fat-free	1 slice	.5	25	18%
Chopped Ham w/natural juices	1 slice	4	55	66%
Corned Beef-98% fat-free	1 slice	.5	15	30%
Corned Beef Loaf, jellied-93% fat-free	1 slice	2	40	45%
Cotto Salami	1 slice	4	55	66%
Cotto Salami-beef	1 slice	3	45	60%
Genoa Salami	1 slice	3	35	77%
Ham-baked w/natural juices-97% fat-free	1 slice	.5	20	23%
Ham-boiled w/natural juices-95% fat-free	1 slice	.5	25	18%
Ham-chopped peppered w/natural juices	1 slice	4	55	66%
Ham-Cracked Black Pepper-95% fat-free	1 slice	1	25	36%
Ham-Honey w/natural juices-95% fat-free	1 slice	1	25	36%
Ham-Lower Salt-95% fat free-water added	1 slice	1	25	36%
Ham-Smoked Cooked-95% fat-free	1 slice	1	25	36%
Ham & Cheese Loaf	1 slice	6	75	72%
Head Cheese	1 slice	4	55	66%
Honey Loaf-95% fat-free	1 slice	1	35	26%
Honey Roll Sausage-beef-90% fat-free	1 slice	2	35	51%
Jalapeno Loaf	1 slice	6	70	77%
Liver Cheese, pork fat wrapped	1 slice	10	115	78%
Luncheon Meat	1 slice	9	100	90%
Luxury Loaf-95% fat-free	1 slice	1	40	23%
New England Brand Sausage-92% fat-free	1 slice	2	30	60%
Old Fashioned Loaf	1 slice	4	65	55%
Olive Loaf	1 slice	4	60	60%
Pastrami-97% fat free	1 slice	.5	15	30%
Peppered Loaf-93% fat-free	1 slice	2	40	45%
Pickle & Pimento Loaf	1 slice	4	65	55%
Picnic Loaf	1 slice	4	60	60%
Salami for Beer	1 slice	5	55	82%

Food and Description	Amount	Fat Grams	Total Calories	% Fat Calories
Salami for Beer-beef	1 slice	6	65	83%
Salami-beef-Machiaeh Brand	1 slice	5	60	75%
Salami-hard	1 slice	3	35	77%
Summer sausage-Thuringer Cervelat	1 slice	6	75	72%
Summer sausage-beef-Thuringer Cervelat	1 slice	6	70	77%
Thin Sliced meats-96% fat free				
Boiled Ham	1 slice	< 1	12	38%
Honey Ham	1 slice	< 1	14	32%
Roast Beef	1 slice	< 1	14	32%
Roast Chicken	1 slice	< 1	14	32%
Roast Turkey	1 slice	< 1	12	38%
Turkey Breast-oven roasted-97% fat-free	1 slice	.5	20	23%
Turkey Breast-smoked-98% fat free	1 slice	.5	20	23%
(Oscar Meyer) Lunchables				
Bologna & American	1 pkg	33	460	65%
Ham & Swiss	1 pkg	19	340	50%
Lean Chicken & Lean Turkey	1 pkg	24	4220	51%
Lean Turkey & Lean Ham	1 pkg	21	390	48%
Salami & Mozzerella	1 pkg	29	420	62%
Pastrami				
Beef	1 oz	8	99	73%
Thin sliced (Carl Buddig)	1 oz	2	40	45%
Turkey	2 oz	3.5	80	39%
Pate-Chicken Liver/canned	1 Tbs	1.7	26	59%
	1 oz	3.7	57	58%
Pate-generic/canned	1 oz	7.9	90	79%
Pate-Goose Liver (de fois gras)/canned	1 Tbs	5.7	60	86%
	1 oz	12	131	82%
smoked-canned	1 oz	12	131	82%
Peppered Loaf/Beef, Pork	1 oz	1.8	42	39%
(Eckrich)	1 slice/1 oz	1	35	26%
Pepperoni/Pork, Beef)	~ 9 oz	110	1248	79%
	1 oz	12	135	80%
(Hormel)	2 slices	7	80	79%
Bits	1 Tbs	3	35	77%
dry	1 oz	13	140	84%
chunk-chub	1 oz	12	140	77%
Leoni Brand	1 oz	12	130	83%
Rosa	1 oz	13	140	84%
Rosa Grande	1 oz	13	140	84%
Pickle Loaf				
(Eckrich)	1oz/1 slice	6	80	68%

Food and Description	Amount	Fat Grams	Total Calories	% Fat Calories
(Hormel)	2 slices	7	102	62%
Pickle and Pimento Loaf/Pork	1 oz	5.99	74	73%
Picnic Loaf/Pork, Beef	1 oz	4.7	66	64%
Polish Sausage/Pork	1 oz	8	92	78%
10" long-1.5" dia	1 sausage	6.5	74	79%
	1 oz	8	92	78%
frozen (Schwan's)	1 link/2.7 oz	24	260	83%
(Hormel)	2 sausages	14	170	74%
(Oscar Meyer)-International	~ 2.5 oz	20	230	78%
Pork/Slender sliced (Eckrich)	1 oz	2	45	40%
Pork Luncheon Meat/(Hormel)-canned	3 oz	21	240	79%
Pork and Beef Luncheon Sausage	~ 1 oz	4.8	60	72%
Potted Meat/(Hormel)	1 Tbs	2	30	60%
(Libby's)	1.83 oz	9	100	81%
Salami/cooked-Beef	1 oz	5.9	74	72%
(Hormel)	2 slices	5	50	90%
cooked-Beef and Pork	1 oz	5.7	71	72%
cooked-Turkey	2 oz	7.8	111	63%
hard (Hormel)	2 slices	7	80	79%
dry	1 oz	10	110	82%
(Health Valley)	3.5 oz	35	400	79%
(Hebrew National)-beef-original deli style	1 oz	7	80	79%
party-dry (Hormel)	1 oz	8	90	80%
Piccolo-dry stick (Hormel)	1 oz	11	120	83%
Salami/Pork-dry or hard	2 slices/ ~1 oz	7	85	74%
Salt Pork/raw	1 oz	22.8	212	97%
Sandwich Spread/Pork, Beef	1 Tbs	3	35	77%
Sausage/Beef-smoked-(Eckrich)	1 oz	9	100	81%
Beef & Pork-smoked links	1 link/~.5 oz	4.9	54	82%
Brown'N Serve-(Hormel)-cooked	2	13	140	84%
uncooked	2	17	180	85%
smoked skinless (Eckrich)	1 oz	16	180	80%
New England Brand-(Eckrich)	1 slice/1 oz	1	35	26%
Patties (Hormel)-canned-hot	1 pattie	13	150	78%
mild	1 pattie	13	150	78%
Pork-fresh-cooked	~ 1 oz	8	100	72%
Pork-(Hormel)				
Little Sizzlers-cooked	2	9	103	79%
Midget Links	2	13	143	82%
Pork-smoked links	1 link/~.5 oz	5	62	73%
Smoked (Eckrich)-Lite	1 link	13	150	78%
	1 oz	6	70	77%

Food and Description	Amount	Fat Grams	Total Calories	% Fat Calories
Smoked (Oscar Meyer)-				
International	1 oz	7	83	76%
Smoked pork (Hormel)	3 oz	27	290	84%
Smoked turkey (Butterball)	1 oz	4	50	72%
Smoked turkey (Louis Rich)	1 oz	3	50	54%
Smoked turkey (Louis Rich)				
w/cheese	1 oz	4	55	66%
Smokie Cheezers (Hormel)	2 sausages	15	168	80%
Smokie Links (Oscar Meyer)	~ 1.5oz	11	125	79%
Smokies-Beef (Oscar Meyer)	~ 1.5 oz	11	125	79%
Smokies-Cheese (Oscar Meyer)	~ 1.5 oz	11	125	79%
Smokies-Little (Oscar Meyer)	9 grams	3	30	90%
Smokies Smoked (Hormel)	2 sausages	14	160	79%
Scrapple	1 oz	4	61	59%
Smok-Y-Links/(Eckrich)				
Beef	2 links	14	160	79%
Cheese	2 links	14	160	79%
Ham	2 links	15	160	84%
Hot	2 links	14	150	84%
Lite	2 links	10	120	75%
Maple-flavored	2 links	14	160	79%
Original	2 links	14	160	79%
Souse	1 slice/1 oz	3.8	51	67%
Spam/(Hormel)-deviled	1 Tbs	3	35	77%
luncheon	1¾ oz	14	150	84%
	2 oz	15	170	79%
smoke-flavored	2 oz	15	170	79%
with cheese chunks	2 oz	15	170	79%
Spam lite (Hormel)	2 oz	12	140	77%
Spreads				
Chicken-canned	1 oz	3	55	49%
Chicken (Hormel)	½ oz	2	30	60%
Chicken (Swanson)-chunky	1 oz	4	60	60%
Chicken (Underwood)-chunky	½ can/			
	2.4 oz	11	150	66%
Corned Beef (Hormel)	½ oz	3	35	77%
(Underwood)	2.25 oz	10	120	75%
Liverwurst (Hormel)	½ oz	3	35	77%
(Underwood)	2.25 oz	16	190	76%
Roast Beef (Hormel)	½ oz	2	31	58%
(Underwood)	2.4 oz	10	140	64%
The Spreadables (Carnation)				
Chicken Salad	2 oz	6	100	54%
Ham Salad	2 oz	6	100	54%

Food and Description	Amount	Fat Grams	Total Calories	% Fat Calories
Tuna Salad	2 oz	6	90	60%
Turkey Salad	2 oz	6	100	54%
Summer Sausage				
Beef	~ 1 oz	7.6	86	80%
Beef & Pork (Eckrich)	1 slice/1 oz	7	90	70%
(Hormel)	2 slices	11	140	71%
beefy dry	1 oz	9	100	81%
Tangy dry chub	1 oz	7	90	70%
Thuringer dry	1 oz	9	90	90%
Turkey	1 slice/1 oz	3.5	52	61%
Thuringer				
Cervelat	1 oz	8.5	98	78%
Old Smokehouse				
chub	1 oz	9	100	81%
dry (Hormel)	1 oz	8	90	80%
sliced	1 oz	9	100	81%
Turkey Breast Meat	~ 1.5 oz	.67	47	13%
(Butterball)				
honey roasted 97% fat free	¾ oz	1	30	30%
oven roasted	1 slice/1 oz	1	30	30%
smoked	1 slice/1 oz	1	35	26%
smoked 97% fat free	¾ oz	1	25	36%
(Eckrich)-Lite-oven roasted	1 oz	1	30	30%
Lite-smoked	1 oz	.5	30	15%
(Hormel)	2 slices	2	60	30%
smoked	2 slices	2	60	30%
(Weaver)	1 slice	< 1	20	23%
Turkey Ham	2 oz	2.88	73	36%
(Butterball)-chopped	1 slice/1 oz	1	35	26%
cold cuts	1 slice/1 oz	1	35	26%
Deli thin	1 oz	1	35	26%
honey cured	1 slice/1 oz	1	35	26%
(Carl Buddig)-Thin sliced	1 oz	2	40	45%
(Weaver)	1 slice	1	23	39%
Turkey Pastrami/(Butterball)				
cold cuts	1 slice/1 oz	1	30	30%
Deli	1 oz	1	35	26%
Slice'N Serve	1 oz	1	35	26%
Turkey Roll/Light and Dark Meat	1 oz	1.98	42	42%
Turkey Roll/Light Meat	1 oz	2	42	43%
Turkey Salami				
(Butterball)	1 slice/1 oz	4	50	72%
Deli	1 oz	4	50	72%
Slice'N Serve	1 oz	4	50	72%

Food and Description	Amount	Fat Grams	Total Calories	% Fat Calories
variety pak	¾ oz	3	40	90%
(Carl Buddig)-Thin sliced	1 oz	2	40	45%
Turkey/Slender sliced (Eckrich)	1 oz	2	45	40%
Thin sliced (Carl Buddig)	1 oz	2	40	45%
Turkey/Smoked (Butterball)-variety pak	¾ oz	1	25	36%
Turkey Spread	~ 2 oz	6	100	54%
Vienna Sausage/canned-beef and pork	1 sausage	4	45	80%
	7 sausages	28	315	80%
(Hormel)-no broth	4 sausages	18	200	81%
(Libby)-in barbeque sauce in Beef Broth	2.5 oz	15	180	75%
5 oz can	3½ links	15	160	84%
9 oz can	3½ links	14	160	79%
canned-chicken (Hormel)	4 sausages	16	180	80%
canned-chicken (Libby)	2 oz	9.6	123	70%
LUPINS				
boiled	½ cup	2	98	18%
raw	½ cup	8	330	22%

M

Food and Description	Amount	Fat Grams	Total Calories	% Fat Calories
MACADAMIA NUT				
dried	1 oz	20.9	199	95%
dry roasted	1 oz	21	193	98%
oil roasted	1 oz	21.7	204	96%
MACARONI (*See* PASTA)				
MACARONI AND CHEESE (*See also* PASTA DINNERS)				
Canned	1 cup	9.6	228	38%
(Franco-American) frozen	7 oz	9	220	37%
(Golden Grain) dry	1.81 oz	2	190	10%
prepared	½ cup	15	300	45%
Standard Home Recipe (USDA)	1 cup	22	430	46%
(Swanson's) frozen	10 oz	21	400	47%
MACARONI SALAD/canned (Joan of Arc)	½ cup	13	200	59%
MACE/ground	1 tsp	.6	8	68%
MACKEREL				
Atlantic				
raw	3 oz	11.8	174	61%

Food and Description	Amount	Fat Grams	Total Calories	% Fat Calories
cooked-dry heat	3 oz	15	223	61%
Jack-canned	1 cup	11.97	296	36%
King-raw	3 oz	1.7	89	17%
Spanish				
cooked-dry heat	3 oz	5	134	34%
raw	3 oz	5	118	38%
MALT (See MILK MIXES and individual FAST FOOD listings)				
MAMEY or MAMMEE APPLE/raw	1	4	431	8%
	~3.5 oz	–	51	–
MANDARIN ORANGE				
canned in juice	1 cup	–	92	–
canned in light syrup	1 cup	.5	125	4%
(Del Monte)	5.5 oz	< 1	100	5%
(Dole)-light syrup	½ cup	< 1	76	6%
(Nutradiet)	½ cup	–	28	–
(S&W)				
natural style	½ cup	–	60	–
sections in heavy syrup	½ cup	< 1	76	6%
MANDARIN TANGERINE JUICE (See TANGERINE JUICE)				
MANGO	1	.57	135	4%
diced/sliced	1 cup	.7	109	6%
MANGO JUICE				
Mango Nectar (Kern's)	6 oz	–	110	–
MANICOTTI/homemade	1 cup	16	365	40%
MANICOTTI W/MEAT SAUCE				
Standard Home Recipe (USDA)	~ 5 oz	11	235	42%
MARGARINE				
(Imperial) Savory Squeeze				
Buttery	1 Tbs	10	90	100%
Garlic & Herb	1 Tbs	10	90	100%
(Land O'Lakes)				
Premium Corn Oil	1 tsp	4	35	100%
Soy oil-regular	1 tsp	4	35	100%
Liquid	1 tsp	3.8	34	100%
Regular-80% fat (hard)	1 Tbs	11	100	100%
	1 Pat	4	35	100%
(soft)	1 Tbs	11	100	100%
Spread-40% fat (soft)	1 Tbs	5.7	50	100%
60% fat (hard)	1 Tbs	9	75	100%
	1 Pat	3	25	100%
(soft)	1 Tbs	9	75	100%
(Touch of Butter) spread/stick	1 Tbs	10	90	100%
LIQUID	1 tsp	3.8	34	100%
(Country Crock)	1 Tbs	9	80	100%

Food and Description	Amount	Fat Grams	Total Calories	% Fat Calories
(Fleischmann's)	1 Tbs	10	90	100%
Squeeze (Parkay)				
Regular	1 Tbs	11	100	100%
Spread	1 Tbs	10	90	100%
REDUCED CALORIE				
(Blue Bonnet)	1 Tbs	6	50	100%
(Fleischmann's)	1 Tbs	6	50	100%
(Imperial)	1 Tbs	6	50	100%
(Mazola)				
Light Corn Oil	1 Tbs	6	50	100%
Regular	1 Tbs	6	50	100%
(Parkay)	1 Tbs	6	50	100%
(Weight Watchers)	1 Tbs	6	50	100%
REGULAR				
(Blue Bonnet) Soft or Stick	1 Tbs	11	100	100%
(Chiffon)				
Soft stick	1 Tbs	11	100	100%
Soft tub	1 Tbs	10	90	100%
(Fleischmann's) Soft or Stick	1 Tbs	11	100	100%
Generic				
Hard	1 Tbs	11	100	100%
	1 Pat	4	35	100%
	4 oz	91	810	100%
Soft	1 Tbs	11	100	100%
	4 oz	92	813	100%
(Gold-N-Sweet)/Canola	1 Tbs	11	100	100%
(Hain)/Safflower	1 Tbs	11	100	100%
(Heartlight)/Canola	1 Tbs	11	100	100%
(Imperial)/soft	1 Tbs	11	100	100%
(Land O'Lakes) Soft or Stick	1 tsp	4	35	100%
(Mazola)	1 Tbs	11	100	100%
(Nucoa) Soft	1 Tbs	11	100	100%
No burn	1 Tbs	11	100	100%
(Parkay) Soft or Stick	1 Tbs	11	100	100%
(Promise)	1 Tbs	10	90	100%
SPREAD				
(Autumn)	1 Tbs	8	80	100%
(Blue Bonnet)				
52% fat	1 Tbs	8	80	100%
75% fat	1 Tbs	11	90	100%
(Fleischmann's)Light Corn Oil				
Soft or Stick	1 Tbs	8	80	100%
Generic				
40% fat/soft	1 Tbs	5.7	50	100%
	4 oz	44	393	100%

Food and Description	Amount	Fat Grams	Total Calories	% Fat Calories
60% fat				
Hard	1 Pat	3	25	100%
	1 Tbs	9	75	100%
	4 oz	69	610	100%
Soft	1 Tbs	9	75	100%
	4 oz	69	613	100%
(Gregg's) Gold-n-Soft-Lite	1 Tbs	7	70	100%
I Can't Believe It's Not Butter	1 Tbs	10	90	100%
(Imperial)-Light	1 Tbs	6	60	100%
(Kraft)-Touch of Butter				
40% fat-Tub	1 Tbs	6	50	100%
50% fat-Stick	1 Tbs	7	60	100%
(Land O'Lakes)				
Stick	1 tsp	4	30	100%
Tub	1 tsp	3	25	100%
(Nucoa)-Heart Beat-corn oil	1 Tbs	3	25	100%
(Parkay)				
50% vegetable oil	1 Tbs	7	60	100%
Light Corn Oil	1 Tbs	8	70	100%
(Promise)/Sunflower oil	1 Tbs	10	90	100%
Extra Light	1 Tbs	6	50	100%
(Shedd's)-Corn Oil	1 Tbs	7	70	100%
Country Crock	1 Tbs	7	70	100%
(Weight Watcher's)-Lite	1 Tbs	6	50	100%
WHIPPED				
(Blue Bonnet)				
Soft	1 Tbs	7	70	100%
Stick	1 Tbs	7	70	100%
(Chiffon)	1 Tbs	8	70	100%
(Fleischmann's)	1 Tbs	7	70	100%
Generic/hard & soft	1 Tbs	7	70	100%
(Miracle Brand)				
Soft	1 Tbs	7	60	100%
Stick	1 Tbs	7	70	100%
(Parkay)				
Soft or Stick	1 Tbs	7	60	100%
MARINADE MIX				
(Durkee)	½ cup	.7	28	23%
(French's)	⅛ pkg	–	10	–
(Kikkoman)	1 oz pkg	–	64	–
MARINARA SAUCE (See SAUCE)				
MARIONBERRIES				
frozen (Schwan's)-no sugar	3.5 oz	–	60	–
MARJORAM/dried	1 tsp	–	2	–

Food and Description	Amount	Fat Grams	Total Calories	% Fat Calories
MARSHMALLOW				
(Campfire)				
large	2	–	40	–
miniature	10	–	17	–
	24	–	40	–
(Kraft)				
Funmallows	1	–	30	–
miniature	10	–	18	–
Jet Puffed	1	–	25	–
miniature	10	–	18	–
Marshmallow Creme-(Kraft)	1 oz	–	90	–
Miniature or large	1 oz	–	94	–
MATZO				
(Goodman's)				
Passover Egg	1 piece	1	132	7%
Passover	1 piece	–	129	
(Manischewitz)				
American	1 board	1.9	115	15%
Egg n/Onion	1 board	1	112	8%
Miniatures	15-20 crackers	.5	90	5%
Passover	1 board	–	129	
Passover Egg	10 crackers	2	108	17%
Passover Egg	1 board	2	132	14%
Thin Salted	1 board	–	100	–
Thin Tea (Daily)	1 board	–	103	–
Thins, dietic	1 board	1	91	10%
Unsalted (Daily)	1 board	–	110	–
Wheat	10 crackers	1	90	10%
Whole Wheat w/bran	1 board	.6	110	5%
MATZO MEAL				
Goodman's Passover	1 cup	1	514	2%
Manischewitz	1 cup	1	510	2%
MAYONNAISE (*See also* SALAD DRESSING)				
Bama-Regular	1 Tbs	11	100	100%
Bennett's-Real	1 Tbs	12	110	98%
Best Foods				
Light	1 Tbs	5	50	90%
Real	1 Tbs	11	100	99%
Estee	1 Tbs	10	100	90%
(Hain)				
Eggless	1 Tbs	12	110	98%
Light	1 Tbs	6	60	90%
Real	1 Tbs	12	110	98%
Safflower	1 Tbs	12	110	98%

Food and Description	Amount	Fat Grams	Total Calories	% Fat Calories
Heart Beat/corn oil	1 Tbs	4	40	90%
Hellman's	1 Tbs	11	100	100%
Hollywood/safflower	1 Tbs	12	110	98%
Kraft				
Cholesterol free	1 Tbs	10	90	100%
Kraft free	1 Tbs	–	12	–
Light	1 Tbs	5	45	100%
Regular	1 Tbs	12	100	100%
Life All Natural/egg-free	1 Tbs	8	70	100%
Miracle Whip Free	1 Tbs	–	20	–
Weight Watchers				
Regular	1 Tbs	4	40	90%
Whipped	1 Tbs	3	35	77%
MEAT SEASONING				
(Durkee)				
Beef Stew				
dry	1 pkg	.5	99	5%
prepared	8 cups	192	3032	57%
Ground Beef				
dry	1 pkg	.9	91	9%
prepared	2 cups	97	1037	81%
Ground Beef w/Onion				
dry	1 pkg		102	4%
prepared	2 cups	96	1318	66%
Hamburger				
dry	1 pkg	5	110	41%
prepared	2 cups	101	1326	69%
Italian Meatball				
dry	1 pkg	.7	22	29%
prepared	2 cups	97	1238	71%
Italian Sloppy Joe				
dry	1 pkg	5	99	46%
prepared	2½ cups	102	1492	62%
Sloppy Joe				
dry	1 pkg	–	118	–
prepared	2½ cups	97	1453	60%
(French's)				
Seasoning Mix dry				
Beef Stew	⅙ pkg	–	25	–
Ground Beef w/Onions	¼ pkg	–	25	–
Hamburger	¼ pkg	–	25	–
Meatball	¼ pkg	–	35	–
Meatloaf	⅛ pkg	–	20	–
Sloppy Joes	⅛ pkg	–	16	–

Food and Description	Amount	Fat Grams	Total Calories	% Fat Calories
(Lipton)				
Microeasy Family Favorites-dry				
Hearty Beef Stew-dry	¼ pkg	.5	70	6%
Homestyle Meatloaf	¼ pkg	1.5	87	16%
(Manwich)				
Sloppy Joe Seasoning Mix-dry	⅙ pkg	.5	20	23%
(McCormick/Schilling)				
Bag'N Season-dry				
Pork Chops	1 pkg	< 1	103	4%
Pot Roast	1 pkg	.6	55	10%
(Oven Fry) coating for Pork-Extra Crispy	¼ pouch	3	120	23%
(Shake & Bake) coatings-For Pork				
Original Barbecue Recipe	¼ pouch	2	80	23%
Original Recipe	¼ pouch	1	80	11%
MEAT SUBSTITUTES (See also VEGETARIAN FOOD)				
Nut Meat	2.5 oz	10	150	60%
Tender Cuts	2.3 oz	1	55	16%
MEAT TENDERIZER/seasoned	1 tsp	–	2	–
MEATLESS LOAF	1 oz	.7	90	7%
MEATLOAF				
Frozen (Banquet) Cookin' Bag	4 oz	4	200	18%
MELBA TOAST (See also CRISPBREAD)				
(Devonsheer)-White				
plain & Veg Toast	1 slice	–	16	–
Garlic, Sesame,				
Onion, Rye, Honey Bran	1 slice	–	12	–
(Lance)-Melba Toast-Oblong	2 slices	–	30	–
Round-garlic	2 slices	1	20	45%
Round-onion	2 slices	1	20	45%
Round-plain	2 slices	1	20	45%
Sesame	2 slices	1	25	36%
(Old London)- Melba Toast				
Pumpernickle	3 slices	< 1	50	9%
Rye	3 slices	< 1	50	9%
Sesame	3 slices	2	50	36%
Sesame-unslated	3 slices	2	50	36%
Wheat	3 slices	< 1	50	9%
White	3 slices	< 1	50	9%
White-Unsalted	3 slices	< 1	50	9%
Whole Grain	3 slices	< 1	50	9%
Whole Grain unsalted	3 slices	< 1	50	9%
(Old London) Snacks -Bacon	5 rounds	1	50	18%
Garlic	5 rounds	1	50	18%
Onion	5 rounds	1	50	18%

Food and Description	Amount	Fat Grams	Total Calories	% Fat Calories
Rye	5 rounds	1	50	18%
Sesame Rounds	5 rounds	2	56	32%
White	5 rounds	1	50	18%
Whole Grain	5 rounds	1	50	18%
MELON (*See* individual listings, such as CANTALOUPE, HONEYDEW, etc.)				
MELON BALLS/frozen	1 cup	.5	58	8%
sweetened	1 cup	.5	245	2%
MEXICAN DINNER/ENTREE (*See also* FROZEN ENTREE/DINNER)				
Beef Enchilada Dinner-frozen				
(El Charrito)	13.75 oz	31	620	45%
(Patio)	13.25 oz	24	514	42%
(Schwan's)	13.45 oz	22	500	40%
Burrito Dinner	12 oz	16	517	28%
Cheese Enchilada Dinner-frozen				
(El Charrito)	13.25 oz	24	570	38%
(Patio)	12.25 oz	9	378	21%
Chicken Enchilada Dinner-frozen				
(El Charrito)	13.75 oz	17	510	30%
Chili Gravy & Beef Enchiladas-frozen				
(Banquet)	7 oz	13	270	43%
Combination Dinner-frozen				
(Patio)	13 oz	21	468	40%
Enchilada Grande Beef Dinner				
(El Charrito)	21 oz	49	950	46%
Fiesta Dinner-frozen				
(Patio)	12.25 oz	20	461	39%
Grande Satillo Dinner-frozen				
(El Charrito)	20.75 oz	34	820	37%
Mexican Hungry Man-frozen				
(Swanson)	20.25 oz	41	820	45%
Mexican-Style-frozen				
(El Charrito)	14.25 oz	35	690	46%
(El Charrito)	20 oz	47	850	50%
(Patio)	13.25 oz	24	533	41%
(Van de Kamp's)	½ pkg	10	220	41%
Mexican-Style-frozen				
(Banquet)	10 oz	9	294	28%
Mexican-Style Combination-frozen				
(Swanson)	14.25 oz	24	520	42%
Pasta Mexicali-frozen				
(Stouffer's)	10 oz	31	490	57%
Queso Dinner-frozen				
(El Charrito)	13.25 oz	16	490	29%

Food and Description	Amount	Fat Grams	Total Calories	% Fat Calories
Satillo Dinner-frozen				
(El Charrito)	13.25 oz	24	570	38%
Supreme Enchilada Dinner-frozen				
(Schwan's)	21 oz	39	870	40%
MEXICAN FOOD				
ACAPULCO DIP (Ortega)	1 oz	–	8	–
BEAN DIP				
Jalapeno (Hain)	4 Tbs	1	70	13%
Jalapeno-Flavored (Wise)	2 Tbs	–	25	–
Mexican (Hain)	4 Tbs	1	60	15%
Onion	4 Tbs	1	70	13%
BURRADAS				
Beef & Bean/frozen (Schwan's)	5.8 oz	18	390	42%
BURRITOS				
Beef				
frozen				
(El Charrito)				
Grande	6 oz	16	430	34%
Green Chili	5 oz	16	370	39%
Green Chili Grande	6 oz	14	410	31%
Jalapeno Grande	6 oz	15	410	33%
Red Chili	5 oz	18	380	43%
Red Chili Grande	6 oz	15	410	33%
Red Hot	5 oz	17	340	45%
Red Hot Beef & Bean	5 oz	18	540	30%
(Hormel)	1	8	205	35%
Burrito Grande	5.5 oz	16	380	38%
(Patio)				
Beef & Bean	5 oz	16	361	40%
Beef & Bean Green Chili	5 oz	12	330	33%
Beef & Bean Red Chili	5 oz	13	333	35%
Red Hot Burritos	5 oz	15	352	38%
(Schwan's)beef & bean	4 oz	7	270	23%
frozen				
(Weight Watchers)	7.62 oz	12	310	35%
Burrito Filling/mix (Del Monte)	½ cup	1	110	8%
Cheese/frozen(Hormel)	1	5	210	21%
Chicken/frozen (Weight Watchers)	7.62 oz	13	310	38%
Chicken & Rice/frozen (Hormel)	1	4	200	18%
Hot Chili Burrito/frozen (Hormel)	1	8	240	30%
homemade - Beefsteak	6 oz	15	250	54%
CHICKEN NUGGETS				
Chicken Duet Gourmet Nuggets/frozen				
(Swanson)	2.7 oz	12	200	54%

Food and Description	Amount	Fat Grams	Total Calories	% Fat Calories
CHILI & CHILI BEANS				
Beef Chili w/beans				
canned (Chef Boyardee)	7.5 oz	17	330	46%
Chilee Weenee canned (Van Camp's)	1 cup	16	310	47%
Chili				
canned				
Chicken				
(Cimmaron)	7.5 oz	4	190	19%
(Hain)-spicy	7.5 oz	2	130	14%
(Stagg)	7 oz	7	200	32%
Fat-free (Health Valley)	5 oz	–	140	–
Lentil				
(Health Valley)	4 oz	5	110	41%
low sodium	4 oz	6	120	45%
Lite chicken (Dennison's)w/beans	7.5 oz	5	200	23%
no beans	7.5 oz	5	210	21%
No Beans				
(Armour Star)	7.5 oz	29	380	69%
(Hormel)	7.5 oz	28	370	68%
	8⅓ oz	33	430	69%
	10.5 oz	41	540	68%
Hot	7.5 oz	28	370	68%
(Libby's)	7.5 oz	30	390	69%
(Stagg) Steak House	7.5 oz	16	280	51%
(Van Camp's)	1 cup	34	410	75%
(Wolf)	1 cup	27	390	62%
Extra Spicy	1 cup	25	360	63%
plain (Gebhardt)	7.5 oz	32	410	70%
Tempeh (Hain)	7.5 oz	4	160	23%
Vegetarian				
(Hain)	7.5 oz	1	160	6%
reduced sodium	7.5 oz	1	170	5%
(Health Valley)				
mild	4 oz	6	120	45%
spicy	4 oz	6	120	45%
With Beans				
(Armour Star)				
Regular	7.5 oz	26	390	60%
Texas	7.5 oz	26	370	63%
(Dennison's)				
Chunky	7.5 oz	14	310	41%
Cook Off	7.5 oz	19	340	51%
(Cimmaron) Hot	7.5 oz	9	230	35%
(Estee)	7.5 oz	20	370	49%

Food and Description	Amount	Fat Grams	Total Calories	% Fat Calories
(Featherweight)	7.5 oz	13	270	43%
(Heinz) Hot	7¾ oz	16	330	44%
(Hormel)	7.5 oz	17	310	49%
	8 oz	17	320	48%
Hot	7.5 oz	16	310	47%
(Libby's)	7.5 oz	13	270	43%
	8 oz	14	290	43%
(Stagg)				
Chili Laredo	7.5 oz	15	290	47%
Country Chili	7.5 oz	14	280	45%
(Van Camp's)	1 cup	23	350	59%
(Wolf)	1 cup	22	350	57%
Extra Spicy	1 cup	21	330	57%
frozen				
(Kraft) w/beef & beans	9.7 oz	22	380	52%
(Stouffer's)-The Right Course				
vegetarian	9.75 oz	7	280	23%
homemade	1 cup	15	400	34%
microwave				
no beans (Hormel)	10.5 oz	22	380	52%
w/beans (Impromptu)	10 oz	10	330	27%
mixes				
(Durkee)				
dry	1 pkt	1.6	148	10%
prepared	1 cup	25	465	48%
(Durkee)-Texas Chili Seasoning Mix				
dry	1 pkt	4	151	24%
prepared	1 cup	51	772	60%
(Kraft)-prepared - Good Times				
Chili Fixin's Original w/beans	4 oz	1	80	11%
Chili Fixin's Original w/o beans	4 oz	–	50	–
Chili Fixin's Texas Style w/beans	4 oz	1	90	10%
Chili Fixin's Texas Style w/o beans	4 oz	1	60	15%
Manwich Chili Fixins (Hunt's)				
sauce only	5.3 oz	1	110	8%
w/regular ground beef	8 oz	14	290	43%
Chili Beans/canned				
Caliente Style-dry				
(Joan of Arc/Green Giant)	½ cup	1	100	9%
in Chili Gravy				
(Dennison's)	7.5 oz	1	180	5%
(Luck's) Hot-pintos	7.5 oz	2	200	9%
in Sauce (Hormel)	5 oz	3	130	21%
(La Loma)	½ cup	4	120	30%

Food and Description	Amount	Fat Grams	Total Calories	% Fat Calories
Mexican Style (Van Camp/s)	1 cup	2	210	9%
(S&W)	½ cup	1	130	7%
Chili con Carne				
canned (Heinz)	7¾ oz	21	350	54%
canned with beans				
(Chef Boyardee)				
EZO	7 oz	20	340	53%
Hot	7 oz	21	350	54%
(Dennison's)	7.5 oz	15	310	44%
	8 oz	17	340	45%
Chunky	7.5 oz	14	310	41%
EZO	7 oz	19	330	52%
Hot	7 oz	15	290	47%
Hot	7.5 oz	16	310	47%
	8 oz	19	350	49%
Without beans	7.5 oz	19	300	57%
	9.5 oz	24	380	57%
frozen w/beans (Stouffer's)	8.75 oz	10	260	35%
Microwave				
with beans				
(Dennison's)	7.5 oz	13	290	40%
Chunky	7.5 oz	13	280	42%
Hot	7.5 oz	15	310	44%
with beans	7⅜ oz	11	250	40%
(Lunch Bucket)	8.5 oz	16	340	42%
hot	8.5 oz	16	340	42%
(Swanson)				
frozen Homestyle Recipe	8.25 oz	10	270	33%
without beans				
(Dennison's)	7.5 oz	19	310	55%
(Hormel)	8.25 oz	28	380	66%
Chili Dip (La Victoria)	1 Tbs	–	6	–
Chili Hot Dog Sauce				
(Chef Boyardee)	1 oz	1	30	30%
(Wolf)	⅙ cup	2	40	45%
Chili Mac (*See* PASTA DISHES)				
Chili Makin's				
original (S&W)	½ cup	1	100	9%
Chili Sauce				
(Del Monte)	¼ cup	1	70	13%
(Heinz)	1 Tbs	–	17	–
Tamalitos in Chili Gravy				
canned (Dennison's)	7.5 oz	16	310	47%

Food and Description	Amount	Fat Grams	Total Calories	% Fat Calories
CHIMICHANGAS				
Beef-homemade with cheese	4 oz	15.6	282	50%
DULCITA				
frozen (Hormel)				
Apple	4 oz	10	290	31%
Cherry	4 oz	9	300	27%
ENCHILADAS				
Beef/Box mix				
(International Lites)				
Enchilada Acapulco-prepared	10 oz	8	250	29%
Beef/ frozen				
(Banquet)	8 oz	8	264	27%
(El Charrito)	11 oz	31	560	50%
w/cheese	16.25 oz	42	880	43%
2 Grande	16.25 oz	35	800	39%
4 Grande	16.25 oz	47	890	48%
(Hormel)	1	5	140	32%
(Old El Paso)	2	10	170	53%
Ranchero (Weight Watchers)	9.12 oz	13	300	39%
(Schwan's)	11.25 oz	16	420	34%
(Van de Kamp's)				
Beef Enchilada	1	12	270	40%
Beef Enchilada Family Pack	¼ pkg	5	150	30%
Beef, Shredded	1	14	360	35%
Cheese/frozen				
(3) El Charrito)	11 oz	20	470	38%
(6) (El Charrito)	16.25 oz	30	780	35%
(Hormel)	1	6	151	36%
(Kraft)	9.8 oz	20	390	46%
(Van de Kamp's)				
Cheese Enchilada	1	15	300	45%
Cheese Enchilada Dinner	½ pkg	9	220	37%
Cheese Enchilada Family Pack	¼ pkg	10	200	45%
Cheese Enchilada Ranchero	½ pkg	12	260	42%
Ranchero (Weight Watchers)	8.87 oz	18	360	45%
Chicken/frozen				
(El Charrito)	11 oz	13	440	27%
(Van de Kamp's)				
Chicken Enchilada	½ pkg	11	260	38%
Chicken Enchilada Suiza	½ pkg	10	230	39%
(Weight Watchers)				
Chicken Enchilada Suiza	9.37 oz	15	330	41%
Chicken Ranchero	7.62 oz	13	310	38%
ENCHILADA SAUCE				
(La Victoria)	1 Tbs	5	80	56%

Food and Description	Amount	Fat Grams	Total Calories	% Fat Calories
(Rosarita)	3 oz	< 1	19	24%
green chili (Old El Paso)	¼ cup	–	18	–
hot				
(Del Monte)	¼ cup	–	45	–
(El Molino)	2 Tbs	1	16	56%
(Old El Paso)	¼ cup	1	30	30%
(Ortega)	1 oz	–	12	–
mild				
(Del Monte)	¼ cup	–	45	–
(Old El Paso)	¼ cup	1	25	36%
(Ortega)	1 oz	–	12	–
mix (Durkee)	1 pkg	1.8	89	18%
FAJITAS				
Beef/ frozen (Weight Watchers)	6.75 oz	7	250	25%
Chicken/frozen (Weight Watchers)	6.75 oz	5	230	20%
FLAUTA				
frozen (Schwan's)				
apple	2 oz	3	140	19%
cherry	2 oz	3	140	19%
GAZPACHO (*See* SOUP)				
GREEN CHILI SAUCE				
mild (El Molino)	2 Tbs	–	10	–
GREEN CHILIES				
whole	1 chili	–	8	–
(Del Monte)	½ cup	–	20	–
whole, sliced, diced, strips (Ortega)	1 oz	–	10	–
HOT PEPPERS				
(Ortega) whole, diced	1 oz	–	8	–
(Vlasic) Mexican tiny hot	1 pepper	–	6	–
JALAPENO PEPPERS	2 peppers	1	14	64%
(Del Monte)	½ cup	1	30	30%
(La Victoria)				
Marinated	1 Tbs	–	4	–
Nacho	1 Tbs	–	2	–
(Ortega) whole, diced	1 oz	–	10	–
(Vlasic) Mexican Hot	1 pepper	–	8	–
MEXICAN CRISPS (Old El Paso)	5 crisps	9	150	54%
MEXICAN RICE (Old El Paso)	½ cup	2	140	13%
MEXICALI DOGS				
frozen (Hormel)	5 oz	21	400	47%
MEXICAN FIESTA				
box mix-prepared				
(Rice-A-Roni) Savory Calssics	1 serving	4	170	21%
MEXICORN				
w/peppers - canned	½ cup	1	80	11%

Food and Description	Amount	Fat Grams	Total Calories	% Fat Calories
NACHOS				
Muy Fresco (Real Fresh)				
frozen-microwave	3.5 oz	9	140	51%
PICANTE SALSA				
(Old El Paso)	2 Tbs	–	10	–
(Ortega)	1 oz	–	10	–
PICANTE SAUCE				
(Old El Paso)	2 Tbs	–	8	–
(Wise)	2 Tbs	–	12	–
PICANTE STYLE PINTO BEANS				
dry	½ cup	1	100	9%
REFRIED BEANS				
Canned				
(Del Monte)				
plain	½ cup	2	130	14%
(Gebhardt)	4 oz	2	130	14%
(Little Pancho)				
w/green chili	½ cup	–	80	
(Old El Paso)	1/4 cup	1	50	18%
(Rosarita)				
plain	4 oz	2	130	14%
spicy	4 oz	2	120	15%
vegetarian	4 oz	2	100	18%
w/green chiles	4 oz	2	120	15%
Spicy (Del Monte)	½ cup	2	130	14%
vegetarian (Old El Paso)	½ cup	1	90	10%
w/green chilis (Old El Paso)	½ cup	2	100	18%
w/ sausage (Old El Paso)	½ cup	16	360	40%
SALSA				
(Del Monte)				
Burrito, & Rojo mild	¼ cup	–	20	–
Green Chili-mild	¼ cup	–	20	–
Picante				
hot	¼ cup	–	20	–
Picant				
hot chunky	¼ cup	–	15	–
(Hain)				
hot	¼ cup	–	22	–
mild	¼ cup	–	20	–
(La Victoria)				
Brava	1 Tbs	–	6	–
Casera	1 Tbs	–	4	–
Green Chili	1 Tbs	–	3	–
Green Jalapena	1 Tbs	–	4	–
Omelette	1 Tbs	–	6	–

Food and Description	Amount	Fat Grams	Total Calories	% Fat Calories
Picante	1 Tbs	–	4	–
Ranchera	1 Tbs	–	6	–
Red Jalapena	1 Tbs	–	6	–
Suprema	1 Tbs	–	4	–
Victoria	1 Tbs	–	4	–
(Ortega)				
Green Chili				
mild	1 oz	–	8	–
medium	1 oz	–	8	–
hot	1 oz	–	10	–
Ranchera	1 oz	–	12	–
Taco				
mild	1 oz	–	10	–
hot	1 oz	–	10	–
Thick 'n Chunky				
(Old El Paso)	2 Tbs	–	6	–
SANCHOS				
frozen (Schwan's) beef & bean	5.8 oz	12	360	30%
SPANISH RICE (See RICE DISHES)				
TACOS				
Beef				
Hamburger Helper (Betty Crocker)				
box mix/dry	⅕ pkg	1	160	6%
box mix/prepared	⅕ recipe	14	340	37%
Standard Home Recipe (USDA)	~ 3 oz	7	153	41%
-w/cheese	~ 3 oz	9	182	45%
Ham/Border Breakfasts				
(Owens) frozen	2 tacos	6	90	60%
Sausage/Border Breakfasts				
(Owens) frozen	2 tacos	12	190	57%
Taco Barquito				
frozen (Schwan's)	5 oz	21	430	44%
Taco Starter				
(Del Monte)	8 oz	1	140	6%
TACO DIP				
(Hain) & sauce	4 Tbs	1	25	36%
(Wise)	2 Tbs	–	12	–
TACO SAUCE				
(Del Monte) hot, mild	¼ cup	–	15	–
(El Molino) red mild	2 Tbs	–	10	–
(La Victoria)				
Green	1 Tbs	–	4	–
Red	1 Tbs	–	6	–
(Ortega)				
hot, mild	1 oz	–	12	–

Food and Description	Amount	Fat Grams	Total Calories	% Fat Calories
Western Style	1 oz	–	8	–
(Old El Paso)	2 Tbs	–	10	–
TACO SEASONING				
(Durkee)	1 pkg	1	67	13%
(Ortega)				
mild	1 oz	1	90	10%
prepared as directed	1 oz	4	60	60%
(Old El Paso)	1 pkg	1	100	9%
TACO SHELLS				
Mini (Old El Paso)	3 shells	4	70	51%
Regular				
(Old El Paso)	1 shell	3	55	49%
(Ortega)	1 shell	2	50	36%
(Rosarita)	1 shell	2	45	40%
Super				
(Old El Paso)	1 shell	6	100	54%
Taco Salad Shell				
(Azteca)	1 shell	12	200	54%
TAMALES				
Beef				
canned				
(Gebhardt)	2	19	270	63%
(Hormel)	2	10	140	64%
(Van Camp's)	8 oz	16	290	50%
(Wolf)	1 cup	24	350	62%
frozen				
(Old El Paso)	2	12	190	57%
(Hormel)	1	7	140	45%
(Schwan's)	1	3	80	34%
homemade	~ 2.5 oz	9.5	183	48%
Beef-Hot 'N Spicy				
canned (Hormel)	2	10	140	64%
TAQUITOS				
Beef/frozen shredded				
(Van de Kamp's)	8 oz	25	490	46%
TOMATILLO ENTERO				
(La Victoria)	1 Tbs	–	6	–
TOMATOES & JALAPENOS				
(Ortega)	1 oz	–	8	–
TORTILLA/CORN CHIPS (*See also* CORN CHIPS)				
(Arizona Sonoran) Rounds	1 oz	8	139	52%
(Arizona) Traditional Rounds	1 oz	6	137	39%
(Azteca) Buenitos	1 oz	7	140	45%
(Doritos)				
Nacho Cheese	1 oz	7	140	45%

Food and Description	Amount	Fat Grams	Total Calories	% Fat Calories
Taco Flavor	1 oz	7	140	45%
Traditional	1 oz	6	140	39%
(Cool Ranch)	1 oz	7	140	45%
(Salsa Rio)	1 oz	7	140	45%
(Doritos) Lights				
all flavors	1 oz	4	110	33%
(Cool Ranch)	1 oz	4	120	30%
(Eagle) Cantina Tortilla				
Nacho	1 oz	8	150	48%
Regular	1 oz	8	150	48%
(Fritos)				
Bar-B-Q Corn Chips	1 oz	9	150	54%
Chili Cheese	1 oz	10	160	56%
Crisp 'N Thin	1 oz	10	160	56%
Dip Size	1 oz	9	150	54%
original	1 oz	9	150	54%
Wild'N Mild	1 oz	9	150	54%
(Hain)				
Sesame	1 oz	7	140	45%
no salt	1 oz	7	140	45%
Sesame Cheese	1 oz	8	160	45%
Taco Style-no salt	1 oz	11	160	62%
(Health Valley)	1 oz	8	130	55%
unsalted	1 oz	8	130	55%
(La Famous) Tortilla Chips	1 oz	7	140	45%
no salt	1 oz	7	140	45%
(Laura Scudder's)				
Corn Chips-all flavors	1 oz	10	160	56%
Tortilla Chips	1 oz	7	140	45%
Strips	1 oz	7	140	45%
(Mi Ranchito)				
Traditional & Supreme Lights	1 oz	6	140	39%
(Planters)				
Corn chips	1 oz	10	160	56%
Tortilla chips				
nacho	1 oz	8	150	48%
(Suncheros)-Keebler/all flavors	1 oz	9	150	54%
(Tostitos)				
Jalapeno and Cheese	1 oz	8	150	48%
Original	1 oz	8	140	51%
Sharp Nacho CHeese	1 oz	8	150	48%
(Wise) Bravos-Nacho Cheese Flavor	1 oz	8	150	48%
TORTILLA STRIPS				
Restaurant Style (Eagle)	1 oz	6	150	42%

Food and Description	Amount	Fat Grams	Total Calories	% Fat Calories
TORTILLAS				
Corn				
(Azteca)	1	–	45	–
(El Charrito)	2	1	95	10%
(Old El Paso)	1	1	60	15%
Flour				
(Azteca)				
7"	1	2	85	21%
9"	1	3	130	21%
(El Charrito)	2	4	170	21%
(Old El Paso)	1	3	150	18%
Mix				
Corn Masa Harina De Maiz				
(Quaker)	1 cup	5	411	11%
Wheat Masa Trigo				
(Quaker)	1 cup	12	445	24%
TOSTACO SHELLS				
Corn (Old El Paso)	1 shell	5	100	45%
TOSTADA				
Beef				
frozen Supreme				
(Van de Kamp's)	8.5 oz	30	530	51%
homemade	~3 oz	7	153	41%
homemade-w/cheese	~3 oz	9	182	45%
TOSTADA SHELLS				
Corn				
Regular				
(Old El Passo)	2 shells	6	110	49%
(Ortega)	1 shell	2	50	36%
MILK				
Buffalo	1 cup	17	236	65%
Buttermilk				
cultured	1 cup	2	99	18%
dry	1 Tbs	–	25	–
low-fat 1½% (Borden)				
Golden Churn	1 cup	4	120	30%
Carob-Chocolate Milk 1%	1 cup	3	160	17%
Chocolate				
lowfat 2%	1 cup	5	179	25%
(Borden)-Dutch Brand	1 cup	5	180	25%
(Carnation)	1 cup	4	170	21%
(Hershey)	1 cup	5	180	25%
Chocolate-Flavored				
Box Drink	1 cup	2	150	12%
(La Parisian) Light Bavarian				

Food and Description	Amount	Fat Grams	Total Calories	% Fat Calories
Fudge Creme Cooler	1 cup	5	130	35%
lowfat 1%	1 cup	2.5	158	142
(Land O' Lakes)	1 cup	3	160	17%
lowfat ½%-(Pevely)	1 cup	1	97	9%
powder (2 Tbs) + water	6 oz	1	100	9%
powder (2 Tbs) + whole milk	8 oz	9	250	32%
(Quik)-Lite	8 oz	5	130	35%
skim (Land O'Lakes)	8 oz	–	140	–
whole	1 cup	8.5	208	37%
(Meadow Gold)	1 cup	8	210	34%
(Nestle)	1 cup	9	210	39%
(Pevely)	1 cup	8	210	34%
Cocoa/Hot Chocolate/with whole milk	8 oz	9	218	37%
Condensed/canned-sweetened	¼ cup	6.6	244	24%
(Carnation)	1 oz	3	123	22%
	3.5 oz	8.7	321	24%
	⅓ cup	9	318	26%
(Dairy Sweet)	⅓ cup	9	320	25%
(Eagle Brand)	⅓ cup	9	320	25%
Dry				
(Milkman)-low-fat mixed w/water	8 oz	–	190	–
	1 quart	5	380	12%
nonfat (Alba)-mixed w/water	8 oz	–	80	–
skim	¼ cup	–	100	–
prepared w/water	8 oz	–	80	–
whole	¼ cup	8.5	159	48%
Eggnog/canned				
(Borden)	4 oz	9	160	51%
commercial	8 oz	19	342	50%
(Land O'Lakes)	8 oz	15	123	11%
Lite (Carnation)	8 oz	8	320	23%
mix-dry	2 tsp	–	110	–
mix (2 heaping tsp) + whole milk	8 oz	8	260	28%
mix-(PDQ) 2/3 tsp + whole milk	8 oz	5	230	20%
Evaporated				
canned whole	¼ cup	4.8	84	51%
canned-lowfat	¼ cup	1.5	55	25%
canned-skim	¼ cup	–	50	–
(Carnation)-whole	3.5 oz	7.6	134	51%
	½ cup	10	170	53%
(Carnation)-lowfat	3.5 oz	1.9	85	20%
	½ cup	3	110	25%
(Carnation)-skim	3.5 oz	–	80	–

Food and Description	Amount	Fat Grams	Total Calories	% Fat Calories
	½ cup	–	100	–
(Milnot)-whole	½ cup	8	150	48%
(Pet)				
whole	½ cup	10	170	53%
Light	½ cup	–	100	–
Goat	8 oz	10	168	54%
canned (Meyenberg)-evaporated	8 oz	8	160	45%
carton				
refrigerated	8 oz	8	150	48%
powder mixed w/water	8 oz	8	150	48%
Human	2 oz	2	42	43%
Lactaid				
lowfat	1 cup	5	120	38%
nonfat	1 cup	–	90	–
Regular				
Lowfat 2%	1 cup	5	121	37%
w/nonfat milk solids added	1 cup	4.7	125	34%
(Borden)-Hi-Protein	1 cup	5	140	32%
(Land O'Lakes)	1 cup	5	120	38%
(Viva)-w/extra calcium	1 cup	5	120	38%
Lowfat 1%	1 cup	2.6	105	22%
w/nonfat milk solids added	1 cup	2.4	104	21%
(Borden) w/L. Acidophilus	1 cup	2	100	18%
(Land O'Lakes)	1 cup	3	100	27%
Lowfat ½%-(Pevely)	1 cup	1	90	10%
Skim	1 cup	.6	100	6%
w/nonfat milk solids added	1 cup	.6	90	6%
(Borden)				
Skim-Line				
protein fortified	1 cup	1	100	9%
vitamins A & D	1 cup	.6	90	6%
Whole	1 cup	8	150	48%
(Borden)				
Vitamin D	1 cup	8	150	48%
w/added calcium-Hi Calcium	1 cup	8	150	48%
(Real)-Real Fresh milk w/vitamins				
A & D-ready to chill box	1 cup	8	150	48%
Soybean "Milk"	8 oz	4.6	79	52%
MILK MIXES				
Carob Mix				
dry	1 Tbs	< 1	45	10%
w/8 oz whole milk	8 oz	9	195	42%
(El Molino)				
dry	1 Tbs	< 1	40	11%

Food and Description	Amount	Fat Grams	Total Calories	% Fat Calories
w/8 oz whole milk	8 oz	9	190	43%
Chocolate				
(Choco Milk)/dry mix	1 oz	1	110	8%
w/8 oz whole milk	8 oz	10	264	34%
Chocolate syrup	2 Tbs	.5	82	6%
+ whole milk	8 oz	8.5	232	33%
Chocolate-flavored syrup				
(Nestle Quik)	1.22 oz	1	100	9%
+ whole milk	8 oz	9	240	34%
+ 2% milk	8 oz	6	220	25%
+ 1% milk	8 oz	4	200	18%
+ skim milk	8 oz	1.6	180	8%
(Estee)-syrup	1 Tbs	–	6	–
(PDQ) 3-4 tsp w/whole milk	8 oz	5	230	20%
(Quik)-chocolate				
dry	3/4 oz/			
	~2½ tsp	1	90	10%
w/8 oz whole milk	8 oz	9	240	34%
w/8 oz 2% milk	8 oz	6	210	26%
w/8 oz 1% milk	8 oz	4	190	18%
w/8 oz skim milk	8 oz	1.6	180	8%
sugar free-dry	1 heaping tsp	.5	18	25%
w/8 oz 2% milk	8 oz	5.5	138	36%
Cocoa				
(Alba)				
Chocolate Marsh	1 pkt	–	60	–
Milk Chocolate	1 pkt	–	60	–
Mocha	1 pkt	–	60	–
(Baker's)	1 oz	2	120	15%
(Carnation)				
Choc Fudge-dry	1 oz	1	110	8%
diet hot cocoa mix	1 env		25	18%
milk chocolate-dry	1 oz	1	110	8%
mocha-sugar-free-dry	1 oz	.5	50	9%
natural mint-dry	1 oz	1	110	8%
rich chocolate-dry	1 oz	1	110	8%
sugar-free-dry	1 oz	.5	50	9%
rich choc w/marsh-dry	1 oz	1	110	8%
70 calorie-dry	3.5 oz	1	353	3%
	3 tsp	–	70	–
With chocolate marsh.	1 pkt	1	110	8%
(Ovaltine)-sugar free-dry	1 pkt	1	40	23%
(Swiss Miss)-instant				
Amaretto Creme	1 pkt	4	140	26%

Food and Description	Amount	Fat Grams	Total Calories	% Fat Calories
Bavarian Chocolate	1 pkt	3	110	25%
Chocolate Creme	1 pkt	4	110	33%
Chocolate Mint	1 pkt	4	145	25%
Chocolate Mocha Creme	1 pkt	4	140	26%
Cocoa/diet	1 env		20	23%
Double Rich	1 pkt	3	110	25%
Lite	1 pkt		70	6%
Milk Chocolate	1 pkt	3	110	25%
Mini Marshmallow	1 pkt	3	110	25%
sugar free	1 pkt	1	50	18%
sugar free-w/mini marshmallows	1 pkt	1	50	18%
(Weight Watchers)-chocolate & marshmallow	1 pkt	–	60	–
Malted (Carnation)				
chocolate-dry	3.5 oz	3.8	375	9%
	3 Heaping Tbs	.8	79	9%
original-dry	3.5 oz	8.5	411	19%
	3 Heaping Tbs	2	90	20%
Malted/chocolate powder	1 Heaping Tbs	1	85	11%
+ whole milk	8 oz	9	235	35%
(Ovaltine)-classic-Traditional Chocolate Malt				
dry	3/4 oz	–	80	–
w/2% milk	8 oz	5	210	21%
Rich Chocolate-dry	3/4 oz	–	80	–
w/2% milk	8 oz	5	210	21%
(PDQ) 3-4 tsp w/whole milk	8 oz	5	180	25%
(Quik) strawberry				
dry	3/4 oz/ ~2½ tsp	–	80	–
w/8 oz whole milk	8 oz	8	230	31%
w/8 oz 2% milk	8 oz	5	200	23%
w/8 oz 1% milk	8 oz	3	180	15%
w/8 oz skim milk	8 oz	.6	170	3%

MILK SHAKE (*See also* FAST FOOD)
canned

(Real) Sport Shake				
chocolate	10 oz	10	310	29%
strawberry	10 oz	10	270	33%
(Frostee)				
chocolate-flavored drink	1 cup	8	200	36%

Food and Description	Amount	Fat Grams	Total Calories	% Fat Calories
strawberry-flavored drink	1 cup	7	180	35%
frozen				
(Micro Magic)				
chocolate	11.5 oz	8	340	21%
strawberry	11.5 oz	9	340	24%
vanilla	11.5 oz	13	380	31%
mix				
(Alba 77) Fit'N Frosty				
chocolate	1 pkt	1	70	13%
chocolate marshmallow	1 pkt	1	70	13%
double fudge	1 pkt	1	70	13%
strawberry	1 pkt	–	70	–
vanilla	1 pkt	–	70	–
(Weight Watchers)				
choc fudge	1 pkt	1	70	13%
orange sherbet	1 pkt	–	70	–
regular				
chocolate	10 oz	10	360	25%
strawberry	10 oz	9	350	23%
vanilla	10 oz	9	340	27%
MILK SUBSTITUTES - Includes no milk fats				
Filled hydrogenated vegetable oils				
w/milk solids	1 cup	8	154	47%
Filled-w/lauric oils & milk solids	1 cup	8	153	47%
Imitation w/hydrogenated				
vegetable oils	1 cup	8	150	48%
Imitation w/lauric acid oils	1 cup	8	150	48%
Reindeer	8 oz	48.6	580	75%
Rennin Products (Coagulates milk				
used in making cheese)	1 tablet	–	1	–
	1 pkg	–	12	–
Sheep	8 oz	17	264	58%
MILKFISH/raw	3 oz	6	125	43%
MILLET (See also FLOUR)				
Whole grain	4 oz	3	371	7%
MINERAL WATER (See SODA)				
MINESTRONE SOUP (See SOUP)				
MISO PASTE	½ cup	8	285	25%
MOLASSES				
Barbados	1 Tbs	–	54	–
	1 oz	–	111	–
	1 cup	–	889	–

Food and Description	Amount	Fat Grams	Total Calories	% Fat Calories
Blackstrap (Plantation)				
3rd extraction	1 Tbs	–	43	–
	1 oz	–	87	–
	1 cup	–	699	–
Brer Rabbit				
Dark	1 Tbs	–	60	–
Light	1 Tbs	–	60	–
Light-Ist extraction	1 Tbs	–	50	–
	1 oz	–	103	–
	1 cup	–	827	–
Medium-2nd extraction	1 Tbs	–	46	–
	1 oz	–	95	–
	1 cup	–	761	–
Mott's				
Grandma's Gold Label	1 Tbs	–	70	–
Grandma's Green Label	1 Tbs	–	70	–
MONKFISH/raw	3 oz	1	64	14%
MOOSE/raw-boneless	3 oz	4.8	152	28%
MOTHBEANS				
boiled	½ cup	–	103	–
raw	½ cup	1.5	335	4%
MOUNTAIN YAM/cooked Hawaiian	1 cup	–	119	–
MOUSSE (See PUDDING & MOUSSE)				
MUFFINS				
Apple-homemade	1	7	135	47%
Blueberry				
Frozen				
(Sara Lee)-Free & Light	1	–	120	–
(Weight Watchers)	5 oz	5	170	26%
Standard home recipe (USDA)	~ 1.5 oz	3.7	112	30%
Box mix				
(Betty Crocker)				
Apple Cinnamon	1	4	120	30%
Banana Nut	1	5	120	38%
Carrot Nut	1	5	150	30%
Chocolate Chip	1	6	150	36%
Cinnamon Streusel	1	9	200	41%
Oatmeal Raisin	1	4	140	26%
Strawberry Crown	1	5	150	30%
Streusel Oat Bran	1	8	190	38%
Wild Blueberry	1	4	120	30%
Wild Blueberry light	1		70	6%
(Betty Crocker)-Bake Shop Muffins				
Banana Walnut	1	9	210	39%

Food and Description	Amount	Fat Grams	Total Calories	% Fat Calories
Bluberry Bran	1	7	200	32%
Blueberry Streusel	1	8	210	34%
Dutch Apple Streusel	1	7	200	32%
(Duncan Hines)				
Bakery Style Blueberry	1	6	190	28%
Bakery Style Bran & Honey Nut	1	7	200	32%
Bakery Style Cinnamon Swirl	1	7	200	32%
Bakery Style Cranberry				
Orange Nut	1	8	200	36%
Bakery Style Pecan Crunch	1	11	220	45%
Bran & Honey	1	4	120	38%
Oat bran blueberry	1	5	110	41%
Wild Blueberry	1	3	110	25%
(Hain)-Oat Bran				
apple/cinnamon	1	3	140	19%
banana nut	1	4	140	26%
raspberry spice	1	3	140	19%
(Hostess) 97% fat free				
Apple Streusel	1	1	100	9%
Blueberry	1	1	100	9%
(Krusteaz)				
Blueberry	1	4	160	23%
Oat Bran	1-2.5 oz	6	210	26%
	1-2 oz	5	190	24%
Bran-homemade	1	3.9	104	
Corn-homemade w/degermed cornmeal	~ 1.5 oz	4	128	30%
w/whole-ground cornmeal	~ 1.5 oz	4	115	31%
mix	1	6	145	37%
(Dromedary)	1	5	130	35%
(Flako)	1	4	120	30%
(Dunkin Donuts)				
apple n' spice	1	8	300	24%
banana nut	1	10	310	29%
blueberry	1	8	280	26%
bran w/raisins	1	9	104	69%
corn	1	12	340	32%
cranberry nut	1	9	290	25%
oat-bran	1	11	330	30%
English				
cracked wheat	1	1	158	6%
plain	1	1	140	6%
sourdough	1	1	130	7%
with raisins	1	1	146	6%
whole wheat	1	1.6	130	11%

Food and Description	Amount	Fat Grams	Total Calories	% Fat Calories
(Earth Grains)				
Plain	1	1	150	6%
Raisin	1	1	150	6%
Wheatberry	1	1	150	6%
Whole Wheat	1	2	170	11%
(Oroweat)-Blueberry	1	1	170	5%
Extra Crisp	1	1	130	7%
Health Nut Raisin	1	4	200	18%
Oat Bran	1	1	150	6%
Oat Nut Raisin	1	2	160	11%
Sourdough	1	1	140	6%
(Pepperidge Farm)				
Cinnamon Apple	1	1	140	6%
Cinnamon Chip	1	3	160	17%
Cinnamon Raisin	1	2	150	12%
Plain	1	1	140	6%
Sourdough	1	1	140	6%
Stoneground Wheat	1	1	130	7%
(Roman Meal)-Plain	1	2	145	12%
(Thomas) -Honey Wheat	1	1	120	8%
Plain & Sourdough	1	1	130	7%
Raisin	1	1	150	6%
Frozen Muffins				
(Pepperidge Farm)				
Blueberry	1	7	180	35%
Bran w/raisins	1	7	180	35%
Carrot Walnut	1	4	170	21%
Chocolate Chip	1	8	210	34%
Cinnamon Swirl	1	6	190	28%
Corn	1	7	180	35%
(Sara Lee)				
Corn	1	13	250	47%
Hearty Fruit				
Apple Cinnamon Spice	1	8	220	33%
Banana Nut	1	9	230	35%
Blueberry	1	8	200	36%
Golden Corn	1	13	250	47%
Oat Bran	1	8	220	33%
Oatmeal & Fruit	1	9	230	35%
Raisin Bran	1	7	220	29%
(Health Valley)-Fat Free fruit	1	< 1	65	7%
Oat Bran Almond-Date	1	6	170	32%
Oat Bran Blueberry	1	4	140	26%
Oat Bran Raisin	1	3	140	19%

Food and Description	Amount	Fat Grams	Total Calories	% Fat Calories
Muffin Mix				
(Martha White)-apple cinnamon, blackberry,				
blueberry, orangeberry, raspberry,				
strawberry	1	3	140	19%
bran	1	5	150	30%
Oatmeal	1	3	112	24%
Orange-homemade	1	6	135	30%
Pouch mix-(Robin Hood/Gold Medal)-prepared				
Applesauce	1	5	160	28%
Banana	1	5	150	30%
Blueberry	1	6	170	32%
Corn	1	2	130	14%
Honey Bran	1	6	170	32%
Toaster Muffins-(Pillsbury)				
Apple Spice	1	5	130	35%
Banana Nut	1	6	130	42%
Old Fashioned Corn	1	5	120	38%
Raisin Bran	1	5	120	38%
Wild Maine Blueberry	1	3	120	23%
(Winchell Donuts) Muffins				
Apple Spice	1	11	327	30%
Banana Nut	1	12	327	33%
Blueberry	1	10	263	34%
Bran	1	13	353	33%
Cherry	1	10	317	28%
Corn	1	13	347	34%
(Wonder) Muffins & Rounds				
English	1	1	130	7%
Hi Fiber Cinnamon Raisin English	1	1	110	8%
Hi Fiber English	1	1	110	8%
Hi Fiber Multi-Grain English	1	1	120	8%
Raisin Rounds	1	2	140	13%
Sour Dough	1	1	130	7%
MULBERRY	1 cup	.55	61	8%
MULLET/striped				
cooked-dry heat	3 oz	4	127	28%
raw	3 oz	3	99	27%
MUNG BEANS				
boiled	6 oz	–	107	–
raw	½ cup	1	361	3%
Sprouts				
(Arrowhead Mills)	½ cup	–	25	–
canned	½ cup	–	8	–
cooked	½ cup	–	13	–

Food and Description	Amount	Fat Grams	Total Calories	% Fat Calories
raw	4 oz	–	40	–
raw	½ cup	–	16	–
stir-fried	½ cup	–	31	–
MUNGO BEANS/boiled	½ cup	–	95	–
MUSHROOM				
canned				
(B&B)	2 oz	1	25	36%
(Libby's)	1 oz	–	70	–
marinated (Cara Mia)	1 oz	1	13	–
Oriental Straw	2 oz	–	12	–
pieces & stems buttons (Green Giant)	½ cup	–	25	–
seasoned whole (Cara Mia)	1 oz	–	7	–
fresh-boiled	½ cup	–	21	–
frozen (Freshlike)	3.5 oz	–	30	–
raw	1	–	5	–
raw/pieces	½ cup	–	9	–
sauteed or fried	10 Small	10	100	9%
Shiitake Mushroom/cooked	4	–	40	–
canned	4 oz	–	45	–
dried	1	–	11	–
MUSHROOM DISHES				
Mushrooms breaded-frozen (Ore Ida)	2⅔ oz	8	140	51%
Mushrooms w/butter sauce-canned	2 oz	1	30	30%
MUSHROOM SOUP (*See* SOUP)				
MUSKELLUNGE (North American Pike)				
raw	3 oz	2	93	19%
MUSSEL				
Blue				
cooked-moist heat	3 oz	3.8	147	23%
raw	3 oz	1.9	73	23%
	1 cup	3	129	21%
MUSTARD				
Brown				
(Heinz)	1 tsp	< 1	8	56%
(Nabisco)	1 tsp	–	4	–
Dip'N Spread (French's)	1 Tbs	1	40	23%
Grey Poupon Dijon				
(Nabisco)	1 tsp	1	18	50%
	1 Tbs	2	30	60%
(Hain)				
stone ground	1 Tbs	1	14	64%
no salt	1 Tbs	1	14	64%
(Heinz)				
mild	1 tsp	–	5	–

Food and Description	Amount	Fat Grams	Total Calories	% Fat Calories
pourable (Kraft)	1 tsp	–	5	–
pure prepared	1 Tbs	–	4	–
Prepared (French's)				
Bold & Spicy	1 Tbs	–	6	–
Dijon	1 Tbs	1	9	100%
Meford	1 Tbs	1	16	56%
w/Horseradish	1 Tbs	1	16	56%
w/Onion	1 Tbs	–	8	–
yellow	1 Tbs	1	10	90%
(Gulden's)				
Creamy Mild	1 Tbs	–	6	–
Diablo	1 Tbs	–	8	–
Spicy Brown	1 Tbs	1	9	100%
MUSTARD, DRIED	1 tsp		12	38%
MUSTARD GREENS				
fresh-boiled	½ cup	–	11	–
frozen-boiled	½ cup	–	14	–
frozen (Pictsweet)	3.3 oz	–	20	–
raw	½ cup	–	7	–
MUSTARD SAUCE (*See* SAUCE)				
MUSTARD SEED/yellow	1 tsp	1	15	60%
MUSTARD SPINACH				
fresh-boiled	½ cup	–	14	–
raw	½ cup	–	17	–

N

Food and Description	Amount	Fat Grams	Total Calories	% Fat Calories
NATTO	½ cup	9.7	187	47%
NAVY BEAN				
boiled	½ cup	.5	129	4%
canned	½ cup	.57	148	4%
(Joan of Arc)	½ cup	< 1	100	5%
Old Fashioned (Ranch Style)	7.5 oz	2	160	7%
Seasoned w/Pork (Luck's)	7.5 oz	7	230	27%
raw	½ cup	1.5	345	4%
sprouts raw	½ cup	–	35	–

Food and Description	Amount	Fat Grams	Total Calories	% Fat Calories
NAVY BEAN SOUP (*See* SOUP)				
NECTARINE/fresh	1	.7	67	9%
NEWBURG SAUCE (*See* SAUCE)				
NON-DAIRY FROZEN DESSERT (*See* FROZEN NON-DAIRY DESSERT)				
NOODLE (*See* PASTA)				
NOODLE SOUP (*See* SOUP)				
NUTMEG/ground	1 tsp	.8	11	66%
NUTRITIONAL SUPPLEMENT (*See also* BREAKFAST BAR, BREAKFAST DRINK)				
DIET				
(Sego) Liquid Diet Food				
Chocolate	10 oz can	1	225	4%
Very chocolate	10 oz can	1	225	4%
Very chocolate malt	10 oz can	1	225	4%
Very dutch	10 oz can	1	225	4%
Very strawberry	10 oz can	5	225	20%
Very vanilla	10 oz can	5	225	20%
Shake Mix (Weight Watchers)				
Chocolate fudge	1 pkt	1	70	13%
Orange sherbet	1 pkt	–	70	–
REGULAR				
Ensure (Ross)				
Black Walnut	8 oz	8.8	250	32%
Chocolate	8 oz	8.8	250	32%
Coffee	8 oz	8.8	250	32%
Eggnog	8 oz	8.8	250	32%
Plus chocolate	8 oz	12.6	355	32%
Plus coffee	8 oz	12.6	355	32%
Plus eggnog	8 oz	12.6	355	32%
Plus strawberry	8 oz	12.6	355	32%
Plus vanilla	8 oz	12.6	355	32%
Strawberry	8 oz	8.8	250	32%
Vanilla	8 oz	8.8	250	32%
(Joe Weider's)				
Carbo Energgizer	6 oz	–	140	–
90 Plus sugar-free	8 oz	1	100	9%
(MLO)Energy Shake-Vanilla				
Dry	2 Tbs	1	110	8%
w/8 oz non-fat milk	1 serving	1	200	5%
NUTS, FORMULATED				
wheat based				
Macadamia-flavored	1 oz	16	176	82%
other flavors	1 oz	18	184	88%
unflavored	1 oz	16	177	81%

Food and Description	Amount	Fat Grams	Total Calories	% Fat Calories
NUTS, MIXED (*See also* Individual Names)				
Mixed Nuts				
(Eagle)	1 oz	16	180	80%
Deluxe	1 oz	17	180	85%
(Planters)				
dry roasted	1 oz	14	160	79%
unsalted	1 oz	15	170	79%
oil roasted	1 oz	16	180	80%
Deluxe	1 oz	17	180	85%
Unslated	1 oz	16	180	80%
select mix				
cashews w/almonds & peanuts	1 oz	14	170	74%
cashews w/almonds & pecans	1 oz	16	180	80%
cashews w/pecans & peanuts	1 oz	16	180	80%
Mixed Nuts With Peanuts				
dry roasted	1 oz	14.6	169	78%
(Guy's)	1 oz	16	180	80%
oil roasted	1 oz	16	175	82%
Mixed Nuts Without Peanuts				
oil roasted	1 oz	15.95	175	82%

O

Food and Description	Amount	Fat Grams	Total Calories	% Fat Calories
OCEAN PERCH, ATLANTIC (*See also* FROZEN ENTREE/DINNER)				
breaded & fried	3 oz	11	185	54%
cooked-dry heat	3 oz	1.8	103	16%
raw	3 oz	1	80	11%
Mixed				
cooked-dry heat	3 oz	1	77	12%
frozen-raw				
(Gorton's)	5 oz	1	110	8%
OCTOBER BEANS				
canned				
Seasoned w/Pork (Luck's)	7.25 oz	6	220	25%
	7.5 oz	7	230	27%

Food and Description	Amount	Fat Grams	Total Calories	% Fat Calories
OCTOPUS/raw	3 oz	.88	70	11%

OILS (*See also* FAT)

[NOTE: All types of oil have the same number of calories (120 calories per tablespoon) and the same number of fat grams (14 fat grams per tablespoon). The difference lies in the type of fat making up the fat grams; i.e., saturated fat vs unsaturated (monounsaturated and polyunsaturated). Check your labels for breakdown. The following chart of the most commonly used fats and oils shows the percent of saturated fats and unsaturated fats contained by each.]

REMEMBER—NO VEGETABLE OIL CONTAINS CHOLESTEROL!

OIL/FAT	% SATURATED	% UNSATURATED
CANOLA	6%	94%
ALMOND	8%	92%
LINSEED	9%	91%
SAFFLOWER	9%	91%
SUNFLOWER	11%	89%
WALNUT	11%	89%
CORN	13%	87%
SESAME	13%	87%
OLIVE	14%	86%
SOYBEAN	15%	85%
MARGARINE (NO TROPICAL OILS)	18%	82%
PEANUT	18%	82%
WHEAT GERM	19%	81%
SHORTENING (VEGETABLE)	26%	74%
COTTONSEED	27%	73%
CHICKEN FAT	30%	70%
LARD	41%	59%
SHORTENING (ANIMAL FAT)	44%	56%
BEEF TALLOW	51%	49%
PALM	51%	49%
BUTTER	66%	34%
PALM KERNEL	81%	19%
COCONUT	92%	8%

OKRA				
canned	½ cup	–	25	–
fresh-boiled	½ cup	–	25	–
frozen-cooked	½ cup	–	34	–
frozen-cut				
(Freshlike)	3.3 oz	–	25	–
(Pictsweet)	3.3 oz	–	25	–
frozen-whole (Freshlike)	3.3 oz	–	30	–

Food and Description	Amount	Fat Grams	Total Calories	% Fat Calories
(Pictsweet)-Express-				
Microwave	2.5 oz	–	20	–
raw	½ cup	–	19	–
OKRA DISHES				
Okra breaded				
frozen				
(Ore Ida)	3 oz	10	170	53%
OLIVE				
Pickled/canned or bottled				
Green	10 Small	3.6	33	98%
	10 Large	4.9	45	98%
	10 Giant	8	76	95%
Pitted Ripe				
(Early California)-all sizes	~1 oz	3	30	90%
(Janet Lee)	8 small	3	30	90%
	7 medium	3	30	90%
	6 large	3	30	90%
(S&W)				
jumbo	3.5 oz	18	163	99%
large	3.5 oz	18	163	99%
xtra large	3.5 oz	18	163	99%
Ripe-Ascolano	10 Xtra lg	6.5	61	96%
	10 Mammoth	7.7	72	96%
	10 Giant	9.5	89	96%
	10 Jumbo	11	105	94%
sliced	1 cup	18.6	174	94%
Ripe-Manzanillo	10 Small	4	38	95%
	10 Medium	4.7	44	96%
	10 Large	5.5	51	97%
	10 Xtra lg	6.5	61	96%
sliced	1 cup	18.6	174	96%
Ripe-Mission	10 Small	5.9	54	98%
	10 Medium	6.9	63	99%
	10 Large	8	73	99%
	10 Xtra lg	9.5	87	98%
sliced	1 cup	27	248	98%
Ripe (S&W)				
large	3.5 oz	18	163	99%
xtra large	3.5 oz	18	163	99%
Ripe-Sevillano	10 Giant	6.5	64	91%
	10 Jumbo	7.8	76	92%
	10 Colossal	9.7	95	92%
	10 SuperCol	11.6	114	92%
sliced	1 cup	12.8	126	91%

Food and Description	Amount	Fat Grams	Total Calories	% Fat Calories
Ripe-salt cured/Greek style	10 Medium	6.9	65	96%
	10 Xtra Lg	9.5	89	96%
OLIVE LOAF (*See* LUNCHEON MEAT)				
ONION				
canned-French Fried Onions				
(Durkee)	1 oz	15	175	77%
canned (S&W)	½ cup	–	35	–
cooked	1 cup	–	60	–
Dehydrated Flakes	1 Tbs	–	16	–
frozen				
chopped (Ore Ida)	2 oz	–	20	–
diced (Freshlike)	1 oz	–	8	–
small whole (Birds Eye)	½ cup	–	40	–
	¼ cup	–	45	–
whole (Freshlike)	3.3 oz	–	95	–
Green-spring	5 Large	–	10	–
(Heinz)-sweet onions	1	–	40	–
raw/chopped	1 Tbs	–	3	–
	½ cup	–	27	–
(Vlasic)-Lightly Spiced Cocktail	1 oz	–	4	–
ONION DISHES				
Chopped Onions/frozen (Ore Ida)	2 oz	–	20	–
Onions in cream sauce/frozen				
(Birds Eye)	3 oz	6	110	49%
Onion Rings/frozen breaded				
pan fried heated in oven	7 rings	18.69	285	59%
Onion Ringers/frozen (Ore Ida)	2 oz	7	140	45%
Small Onions w/cream sauce/frozen				
(Birds Eye)	3 oz	6	110	49%
ONION POWDER	1 tsp	–	7	–
ONION SOUP (*See* SOUP)				
OPOSSUM/braised or roasted	3 oz	8	190	38%
ORANGE (*See also* MANDARIN ORANGE)				
Oranges	1	–	62	–
Oranges/Navels	1	–	65	–
Oranges/Valencias	1	–	59	–
ORANGE-APRICOT DRINK				
Canned	8 oz	–	128	–
(Tropicana) Twister	8 oz	–	114	–
ORANGE-BANANA JUICE				
(Chiquita)	6 oz		100	5%
(Smucker's)	8 oz	–	120	–
ORANGE-CRANBERRY DRINK				
(Tropicana) Twister	8 oz	–	114	–

Food and Description	Amount	Fat Grams	Total Calories	% Fat Calories
ORANGE DRINK				
(Bama)	8.45 oz	–	120	–
(Hawaiian Punch)	6 oz	–	100	–
(Juice Works)	6 oz	–	90	–
Orange Drink Miix (Crystal Light)-mix diet	8 oz	–	4	–
Orange Flavor Breakfast Drink (Tang)	4 oz	–	60	–
	6 oz	–	90	–
(Tang) sugar-free	6 oz	–	6	–
Orange Flavor Drink w/orange pulp from frozen concentrate	6 oz	–	91	–
Orange Fruit Juice Blend (Mott's)	10 oz	–	144	–
Orange-Squeezit (Betty Crocker)	6.75 oz	–	110	–
(Tropicana)-single serve	10 oz	–	132	–
ORANGE-GRAPEFRUIT JUICE				
canned (sweetened)	8 oz	–	107	–
(Kraft) Pure 100%	6 oz	–	80	–
ORANGE JUICE				
canned/sweetened	8 oz	–	119	–
canned/unsweetened	8 oz	–	104	–
(Del Monte)	6 oz	–	80	–
fresh	8 oz	.5	111	4%
from frozen conc.	1 cup	–	112	–
frozen (Birds Eye)	6 oz	–	80	–
frozen-undiluted	6 oz	–	340	1%
(Gold-N-Rich)	6 oz	–	80	–
Juice Bowl (Campbell's)	6 oz	–	90	–
(Kraft) Pure 100%	6 oz	–	80	–
(Libby's)-unsweetened	6 oz	–	80	–
(Mott's)blend	9.5 oz	–	139	–
(S&W)	6 oz	–	83	–
(Sippin Pak)from concentrate	8.45 oz	–	110	–
(Sunkist)-fresh squeezed	6 oz	–	77	–
(Tree Top)	6 oz	–	90	–
(Tropicana)	6 oz	–	75	–
	8 oz	–	109	–
from concentrate	8 oz	–	112	–
	6 oz	–	84	–
ORANGE-LEMON DRINK	8 oz	–	124	–
ORANGE-PASSION FRUIT DRINK				
(Tropicana) Twister	8 oz	–	89	–

Food and Description	Amount	Fat Grams	Total Calories	% Fat Calories
ORANGE PEEL				
candied	1 oz	–	90	–
fresh	1 Tbs	–	–	–
ORANGE-PINEAPPLE JUICE				
(Kraft) Pure 100%	6 oz	–	80	–
(Tropicana)	8 oz	–	111	–
unsweetened	6 oz	–	80	–
ORANGE PUNCH				
Orange Mountain Berry Punch	8.45 oz	–	110	–
ORANGE-STRAWBERRY-BANANA DRINK				
(Tropicana) Twister	8 oz	–	90	–
ORANGE-STRAWBERRY-BANANA JUICE				
(Tropicana)	6 oz	–	106	–
OREGANO/ground	1 tsp	–	5	–
ORIENTAL FOOD				
BEEF MANDARIN				
Frozen (Van de Kamp's)	11 oz	10	310	29%
BEEF PEPPER ORIENTAL				
canned	¾ cup	2	80	23%
(BETTY CROCKER)				
Chicken Helper - prepared box mix				
Teriyaki Chicken	1 serving	23	480	43%
(BOOTH) LIGHT ENTREE				
Shrimp Oriental/frozen	10 oz	3	190	14%
CHOP SUEY				
Standard Home Recipe (USDA)				
w/beef w/o noodles	1 cup	17	300	51%
w/beef & pork	1 cup	17	300	51%
CHOW MEIN-BEEF				
Canned	¾ cup	1	70	13%
Standard Home Recipe (USDA)	1 cup	17	300	51%
CHOW MEIN-CHICKEN				
canned	¾ cup	3	80	34%
homemade	¾ cup	10	255	35%
microwave (Kid's Kitchen)				
box mix	7.5 oz	1	90	10%
CHOW MEIN-PORK				
homemade w/noodles	1 cup	24.7	432	51%
homemade without noodles	¾ cup	14	223	57%
CHOW MEIN-SHRIMP				
homemade w/noodles	¾ cup	3.9	141	25%
(CHUN KING)				
Divider Pak Entrees/Canned-Prepared				
Beef Chow Mein				
40 oz package	7 oz	2	100	18%

Food and Description	Amount	Fat Grams	Total Calories	% Fat Calories
24 oz package	8 oz	2	110	16%
Beef Pepper Oriental	7 oz	4	110	33%
Chicken Chow Mein				
40 oz package	7 oz	4	110	33%
24 oz package	8 oz	4	120	30%
Pork Chow Mein	7 oz	4	120	30%
Shrimp Chow Mein	7 oz	2	100	18%
Egg Rolls & Side Dishes/Frozen				
Chicken Egg Rolls	3.5 oz	7	210	30%
Chinese Pea Pods	1.5 oz	–	16	–
Fried Rice w/Chicken	8 oz	4	254	14%
Fried Rice w/Pork	8 oz	5	263	17%
Meat & Shrimp Egg Rolls	3.5 oz	8	214	34%
Pork Restaurant Style				
Egg Rolls	3 oz	6	172	31%
Shrimp Egg Rolls	3.5 oz	6	189	29%
Entrees/Frozen				
Beef Pepper Oriental	13 oz	3	309	9%
Beef Terijaki	13 oz	2	379	5%
Chicken Chow Mein	13 oz	5	361	13%
Crunchy Walnut Chicken	13 oz	5	117	39%
Hunan Pork	13 oz	6	324	17%
Imperial Chicken	13 oz	1	294	3%
Sweet & Sour Pork	13 oz	4	394	9%
Szechuan Beef	13 oz	2	331	5%
Stir-Fry Entrees/Canned-Prepared				
Chow Mein w/beef	6 oz	19	290	59%
Chow Mein w/chicken	6 oz	11	220	45%
Egg Foo Young	5 oz	8	140	51%
Pepper Steak	6 oz	17	250	61%
Sukiyaki	6 oz	17	260	59%
EGGROLL				
homemade w/no meat	2.25 oz	5.9	102	52%
FRIED RICE (*See* RICE DISHES)				
(HUNT'S) MINUTE GOURMET				
Sweet & Sour Chicken/box mix	7.8 oz	4	300	12%
(IMPROMTU LITE) microwave box mix				
Sweet & Sour Chicken	9 oz	3	290	9%
(INTERNATIONAL LITES)				
Microwavable Box				
Beef Peking	10 oz	3	230	12%
Chicken Peking	10 oz	3	230	12%
(JENO'S)				
frozen				
Chicken egg rolls	3 oz	9	190	43%

Food and Description	Amount	Fat Grams	Total Calories	% Fat Calories
Shrimp & Cheese Egg Rolls	3 oz/ ~ 6 rolls	8	190	38%
(LA CHOY)				
Canned				
Bi-Packs/prepared as directed				
Beef Chow Mein	¾ cup	1	70	13%
Beef Pepper Oriental	¾ cup	3	100	27%
Chicken Chow Mein	¾ cup	3	80	34%
Pork Chow Mein	¾ cup	4	80	45%
Shrimp Chow Mein	¾ cup	1	70	13%
Sukiyaki	¾ cup	1	70	13%
Vegetable Chow Mein	¾ cup	2	50	36%
Chow Meins				
Beef	¾ cup	1	60	15%
Chicken	¾ cup	2	70	26%
Meatless	¾ cup	1	35	26%
Shrimp	¾ cup	1	45	20%
Entrees				
Beef Pepper Oriental	¾ cup	2	90	20%
Sweet & Sour Oriental				
w/chicken	¾ cup	2	240	8%
w/pork	¾ cup	4	250	14%
(LEAN CUISINE)				
Chicken Chow Mein	11.25 oz	5	250	18%
Chicken Oriental w/egg noodles	~ 9 oz	6	240	23%
(LEAN POCKETS)				
Chicken Oriental/frozen	1	6	250	22%
ORIENTAL BEEF				
Box-prepared				
(Hunt's Minute Gourmet)	6.4 oz	14	290	43%
Frozen				
(Lean Cuisine)	8.5 oz	7	250	25%
(The Gourmet)	1 serving	9	290	29%
(ORIENTAL CLASSICS)				
Box mix				
Sweet & Sour Chicken Dinner	¼ pkg	7	470	13%
Stir Fried Rice Dinner	1 serving	14	430	29%
(SCHWAN'S) HOME DELIVERY				
Pork Egg Roll/frozen	2 oz	5	120	38%
Shrimp Egg Roll	2 oz	2	90	20%
SUSHI-homemade w/vegetables	4.5 oz	–	181	–
SWEET & SOUR CHICKEN				
canned-prepared	¾ cup	2	120	15%
SWEET & SOUR PORK				
frozen (Van de Kamp's)	11 oz	15	430	31%

Food and Description	Amount	Fat Grams	Total Calories	% Fat Calories
homemade	¾ cup	7.7	187	37%
SZECHWAN CHICKEN/				
(International Lites)				
microwavable - box prepared	10 oz	5	270	17%
TERIYAKI CHICKEN				
canned-prepared	¾ cup	2	85	21%
(Hormel) Chicken By George				
Gourmet Entree	5 oz	4	180	20%
TERIYAKI SHRIMP				
homemade	¾ cup	1	174	5%
(TYSON)				
Gourmet Selection Entrees				
Chicken Oriental	10.25 oz	7	270	23%
Peking Chicken	10 oz	20	390	46%
Sweet & Sour Chicken	11 oz	16	440	33%
Teriyaki Chicken	11 oz	2	130	14%
Teriyaki Chicken Wings	11 oz	14	220	57%
WON TON SOUP *(See* SOUP)				
ORIENTAL FOOD SEASONINGS				
(Durkee)				
Chop Suey-dry	1 pkg	2	128	14%
prepared	3½ cups	42	1113	34%
Fried Rice				
dry	1 pkg	1	62	15%
prepared	2 cups	1.5	430	9%
Sweet & Sour Sauce				
prepared	1 cup	5.7	230	22%
(Kikkoman)				
Baste & Glaze				
Teriyaki	1 tsp	< 1	9	50%
(La Choy)				
Teriyaki Marinade & Sauce	1 oz	–	30	–
(S&B Sunbird)				
Oriental Seasonings/dry				
Beef & Broccoli	1 pkg	–	97	–
Chinese Barbeque	1 pkg	1	54	17%
Chop Suey	1 pkg	.6	85	6%
Chow Mein	1 pkg	.57	84	6%
Fried Rice	1 pkg	–	57	–
Oriental Chicken	1 pkg	7	140	45%
Stir Fry	1 pkg	.5	75	6%
Sukiyaki	1 pkg	.9	84	10%
Sweet & Sour	1 pkg	–	85	–
Tomato Beef	1 pkg	1	131	7%
Teriyaki Marinade	1 pkg	1	100	9%

Food and Description	Amount	Fat Grams	Total Calories	% Fat Calories
OYSTER				
Eastern				
meat only	1 cup	4	160	23%
battered & fried	3 oz	10	181	50%
	6 Medium	11	175	57%
breaded & fried	3 oz	10.7	167	58%
	6 Medium	11	173	57%
canned	3 oz	2	58	31%
whole(S&W)	2 oz	3	95	28%
raw	6 Medium	2	58	31%
steamed	3 oz	4	117	31%
	6 Medium			
	~ 1.5 oz	2	58	31%
Pacific/Western				
canned	6-9 Medium/			
	12 oz	7.5	309	22%
	1 cup	5	218	21%
raw	3 oz	2	69	26%

OYSTER STEW (*See* SOUP)

P

Food and Description	Amount	Fat Grams	Total Calories	% Fat Calories
PANCAKE				
BUCKWHEAT				
Box mix w/whole milk	1	2	55	33%
(Aunt Jemima)	3	8	230	31%
FROZEN				
(Aunt Jemima)				
Blueberry	3	4	200	18%
Buttermilk	3	2	180	10%
Original	3	2	180	10%
(Downyflake)				
Blueberry	2	7	170	37%
(Great Starts)				
w/blueberry sauce	7 oz	10	410	22%
w/lite links	5.5 oz	16	350	41%
w/sausages	6 oz	22	460	43%
w/strawberries	6 oz	11	430	23%

Food and Description	Amount	Fat Grams	Total Calories	% Fat Calories
whole wheat w/lite links	5.5 oz	16	350	41%
(Krusteaz)				
Blueberry	3	5	300	15%
Buttermilk	3	5	290	16%
Whole Wheat N Honey	3	4	250	14%
(Morningstar Farms)-plain	3.5 oz	5	232	19%
(Swanson)				
Budget Breakfast	3.5 oz	12	290	37%
FROZEN MICROWAVEABLE				
(Aunt Jemima)				
Blueberry	3	4	220	16%
Buttermilk	3	4	240	15%
Original	3	4	210	17%
(Krusteaz)				
Blueberry	1	2	100	18%
Buttermilk	1	2	96	9%
Whole Wheat	1	1	83	11%
(Microwave Morning)				
w/whipped maple flavored topping	4.7 oz	13	380	31%
(Pillsbury)				
Blueberry	3	4	250	14%
Buttermilk	3	4	60	14%
Harvest Wheat	3	4	240	15%
Original	3	4	240	15%
w/oatbran	3	4	260	14%
(Weight Watchers)				
w/blueberry topping	1 pkg	4	260	14%
w/links	4.5 oz	10	240	38%
w/strawberry topping	1 pkg	4	230	16%
PANCAKE/WAFFLE MIX				
(Arrowhead Mills)				
Blue Heaven	½ cup	2	200	9%
Buckwheat	½ cup	2	270	7%
Griddle Lite	½ cup	3	260	10%
Multi-grain	½ cup	2	350	5%
(Aunt Jemima)				
Buttermilk Pancake & Waffle	3	8	220	33%
Complete Pancake & Waffle	3	4	250	14%
Complete Buttermilk	3	3	230	12%
Lite	3	2	130	14%
Original Pancake & Waffle	3	7	200	32%
No colesterol version	3	4	170	21%

Food and Description	Amount	Fat Grams	Total Calories	% Fat Calories
Pancake Express				
Blueberry	3	4	230	16%
Buttermilk	3	3	230	12%
Lite	3	2	130	14%
Original	3	3	240	11%
Whole Wheat	3	9	270	30%
(Betty Crocker)				
Buttermilk	3	10	280	32%
Complete	3	3	210	13%
(Bisquick)				
Shake'N Pour				
Blueberry	3	3	270	10%
Buttermilk	3	3	250	11%
Original	3	4	260	14%
Blue Corn Pancake & Waffle	⅓ cup	2	200	9%
(Estee)	3	–	100	–
Buckwheat	½ cup	3	235	12%
(Rich Earth)	½ cup	2	190	10%
7-Grain Buttermilk	½ cup	2	200	9%
Stone Ground Whole Wheat	½ cup	2	220	8%
Unbleached Wheat & Soya	½ cup	2	235	8%
(Featherweight)	3	1	130	7%
(Health Valley)				
Buttermilk & Biscuit/dry	1 oz	1	100	9%
(Hungry Jack)				
Blueberry	3	15	320	42%
Buttermilk	3	11	240	41%
Buttermilk Complete Packets	3	3	180	15%
Extra Lights	3	7	240	26%
Complete	3	2	190	10%
Panshakes	3	6	250	22%
(Krusteaz)				
Blueberry	3	4	205	18%
Buttermilk	3	3	200	14%
Complete whole wheat/honey	3	1	215	4%
Complete Oat Bran	3	2	200	9%
Lite	3	1	130	7%
Martha White/FlapStax	1	2	100	18%
Light Crust Pancake/dry mix	2 oz	3	120	23%
Robin Hood/(Gold Medal)				
Pouch mix				
Buttermilk-prepared	⅛ mixture	2	100	18%
Standard Home Recipe (USDA)				
Buckwheat (6" dia)	3	9	410	20%

Food and Description	Amount	Fat Grams	Total Calories	% Fat Calories
Buttermilk (6" dia)	3	15	490	28%
Plain (4" dia)	1	2	62	29%
(6" dia)	1	5	169	27%
PANCAKE/WAFFLE SYRUP (*See also* SYRUP)				
(Aunt Jemima)				
Butter Lite	2 Tbs	–	50	–
Lite	2 Tbs	–	50	–
Regular	2 Tbs	–	110	–
(Cary's) Low-cal	1 Tbs	–	6	–
(Estee)/all flavors	1 Tbs	–	4	–
(Featherweight)-Lite				
All flavors	1 Tbs	–	16	–
(Golden Griddle)	1 Tbs	–	55	–
(Karo)-Pancake	1 Tbs	–	60	–
(Log Cabin)				
Buttered	2 Tbs	–	100	–
Country Kitchen	2 Tbs	–	100	–
Lite	2 Tbs	–	50	–
Maple Honey	2 Tbs	–	100	–
Regular	2 Tbs	–	100	–
(Mrs. Butterworth's)-Lite	2 Tbs	–	60	–
(Nabisco)-Vermont Maid	1 Tbs	–	50	–
(Nutradiet)				
Blueberry	1 tsp	–	4	–
Maple Flavored	1 tsp	–	4	–
Strawberry	1 tsp	–	4	–
(Smucker's)				
All fruit flavors	1 Tbs	–	50	–
PAPAW/fresh	½ lb	2	194	84%
PAPAYA/fresh	1	.5	117	4%
(Del Monte)	⅓ med/ ⅔ cup pulp	–	60	–
PAPAYA JUICE				
Papaya Delight/bottled	6 oz	–	90	–
Papaya Juice/canned	8 oz	–	120	–
Papaya Nectar	8 oz	–	142	–
(Kern's)	6 oz	–	110	–
(Knudsen)	8 oz	–	100	–
(Libby's)	6 oz	–	110	–
PAPAYA-PINEAPPLE JUICE				
Nectar (Kern's)	6 oz	–	110	–
PAPAYA PUNCH				
(Tropicana) single serve	8 oz	–	110	–
PAPRIKA	1 tsp	–	6	–

Food and Description	Amount	Fat Grams	Total Calories	% Fat Calories
PARSLEY	10 sprigs	–	3	–
	½ cup	–	10	–
dried	1 tsp	–	1	–
freeze-dried	Any Amount	–	–	–
PARSNIP				
fresh-cooked	½ cup	–	63	–
raw	½ cup	–	50	–
PASSION FRUIT				
fresh	1	–	18	–
	½ lb	–	106	–
PASSION FRUIT JUICE				
fresh				
purple	1 cup	–	126	–
yellow	1 cup	–	149	–
Passionfruit Delight/bottled	6 oz	–	90	–
PASSION FRUIT-ORANGE-GUAVA JUICE				
from frozen conc.	6 oz	–	80	–
PASSION FRUIT-ORANGE JUICE				
from frozen conc.	6 oz	–	80	–
Passionfruit-Orange Nectar (Kern's)	6 oz	–	120	–
PASTA				
(American Beauty)				
Coiled Vermicelli-dry	2 oz	1	210	4%
Curly Roni-dry	2 oz	1	210	4%
Elbo Roni-dry	2 oz	1	210	4%
Extra Wide Egg Noodles-dry	2 oz	3	220	12%
Fettuccine-dry	2 oz	3	220	12%
Fine Egg Noodles-dry	2 oz	3	220	12%
Krinkly Egg Noodles-dry	2 oz	3	220	12%
Lasagne-dry	2 oz	1	210	4%
Long Spaghetti-dry	2 oz	1	210	4%
Mostaccioli-dry	2 oz	1	210	4%
Rainbow Shells-dry	2 oz	1	210	4%
Rainbow Twirls-dry	2 oz	1	210	4%
Roni Mac-dry	2 oz	1	210	4%
Rotini-dry	2 oz	1	210	4%
Salad Mac-dry	2 oz	1	210	4%
Shell Roni-dry	2 oz	1	210	4%
Shell Ronni-Large-dry	2 oz	1	210	4%
Spaghetti-dry	2 oz	1	210	4%
Thin Spaghetti-dry	2 oz	1	210	4%
Vermicelli-dry	2 oz	1	210	4%
Wide Egg Noodles-dry	2 oz	3	220	12%
Couscous (Near East)-dry	1.25 oz	–	120	–

Food and Description	Amount	Fat Grams	Total Calories	% Fat Calories
(Creamette)				
Egg Noodles				
Homestyle/dry	2 oz	3	220	12%
Pennsylvania Dutch				
Broad/dry	2 oz	3	220	12%
Egg Noodle Dumpling	2 oz	4	220	16%
Enriched Egg Noodles-dry	2 oz	3	220	12%
Enriched Elbow Macaroni-dry	2 oz	1	210	4%
Enriched Fettuccine-dry	2 oz	1	210	4%
Enriched Lasagna-dry	2 oz	1	210	4%
Enriched Linguini-dry	2 oz	1	210	4%
Enriched Mostaccioli-dry	2 oz	1	210	4%
Enriched Rainbow Rotini-dry	2 oz	1	210	4%
Enriched Rigatoni-dry	2 oz	1	210	4%
Enriched Rotini-ddry	2 oz	1	210	4%
Enriched Spaghetti-dry	2 oz	1	210	4%
Enriched Spinach Macaroni				
Ribbons-dry	2	1	210	4%
Enriched Thin Spaghetti-dry	2 oz	1	210	4%
Enriched Vermicelli-dry	2 oz	1	210	4%
Enriched Wide Egg Noodles-dry	2 oz	3	220	12%
No Egg Yolk Ribbons-dry	2 oz	1	210	4%
Egg Noodles Homestyle (Reames)				
frozen-cooked	½ cup	2	160	11%
Egg Noodle Substitute (Foulds)				
No Yolks/dry	2 oz	2	210	9%
(Golden Grain)				
Egg noodles-dry	2 oz	2	210	9%
Pasta-dry	2 oz	1	200	5%
(Grandma's)				
Wide Egg Noodles				
Country Style				
frozen	4 oz	2	175	10%
(Health Valley)				
Elbows				
whole wheat-dry	2 oz	1	202	5%
whole wheat w/4 veg-dry	2 oz	1	202	5%
Lasagna				
spinach-dry	2 oz	1	170	5%
whole wheat-dry	2 oz	1	170	5%
Spaghetti				
whole wheat-dry	2 oz	1	170	5%
whole wheat amaranth-dry	2 oz	1	200	5%
whole wheat w/spinach-dry	2 oz	1	170	5%

Food and Description	Amount	Fat Grams	Total Calories	% Fat Calories
Macaroni				
enriched/unenriched				
cooked-firm	1 cup	1	190	5%
tender-cold	1 cup	< 1	115	4%
tender-hot	1 cup	1	155	6%
dry	8 oz	2.7	838	3%
Matzo Farfel/Farfal				
(Manischewitz)	1 cup	.8	180	4%
(Mueller's)				
Egg Noodles-dry	2 oz	3	220	12%
Golden Rich Egg Noodles-dry	2 oz	3	220	12%
Lasagna-dry	2 oz	1	210	4%
Macaroni-dry	2 oz	1	210	4%
Spaghetti-dry	2 oz	1	210	4%
Tri-Color Twists-dry	2 oz	1	210	4%
Noodles				
chow mein				
canned	1 cup	11	220	45%
dry-(La Choy)	½ cup	8	150	48%
egg				
cooked	1 cup	2	200	9%
dry	8 oz	10	881	10%
flakes				
Goodman's)-dry	2 oz	3	220	12%
frozen				
(Reames)	2 oz	2	160	11%
spinach				
(Ronzoni)-dry	2 oz	2	210	9%
Oriental Noodles				
Chinese (Chun King)				
canned	1 oz	7	140	45%
chow funn				
wheat-dry	1 oz	< 1	102	4%
saimin				
wheat-dry	1 oz	–	95	–
soba				
buckwheat-dry	1 oz	1	100	9%
Pastini				
carrot-dry	4 oz	2	420	4%
egg-dry	1 cup	7	651	10%
spinach-dry	4 oz	2	415	4%
(Pritikin)				
Ribbon Pasta				
whole wheat-dry	2 oz	2	220	8%

Food and Description	Amount	Fat Grams	Total Calories	% Fat Calories
Spaghetti				
whole wheat-dry	2 oz	2	220	8%
(Ronzoni)				
Egg Noodles				
dry	2 oz	2	210	9%
Spinach-dry	2 oz	3	220	12%
Macaroni-dry	2 oz	< 1	210	2%
Medium Shells-dry	2 oz	1	210	4%
Spinach Macaroni-dry	2 oz	< 1	210	2%
Tri-color Rotini-dry	2 oz	1	210	4%
Spaghetti				
cooked				
firm stage	1 cup	.7	192	3%
tender stage	1 cup	.6	155	4%
dry	8 oz	2.7	888	3%
Spaghetti				
(American Beauty)-dry	2 oz	1	210	4%
(Westbrae Natural)				
plain-dry	2 oz	2	210	9%
Spinach-dry	2 oz	2	210	9%

PASTA DINNER (*See also* FROZEN ENTREE/DINNER and individual listings)
(NOTE: Data for homemade dishes in this table will vary, pending type of ingredients used, i.e. low-fat milk & cheeses.)
(Chef Boy Ar Dee)

Food and Description	Amount	Fat Grams	Total Calories	% Fat Calories
CannedPasta Products				
ABC's & 1,2,3's				
w/Mini Meatballs	7.5 oz	9	230	35%
in Sauce	7.5 oz	1	160	6%
Beef-O-Getti	7.5 oz	9	220	37%
Beefaroni	7.5 oz	8	220	33%
	8 oz	9	260	31%
	8.7 oz	8	250	29%
ChiliMac	7.5 oz	11	230	43%
Dinosaurs in Cheese Flavored Sauce	8.6 oz	1	200	5%
Dinosaurs in Spaghetti Sauce				
w/cheese flavor	7.5 oz	1	155	6%
Dinosaurs w/Meatballs	8.6 oz	11	280	35%
Dinosaurs w/Mini Meatballs	7.5 oz	8	230	31%
Lasagna	7.5 oz	8	240	30%
Lasagna	8 oz	8	250	29%
Macaroni Shells in Tomato Sauce	7.5 oz	1	150	6%
Mini Bites	7.5 oz	12	260	42%
Mini Cannelloni	7.5 oz	7	230	27%
Pac Man in Chicken Sauce	7.5 oz	7	170	37%

Food and Description	Amount	Fat Grams	Total Calories	% Fat Calories
Pac Man in Tomato Sauce	7.5 oz	1	150	6%
Pac Man w/Meatballs	7.5 oz	9	230	35%
Roller Coasters	7.5 oz	9	230	35%
Smurf Beef Raviioli & Pasta in Meat Sauce	7.5 oz	5	230	20%
Smurf Beef in Spaghetti Sauce w/Cheese flavor	7.5 oz	1	150	6%
Smurf Pasta w/Meatballs	7.5 oz	9	240	34%
Spaghetti & Meatballs-25.5 oz	8.5 oz	11	250	40%
Spaghetti & Meatballs w/tomato sauce-15 oz	7.5 oz	9	230	35%
Spaghetti & Meatballs w/tomato sauce-39 oz	7.8 oz	10	240	38%
Spaghetti'n Beef in tomato sauce	7.5 oz	9	240	334%
Tic Tac Toes in Spaghetti Sauce w/cheese flavor	7.5 oz	1	160	6%
Tic Tac Toes w/Mini Meatballs	7.5 oz	9	240	34%
Zooroni w/Meatballs in Sauce	7.5 oz	8	240	30%
Dinner Products				
Lasagna Dinner	5.97 oz	8	280	26%
Spaghetti Dinner w/Condensed Meat Sauce	3.25 oz	6	250	22%
Spaghetti packaged Dinner w/prepared Meat Sauce	4.88 oz	3	240	11%
Spaghetti packaged Dinner w/prepared Mushroom Sauce	4.88 oz	1	210	4%
EZO Products				
ABC's & 1,2,3's in Sauce	7 oz	1	160	6%
ABC's & 1,2,3's w/Meatballs	7 oz	8	230	31%
Beef Stew	7 oz	13	220	53%
Chili Mac	7 oz	9	230	35%
Mini Cannelloni	7.5 oz	9	240	34%
Roller Coasters	7 oz	9	230	35%
Spaghetti'N Beef in Tomato Sauce	7 oz	8	220	33%
EZO Products-Microwave				
ABC's & 123's w/Mini Meatballs	7.5 oz	11	260	38%
Beef Raioli	7.5 oz	4	190	19%
Beefaroni	7.5 oz	7	220	29%
Lasagna	7.5 oz	9	230	35%
	7 oz	8	220	33%
Spaghetti w/Meatballs	7.5 oz	10	240	38%
Tic Tac Toes w/Meatballs	7.5 oz	11	260	38%

Food and Description	Amount	Fat Grams	Total Calories	% Fat Calories
Tic Tac Toes w/Mini Meatballs	7 oz	8	210	34%
Tic Tac Toes in Spaghetti Sauce w/Cheese flavor	7 oz	1	160	6%
LIDO Club Products				
Beef Ravioli	7.5 oz	4	190	19%
Spaghetti Rings & Little Meat Balls	7.5 oz	10	220	41%
Mama Leone's Pasta Suprema				
Beef Ravioli	7.5 oz	7	240	26%
Cheese Ravioli	7.5 oz	2	200	9%
Mini Lasagna	7.5 oz	1	170	5%
Spaghetti in Tomato Saucew	7.5 oz	1	160	6%
Ziti in Meat Falvored Sauce	7.5 oz	4	170	21%
Ravoli Products				
Beef Ravioli in Sauce	8 oz	5	220	21%
	8.7 oz	6	240	23%
Beef Ravioli in Tomato & Meat Sauce	7.5 oz	5	220	21%
Cheese Ravioli in Beef & Tomato Sauce	7.5 oz	3	200	14%
Cheese Ravioli in Tomato Sauce	7.5 oz	5	200	23%
Chicken Ravioli	7.5 oz	4	180	20%
Mini Ravioli-Beef	7.5 oz	5	210	38%
Mini Ravioli-Beef	8 oz	6	230	24%
Mini Ravioli-Chicken	7.5 oz	8	220	33%
(Estee)				
Ravioli Beef	7.5 oz	6	210	26%
Spaghetti & Meatballs	7.5 oz	15	240	56%
(Franco-American)				
Canned Products				
Beef Ravioli's in Meat Sauce	7.5 oz	8	250	29%
Hearty Pasta Beef Ravioli in Meat Sauce	7.5 oz	11	280	35%
Hearty Pasta Macaroni w/Beef in Tomato Sauce	7.5 oz	5	200	23%
Hearty Pasta Twists in Pizza Sauce	7.5 oz	7	220	29%
Macaroni & Cheese	7⅜ oz	5	170	27%
Spaghetti w/Meatballs in Tomato Sauce	7⅜ oz	8	220	33%
Spaghetti in Tomato Sauce w/cheese	7⅜ oz	2	190	10%
Spaghettio's in Tomato & Cheese Sauce	7.5 oz	2	170	7%

Food and Description	Amount	Fat Grams	Total Calories	% Fat Calories
Spaghettio's w/Meatballs in Tomato Sauce	7⅜ oz	8	210	66%
Spaghettio's w/Sliced Beef Franks in Tomato Sauce	7⅜ oz	9	220	37%
Sporty O's	7⅜ oz	8	210	34%
Teddy O's	7.5 oz	2	170	11%
(Golden Grain)				
Lunch-In-One Microwave				
Fettuccine Alfredo	1 package	13	350	33%
Macaroni & Cheese	1 package	10	340	26%
Pasta Broccoli Au Gratin	1 package	10	330	27%
Pasta & Three Cheeses	1 package	12	340	32%
Shells & Creamy Sauce	1 package	12	340	32%
Noodle Roni				
Angel Hair Pasta				
w/herbs-dry	1 serving	2	120	15%
w/herbs-prepared	1 serving	8	200	36%
w/parmesan cheese-dry	1 serving	3	140	19%
w/parmesan cheese-prepared	1 serving	9	210	39%
Broccoli Au Gratin	½ cup	9	190	43%
Broccoli & Mushroom	½ cup	14	240	53%
Chicken & Mushroom	½ cup	4	160	23%
Creamy Chicken	½ cup	8	180	40%
Creamy Garlic	½ cup	17	300	51%
Fettuccine	½ cup	15	250	54%
Herb & Butter	½ cup	7	160	39%
Mild Cheddar	½ cup	9	190	43%
Parmesano	½ cup	14	250	50%
Romanoff	½ cup	10	200	45%
Sour Cream & Scallions	½ cup	15	240	56%
Stroganoff	½ cup	17	350	44%
Vegetable Alfredo	½ cup	14	240	53%
(Green Giant)				
Entrees-frozen				
Lasagna	12 oz	20	490	37%
Macaroni & Cheese	9 oz	10	290	31%
Garden Gourmet-frozen				
Fettucine Primavera	9.5 oz	13	260	45%
Pasta Dijon	9.5 oz	20	300	60%
Rotini Cheddar	9.5 oz	13	280	42%
Pasta Accents-frozen				
Cheddar Cheese Seasoning	½ cup	4	100	36%
Garlic Seasoning	½ cup	4	100	36%
Lemon Butter Seasoning	½ cup	3	80	34%

Food and Description	Amount	Fat Grams	Total Calories	% Fat Calories
Parmesan Cheese Seasoning	½ cup	4	90	40%
Sour Cream & Herb Seasoning	½ cup	6	110	49%
Southwestern Seasoning	½ cup	5	90	50%
(Hain)				
Pasta & Sauce (dry unless noted)				
Creamy Parmesan	¼ pkg	3	150	18%
Creamy Swiss	1 Serving	4	170	21%
Fettuccini Alfredo	1 serving	4	180	20%
-prepared	½ cup	24	350	62%
Italian Herb	1 Serving	2	110	16%
Marinara	1 serving	1	120	8%
Primavera	1 serving	4	140	26%
Tangy Cheddar	1 serving	6	180	30%
(Health Valley)				
Oat Bran Pasta Dinners				
Fettucini Herb Italiano	9 oz	3	320	8%
Fettucini Marinara	9 oz	3	320	8%
Fettucini Primavera	9 oz	3	320	8%
(Heinz)				
Chili-Mac	7.5 oz	12	250	43%
Macaroni'N Beef in Tomato Sauce	7.25 oz	8	200	36%
Macaroni & Cheese	7.5 oz	8	190	38%
Noodles & Beef in Sauce	7.5 oz	8	170	42%
Noodles & Chicken	7.5 oz	7	160	39%
Noodles & Tuna	7.5 oz	5	170	27%
Spaghetti in Tomato Sauce				
w/cheese	7.75 oz	2	160	11%
Spaghetti in Tomato Sauce w/meat	7.5 oz	6	170	32%
(Kid's Kitchen)				
Microwave				
Macaroni & Cheese	7.5 oz	5	170	27%
Macaroni & Chicken	7.5 oz	2	120	15%
(Kraft)				
Dinners				
Egg Noodles w/Cheese Dinner	¾ cup	17	340	45%
Egg Noodles w/Chicken Dinner	¾ cup	9	240	34%
Macaroni & Cheese	¾ cup	13	290	40%
Deluxe	¾ cup	8	260	28%
Family Size	¾ cup	13	290	40%
Micromac-dry	¼ pkg	2	150	12%
Micromac-prepared	½ cup	7	210	30%
Macaroni & Cheese/unprepared				
Dinomac	⅓ box	2	190	9%
Teddy Bears	⅓ box	2	190	9%

Food and Description	Amount	Fat Grams	Total Calories	% Fat Calories
Wild Wheels	⅓ box	2	190	9%
Pasta Salad				
Broccoli & Vegetable	⅙ box	15	210	64%
Garden Primavera	⅙ box	7	170	37%
Light Italian	⅙ box	3	130	21%
Spaghetti Dinner				
American Style	1 cup	7	300	21%
Tangy Italian Style	1 cup	8	310	23%
W/Meat Sauce	1 cup	14	360	35%
Spiral Macaroni & Cheese	¾ cup	17	330	46%
Velveeta Shells & Cheese				
prepared	¾ cup	10	260	35%
Pasta & Cheese				
Cheddar Broccoli/dry	⅕ box	4	140	26%
Fettuccine Alfredo	½ cup	9	180	45%
Herb & Garlic	½ cup	8	180	40%
Parmesan	½ cup	8	180	40%
3-Cheese & Vegetable	½ cup	8	180	40%
Pasta Salad				
Broccoli & Vegetable	½ cup	15	210	64%
Creamy Dill	½ cup	11	200	50%
Garden Primavera	½ cup	7	170	37%
Herb & Garlic	½ cup	12	210	51%
Homestyle	½ cup	16	240	60%
Light Italian	½ cup	3	130	21%
Rancher's Choice	½ cup	16	240	60%
(Lean Cuisine)				
Cheese Canaloni				
frozen	9⅛ oz	10	260	35%
(Little Chef)				
Entree Pasta Italiano Mix				
dry	¼ pkg	–	110	–
w/chicken	1 cup	10	290	31%
w/tofu	1 cup	11	250	40%
(Lipton)				
Hearty Ones Microwave				
Garden Medley	11 oz	4	320	11%
Shells & Cheese	11 oz	7	370	17%
Twists Italiano	11 oz	2	330	5%
Noodles & Sauce				
Alfredo	½ cup	10	220	41%
Alfreado Carbonara	½ cup	11	210	47%
Beef Flavored	½ cup	7	180	35%
Butter	½ cup	10	200	45%

Food and Description	Amount	Fat Grams	Total Calories	% Fat Calories
Butter & Herb	½ cup	9	190	43%
Cheese	½ cup	9	190	43%
Chicken Flavored	½ cup	8	180	40%
Creamy Garlic	½ cup	10	210	43%
Parmesan	½ cup	11	200	50%
Sour Cream & Chives	½ cup	9	200	41%
Stroganoff w/Sour Cream & Mushrooms	½ cup	9	200	41%
(Lunch Bucket)				
Microwave				
Chili Mac	8.5 oz	13	260	45%
Fettucini Marinara	8.5 oz	2	220	8%
Lasagna	10 oz	10	300	30%
Macaroni'N Beef	8.5 oz	11	320	31%
Pasta n'Chicken	8.5 oz	8	220	33%
Spaghetti'N Meat Sauce	8.25 oz	7	250	25%
(Minute Microwave)				
prepared w/butter				
Chicken Flavored Noodles				
family size	½ cup	5	160	23%
single size	½ cup	4	160	23%
Noodles Alfredo				
family size	½ cup	6	170	32%
single size	½ cup	5	160	28%
Parmesan Noodles				
family size	½ cup	6	170	17%
single size	½ cup	5	160	23%
Pasta & Cheddar Cheese				
family size	½ cup	7	160	39%
single size	½ cup	6	160	34%
(Ragu)				
Pasta Meals				
Elbows in Sauce w/Ground Beef, Mushrooms, and Green Peppers	7.5 oz	4	200	18%
Mini Lasagna in Sauce	7.5 oz	1	160	6%
Shells in Sauce w/Ground Beef	7.5 oz	4	190	19%
Spaghetti in Sauce	7.5 oz	1	170	5%
Spaghetti in Sauce w/Ground Beef	7.5 oz	4	210	17%
Twists in Sauce	7.5 oz	1	160	6%
Ramen Noodles				
Beef	½ pkg	7	190	33%
Chicken	½ pkg	7	190	33%
Oriental	½ pkg	7	190	33%

Food and Description	Amount	Fat Grams	Total Calories	% Fat Calories
(Rice-A-Roni) Lunch For One				
Broccoli Au Gratin	1 pkg	10	330	27%
Fettuccine Alfredo	1 pkg	13	350	33%
Macaroni & Cheese	1 pkg	10	340	26%
Pasta & Three Cheeses	1 pkg	12	340	32%
Shells & Creamy Sauce	1 pkg	8	290	25%
(Van Camp's)				
Canned Products				
Chilee Weenee	1 cup	16	310	47%
Noodlee Weenee	1 cup	8	240	30%
Spaghettee Weenee	1 cup	7	240	26%
(Wolf)				
Chili-Mac				
canned	1 cup	20	320	56%
PASTA MIX				
(NOTE: Mixes are prepared as directed unless otherwise stated.)				
(Betty Crocker)				
Presto Pasta				
Creamy Alfredo	¼ pkg	18	370	44%
Ground Beef in Tomato Herb				
Sauce-dry	¼ pkg	8	280	26%
Italian Sausage in Tomato Herb				
Sauce-dry	¼ pkg	8	280	26%
Tomato Mushroom-dry	¼ pkg	6	240	26%
Suddenly Salad				
Caesar	⅙ pkg	8	170	42%
Classic Pasta	⅙ pkg	6	150	36%
Creamy Macaroni	⅙ pkg	10	200	45%
Italian Pasta	⅙ pkg	6	150	36%
Pasta Primavera	⅙ pkg	10	190	47%
Ranch & Bacon	⅙ pkg	11	210	47%
PASTA SAUCE				
(McCormick-Schilling)				
Pasta Prima Sauce Blends				
Herb & Garlic-dry	1 pkg	< 1	65	7%
Marinara-dry	1 pkg	< 1	74	6%
Pesto-dry	1 pkg	< 1	38	12%
Salad Vinaigrette-dry	1 pkg	< 1	78	6%
PASTRAMI (See also LUNCHEON MEAT)				
	1 oz	8	99	73%
PASTRY (See CAKE AND CAKE PASTRY)				
PASTRY SHEET				
Fillo-all purpose dough	1⅓ leaves	–	80	–
(Pepperidge Farm) Puff Pastry Sheets	¼ sheet	17	260	59%

Food and Description	Amount	Fat Grams	Total Calories	% Fat Calories
PASTRY SHELL /frozen				
(Pepperidge Farm)	1 shell	15	210	64%
PASTRY, TOASTER				
(PILLSBURY) BREAKFAST PASTRIES				
Apple	1	9	200	41%
Cinnamon	1	10	200	45%
Strawberry	1	9	190	43%
POP TARTS (KELLOGG'S)				
Frosted blueberry	1	6	210	26%
Frosted brown sugar/cinnamon	1	7	210	30%
Frosted cherry	1	5	200	23%
Frosted chocolate fudge	1	5	200	23%
Frosted cinnamon	1	7	210	30%
Frosted dutch apple	1	6	210	26%
Frosted raspberry	1	5	200	23%
Frosted strawberry	1	5	200	23%
Frosted vanilla cream	1	5	200	23%
Unfrosted blueberry	1	6	210	26%
Unfrosted milk chocolate	1	6	210	26%
Unfrosted raspberry	1	6	210	26%
Unfrosted strawberry	1	6	210	26%
TOASTER MUFFINS (PILLSBURY)				
Apple spice	1	5	130	35%
Banana nut	1	6	130	42%
Old fashioned corn	1	5	120	38%
Raisin bran	1	5	120	38%
Wild Maine blueberry	1	3	120	23%
TOASTER STRUDEL BREAKFAST PASTRY (PILLSBURY)				
Apple spice, Blueberry, Cinnamon,				
Raspberry, Strawberry	1	8	190	38%
Cherry	1	9	190	43%
TOASTETTES PASTRY (NABISCO)				
Apple	1	5	200	23%
Blueberry	1	5	200	23%
Cherry strawberry	1	5	200	23%
Frosted blueberry	1	5	200	23%
Frosted brown sugar cinnamon	1	5	200	23%
Frosted cherry	1	5	200	23%
Frosted fudge	1	6	200	27%
Frosted strawberry	1	5	200	23%
PEA (*See also* PEA DISHES, PEA & CARROT, PIGEON PEA, SNOW PEA)				
Alaska (Early or June)				
canned				
not drained	½ cup	–	67	–
drained	½ cup	–	75	–

Food and Description	Amount	Fat Grams	Total Calories	% Fat Calories
canned				
(Festal)	½ cup	–	70	–
(Green Giant)	½ cup	–	50	–
(S&W)-Petit Pois	½ cup	–	70	–
frozen				
(Green Giant)	½ cup	–	50	–
(Harvest Fresh)	½ cup	–	60	–
Edible Podded				
fresh-cooked	½ cup	–	34	–
frozen-boiled	½ cup	–	54	–
frozen (Chun King)	1.5 oz	–	16	–
frozen (La Choy)	1 pkg	–	70	–
Green Peas				
canned	½ cup	–	59	–
fresh-cooked	½ cup	–	67	–
frozen				
(Birds Eye)	3.3 oz	–	80	–
(Health Valley)	5.5 oz	–	126	–
raw	½ cup	–	63	–
Split Peas				
boiled	½ cup	–	115	–
raw	½ cup	1	348	3%
Sweet Peas (wrinkled peas, sugar peas)				
canned-not drained	½ cup	–	71	–
(Nutradiet)	½ cup	–	40	–
canned-drained	½ cup	–	68	–
(Del Monte)	½ cup	–	60	–
(Green Giant)	½ cup	–	50	–
(Libby)	½ cup	–	60	–
canned				
Garden				
(Freshlike)	½ cup	–	50	–
(Green Giant)-50% Less Salt	½ cup	–	50	–
Mini (Green Giant)	½ cup	–	60	–
Perfection (S&W)	½ cup	–	70	–
Small				
(Del Monte)	½ cup	–	50	–
(Freshlike)	½ cup	–	50	–
frozen				
(Green Giant)	½ cup	–	50	–
(Harvest Fresh)	½ cup	–	50	–
Tender Tiny Peas				
frozen (Birds Eye)	½ cup	–	60	–

Food and Description	Amount	Fat Grams	Total Calories	% Fat Calories
PEA & CARROT				
canned (Nutradiet)	½ cup	–	35	–
Sweet Peas & Sliced Carrots/canned (Freshlike)	½ cup	–	50	–
PEA DISHES (*See also* PEA & CARROT)				
Early Peas in Butter Sauce frozen microwave (Green Giant)	4.5 oz	2	80	23%
Field Peas w/Snaps seasoned w/pork canned (Luck's)	7.5 oz	7	200	32%
Green peas in cream sauce frozen (Birds Eye)	2.6 oz	6	120	45%
Green peas, onions, red pepper, & garlic canned	½ cup	–	57	–
Green Peas & Rice w/mushrooms frozen (Birds Eye)	2.3 oz	–	110	–
Green peas, potatoes in cream sauce frozen (Bird's Eye)	2.6 oz	6	130	42%
Mini Peas, Pea Pods & Water Chestnuts in Butter Sauce frozen (LeSueur)	½ cup	2	80	23%
Peas in Cream Sauce frozen (Green Giant)	½ cup	4	90	40%
Peas in Butter Sauce frozen Micro Quick (Freshlike)	5 oz	2	110	16%
Peas, Pearl Onions in cheese sauce frozen (Birds Eye)	½ cup	5	140	32%
Peas, Pearl Onions, Mushrooms frozen (Pictsweet)-Express microwave	2.5 oz	–	45	–
Peas & potatoes w/cream sauce frozen (Birds Eye)	½ cup	6	127	43%
Peas, Onions, & Carrots in butter sauce frozen (LeSueur)	½ cup	3	80	34%
Peas-Seasoned canned (Del Monte)	½ cup	–	60	–
Sweet Pea Cauliflower Medley frozen (Green Giant) Valley Combinations	½ cup	–	30	–
Sweet Peas in Butter Sauce frozen (Green Giant)	½ cup	2	80	23%
Sweet Peas & Diced Carrots canned (S&W)	½ cup	–	50	–
Sweet Peas & Onions canned (Green Giant)	½ cup	–	50	–

Food and Description	Amount	Fat Grams	Total Calories	% Fat Calories
Sweet Peas & Tiny Pearl Onions				
canned (S&W)	½ cup	1	60	15%
Sweet Peas & Sliced Mushrooms in Butter Sauce				
Vegetable Classics (Del Monte)				
microwave	½ cup	2	60	30%
Sweet Peas & Tiny Onions				
canned (Freshlike)	½ cup	–	60	–
PEA SOUP (See SOUP)				
PEA SPROUT/cooked	½ cup	–	80	–
PEACH				
canned				
in water	1 cup	–	58	–
in juice	1 cup	–	109	–
in heavy syrup	1 cup	–	190	–
(Del Monte)				
Freestone halves or slices	½ cup	–	90	–
Yellow Cling halves				
or slices	½ cup	–	80	–
Lite Freestone	½ cup	–	60	–
Lite yellow cling	½ cup	–	50	–
dried				
cooked halves				
no sugar	½ cup	< 1	100	5%
w/sugar	½ cup	< 1	165	3%
uncooked halves	10 large	1	380	2%
	10 medium	.9	341	2%
	½ cup	.6	191	2%
(Del Monte)	2 oz	–	140	–
(Mariani)	¼ cup	–	140	–
(Sun Maid)	2 oz	–	140	–
fresh	1	–	37	–
slices	1 cup	–	73	–
frozen				
no sugar	3.5 oz	< 1	45	10%
sliced	1 cup	< 1	132	3%
sweetened				
sliced	1 cup	< 1	235	2%
Fruit Cup				
(Del Monte)				
yellow cling peaches, diced	5 oz	–	110	–
(Nutradiet)				
halves	½ cup	–	30	–
sliced	½ cup	–	30	–

Food and Description	Amount	Fat Grams	Total Calories	% Fat Calories
(S&W)				
clingstone				
halves in heavy syrup	½ cup	–	100	–
freestone				
halves in heavy syrup	½ cup	–	100	–
slices in heavy syrup	½ cup	–	100	–
natural	½ cup	–	90	–
yellow cling				
sliced in heavy syrup	½ cup	–	100	–
spiced				
canned in syrup	1 cup	–	180	–
(Del Monte)w/pits	3.5 oz	–	80	–
(S&W) yellow cling				
whole in heavy syrup	½ cup	–	90	–
PEACH BUTTER				
(Smucker's)	1 tsp	–	15	–
PEACH JUICE				
Orchard Peach/frozen concentrate	6 oz	–	90	–
Peach (Dole) Pure & Light	6 oz	–	102	–
(Smucker's)	8 oz	–	120	–
Peach Delight/bottled	6 oz	–	90	–
Peach Nectar/canned	8 oz	–	134	–
(Kern's)	6 oz	–	110	–
Peach, Ripe Nectar (Libby's)	8 oz	–	130	–
PEANUT				
ALL TYPES				
boiled	½ cup	7	102	62%
dried	1 oz	13.97	161	78%
dry roasted	1 oz	13.9	164	76%
Lite	1 oz	9	135	60%
honey roasted	1 oz	13	170	69%
oil roasted	1 oz	13.8	163	76%
	½ cup	35.5	418	76%
BY BRAND NAME				
(Eagle)				
cinnamon roasted	1 oz	13	170	69%
cinnamon honey roasted	1 oz	13	170	69%
dry honey roasted	1 oz	13	170	69%
lightly salted	1 oz	15	170	79%
maple roasted	1 oz	13	170	69%
maple honey roasted	1 oz	13	170	69%
oil honey roasted	1 oz	13	170	69%
salted	1 oz	14	170	74%
Roaster's Choice-salted	1 oz	15	170	79%
(Frito Lay's)	1 oz	15	170	79%

Food and Description	Amount	Fat Grams	Total Calories	% Fat Calories
(Guy's)				
dry roasted	1 oz	14	170	74%
Spanish-salted	1 oz	14	170	74%
(Laura Scudder's)-Virginia	1 oz	15	182	74%
(Little Debbie)				
honey roasted	1.13 oz	13	190	62%
salted	1.25 oz	18	230	70%
(Planters)				
dry roasted				
salted	1 oz	14	160	79%
unsalted	1 oz	14	160	79%
honey roasted	1 oz	13	170	69%
honey/dry roasted	1 oz	13	160	73%
in shell				
salted	1 oz	14	160	79%
unsalted	1 oz	14	160	79%
oil roasted cocktail	1 oz	15	170	79%
unsalted	1 oz	15	170	79%
oil roasted redskin	1 oz	15	170	79%
Sweet "N Crunchy	1 oz	8	140	51%
oil roasted salted	1 oz	15	170	79%
(Weight Watchers)	.7 oz	7	100	63%
	½ cup	36	428	76%
PEANUT, SPANISH	1 oz	13.7	162	76%
	½ cup	36	425	76%
(Laura Scudder's)	1 oz	15	181	75%
(Planters)				
dry roasted	1 oz	14	160	79%
oil roasted	1 oz	15	170	79%
raw	1 oz	12	150	72%
PEANUT, VALENCIA				
oil-roasted	1 oz	14	165	76%
	½ cup	37	424	79%
PEANUT, VIRGINIA				
oil-roasted	1 oz	4.5	161	25%
PEANUT BUTTER				
CHUNKY				
	2 Tbs	16	188	77%
	½ cup	64	760	76%
	1 cup	131.9	1526	78%
(Country Pure)	2 Tbs	16	190	76%
(Erewhon)	2 Tbs	14	190	66%
(Erewhon) No Salt	2 Tbs	14	190	66%
(Estee)	1 Tbs	8	100	72%

Food and Description	Amount	Fat Grams	Total Calories	% Fat Calories
(Featherweight)	1 Tbs	7	90	70%
(Health Valley)	1 Tbs	7	83	76%
No Salt	1 Tbs	7	83	76%
(Nu Made)	2 Tbs	16	190	76%
(Peter Pan)	2 Tbs	16	180	80%
(Smucker's)-Natural	2 Tbs	16	200	72%
CREAMY				
	2 Tbs	16	188	77%
	½ cup	64	760	76%
	1 cup	131.9	1526	78%
(Arrowhead Mills)	2 tbs	16	190	76%
(Country Pure)	2 Tbs	16	190	76%
(Erewhon)	2 Tbs	14	190	66%
(Featherweight)	2 Tbs	15	180	75%
(Health Valley)	1 Tbs	7	83	76%
No Salt	1 Tbs	7	83	76%
(Jif)	2 Tbs	16	190	76%
(Laura Scudder's)				
Roasted				
Honey Nut	2 tbs	16	200	72%
(Nu Made)	2 Tbs	16	190	76%
(Nutradiet)	1 Tbs	8	93	87%
(Peter Pan)	2 Tbs	16	180	80%
no sugar	2 Tbs	17	180	85%
(Skippy)	2 Tbs	17	190	81%
Roasted Honey Nut	2 Tbs	17	190	81%
CRUNCHY				
(Arrowhead Mills)	2 Tbs	16	190	76%
(Bama)	2 Tbs	17	200	77%
(Laura Scudder's)				
Roasted Honey Nut	2 Tbs	16	200	72%
(Skippy)				
Roasted Honey Nut	2 Tbs	17	190	81%
EXTRA CRUNCHY				
(Jif)	2 Tbs	17	190	81%
(Peter Pan)	2 Tbs	16	180	80%
MIXED				
w/fudge (Smucker's)				
Goober Fudge	2 Tbs	13	240	49%
w/honey (Smucker's)				
Goober Honey	2 Tbs	10	180	50%
w/jelly				
(Bama)	2 Tbs	7	150	42%
(Smucker's)				
Goober Grape	2 Tbs	10	180	50%

Food and Description	Amount	Fat Grams	Total Calories	% Fat Calories
Goober Strawberry	2 Tbs	10	180	50%
NO SALT NATURAL				
(Smucker's)	2 Tbs	17	200	77%
NUTTY				
(Laura Scudder's)	2 Tbs	16	200	72%
SMOOTH				
	2 Tbs	16	188	77%
	½ cup	64	759	76%
(Bama)	2 Tbs	17	200	77%
(Laura Scudder's)	2 Tbs	16	200	72%
unsalted	2 Tbs	16	200	72%
(Nutradiet)	1 Tbs	8	93	77%
SUPER CHUNK				
(Skippy)	2 Tbs	17	190	81%
	1 cup	137	1540	80%
PEANUT BUTTER FLAVORED CHIPS				
(Reese's)	¼ cup	13	230	51%
PEANUT FLOUR				
Low Fat	1 oz	6	120	45%
	1 cup	13	257	46%
PEAR				
fresh				
Bartlett	1	1	100	9%
Bosc	1	1	85	11%
D'Anjou	1	1	120	8%
slices	1 cup	.66	97	6%
candied	1 oz	–	86	–
canned				
in water	1 cup	< 1	71	6%
in juice	1 cup	< 1	123	4%
in light syrup	1 cup	< 1	130	4%
in heavy syrup	1 cup	< 1	188	2%
(Del Monte)				
halves or slices	½ cup	–	80	–
Lite halves or slices	½ cup	–	50	–
dried				
cooked	1 cup	.78	325	2%
uncooked	1 cup	1	472	2%
dried				
(Mariani)	¼ cup	–	150	–
(Nutradiet)				
peeled halves	½ cup	–	35	–
peeled quarters	½ cup	–	35	–

Food and Description	Amount	Fat Grams	Total Calories	% Fat Calories
(S&W)				
Bartlett halves in heavy syrup	½ cup	–	100	–
natural-sliced	½ cup	–	80	–
PEAR JUICE				
Pear, Ripe Nectar (Libby's)	8 oz	–	150	–
Pear Nectar				
canned	1 cup	–	149	–
PEAR-PINEAPPLE JUICE				
Pear-Pineapple Nectar (Kern's)	1 cup	–	112	–
PECAN				
(Azar)				
chips	1 oz	21	210	90%
halves	1 oz	21	210	90%
pieces	1 oz	21	210	90%
dried	1 oz	19	190	90%
	1 cup/ halves	73	721	91%
dry roasted	1 oz	18	187	87%
	10 Xtra large	28.7	277	93%
(Eagle)				
honey roasted	1 oz	19	200	86%
in shell	10 large	24.5	236	93%
oil roasted	1 oz	20	195	92%
(Planters)				
chips	1 oz	20	190	95%
halves	1 oz	20	190	95%
pieces	1 oz	20	190	95%
shelled				
chopped	1 cup	84	811	93%
	1 Tbs	5	52	87%
ground	1 cup	67.6	653	93%
halves	10 large	6	62	87%
	10 jumbo	10	96	94%
	10 mammoth	12.8	124	93%
	1 cup	76.9	742	93%
PECAN FLOUR	1 oz	–	93	–
PEPPER/Cherry Type				
Greek Pepperoncini Salad (Vlasic)				
Mild	1 oz	–	4	–
Hot	1 oz	–	10	–
(Heinz)	1	–	8	–
Hot Banana				
(Heinz)	1	–	6	–

Food and Description	Amount	Fat Grams	Total Calories	% Fat Calories
(Vlasic)	1 oz	–	4	–
Hot Chili-Red				
raw	1 pepper	–	18	–
raw/chopped	½ cup	–	17	–
Hot Chili-Green/raw	½ cup	–	16	–
Hot Pepper Rings/Slices (Heinz)	1	–	4	–
Jalapeno				
canned/whole	2 peppers	1	14	64%
chopped	½ cup	1	20	45%
Mild	1 oz	–	8	–
(Heinz)-sweet	1	–	8	–
Sweet (Green & Red)				
raw	1 pepper	–	18	–
raw/chopped	½ cup	–	12	–
freeze-dried	½ cup	–	10	–
	1 Tbs	–	1	–
(Heinz)-rings/slices	1	–	4	–
Sweet Pepper Mementos (Heinz)	1	–	6	–
(Vlasic)-Mexican Hot	1 oz	–	8	–
Mexican Tiny Hot	1 oz	–	6	–
PEPPER DISHES				
Stuffed green pepper w/rice (no meat)				
homemade	~ 5 oz	11.9	198	54%
Stuffed green pepper w/beef & rice				
Standard Home Recipe (USDA)	½ Pepper	13	219	53%
Stuffed green pepper w/beef & bread crumbs				
Standard Home Recipe (USDA)	1 Med Pep.	10.5	325	29%
PEPPER POT SOUP (*See* SOUP)				
PEPPER SEASONING				
black	1 tsp	–	5	–
red				
(cayenne)	1 tsp	–	5	–
white	1 tsp	–	7	–
PEPPERONI (*See* LUNCHEON MEAT)				
PERCH (*See* OCEAN PERCH)				
PERSIMMON				
fresh/native	1	–	32	–
Japanese (or Kaki)				
fresh	1	< 1	118	4%
dried	1	< 1	93	5%
PESTO SAUCE (*See* SAUCE)				
PHEASANT				
breast meat only-raw	~ 6 oz	5.9	243	22%
giblets-raw	3 oz	4	119	30%

Food and Description	Amount	Fat Grams	Total Calories	% Fat Calories
leg meat only-raw	~ 4 oz	4.6	143	29%
meat & skin-raw	~ 1 lb	37	723	46%
meat only-raw	~ ¾ lb	12.8	470	25%
PICANTE SALSA (*See* MEXICAN FOOD and SAUCE)				
PICKLE				
Bread & butter pickles	3 slices	–	16	–
	1 oz	–	25	–
(Claussen)-Dill	1 oz	–	6	–
(Del Monte)-Dill Halves	1 oz	–	3	–
Deli Style Dill halves	1 oz	–	4	–
Dill pickles	1 medium	–	15	–
(Featherweight)-Whole Dill	1	–	4	–
Genuine Dill	1 oz	–	2	–
Gherkin pickles	1 Small	–	22	–
Hamburger Chips	1 oz	–	2	–
Hamburger Dill	1 oz	–	2	–
(Heinz)-Baby Kosher Dill	1 oz	–	4	–
Hot Garlic	1 oz	–	6	–
Kosher	2 oz	–	7	–
halves	1 piece	–	9	–
slices	1 oz	–	3	–
whole	1 oz	–	2	–
Kosher Dill	1 oz	–	4	–
Kosher Dill Chips	1 oz	–	4	–
Kosher Dill Spears	1 oz	–	4	–
Old Fashioned Kosher Chips	1 oz	–	4	–
Old Fashioned Kosher				
Deli Halves	1 oz	–	4	–
Old Fashioned Whole Kosher	1 oz	–	4	–
Picalilli	1 oz	–	30	–
Pickled cucumbers	2 spears	–	13	–
Polish Style Dills	1 oz	–	4	–
Polish Style Dill Spears	1 oz	–	4	–
Polskie Ogorki	1 oz	–	6	–
Processed Dill	1 oz	–	2	–
Sour	1 oz	–	3	–
Sweet Cucumber Slices	1 oz	–	20	–
Sweet Cucumber Stix	1 oz	–	25	–
Sweet Gherkins	1 oz	–	35	–
Sweet Midget Gherkins	1 oz	–	35	–
Sweet Mixed	1 oz	–	40	–
Sweet Pickles	1 oz	–	35	–
Sweet Pickle Slices	1 oz	–	35	–
Sweet Salad Cubes	1 oz	–	30	–

Food and Description	Amount	Fat Grams	Total Calories	% Fat Calories
(Vlasic)				
Bread & Butter Chunks	1 oz	–	25	–
Sweet Butter Chips	1 oz	–	30	–
Sweet Butter Stix	1 oz	–	18	–
Half-The-Salt Pickles				
Hamburger Dill Chips	1 oz	–	2	–
Kosher Crunchy Dills	1 oz	–	4	–
Kosher Dill Spears	1 oz	–	4	–
Sweet Butter Chips	1 oz	–	30	–
Kosher Pickles				
Baby Dills	1 oz	–	4	–
Crunchy Dills	1 oz	–	4	–
Dill Gherkins	1 oz	–	4	–
Dill Spears	1 oz	–	4	–
Snack Chunks	1 oz	–	4	–
No-Garlic Pickles				
Crunchy Dills	1 oz	–	4	–
Dill Spears	1 oz	–	4	–
Original Dills				
Original Dills	1 oz	–	2	–
Polish Snack Chunks	1 oz	–	4	–
Zesty Crunchy Dills	1 oz	–	4	–
Zesty Dill Spears	1 oz	–	4	–
Zesty Dill Snack Chunks	1 oz	–	4	–
Refrigerated Pickles				
Deli Bread & Butter	1 oz	–	25	–
Deli Dill Halves	1 oz	–	4	–
PIE & COBBLER (*See* PIE CRUST, PIE FILLING)				
Apple-frozen-(Banquet)	3.33 oz	11	250	40%
(Mrs. Smith's)-Natural Juice	½ pie	22	420	47%
Streusel	½ pie	16	420	34%
Old Fashioned	⅛ pie	27	530	46%
Apple Raisin	⅛ pie	28	560	45%
Ready to Bake	⅛ pie	17	390	39%
Dutch Apple Crumb	⅛ pie	13	420	28%
Thaw'N'Serve-Lattice	⅛ pie	11	280	35%
(Weight Watchers)	3.5 oz	5	200	23%
homemade (9" dia)	⅙ pie	18	405	40%
Apple cobbler-frozen (Stilwell)	4 oz	4	200	18%
Apple-Dutch (Little Debbie)	2.17 oz	8	230	31%
Apple Crumb-mix (Dromedary)	1 piece	6	237	23%
Apple Streusel/frozen				
(Sara Lee) Free & Light	1 slice	2	170	11%
Banana-frozen-(Banquet)	2.33 oz	10	180	50%

Food and Description	Amount	Fat Grams	Total Calories	% Fat Calories
(Mrs. Smith's)-Thaw'N Serve	⅛ pie	12	240	45%
Banana Cream-homemade (9" dia)	⅙ pie	13	300	39%
Banana Custard-homemade (9" dia)	⅙ pie	14	336	38%
Berry-frozen (Mrs. Smith's)				
Ready To Bake	⅛ pie	16	400	36%
Blackberry-frozen (Banquet)	3.33 oz	11	270	37%
homemade (9" dia)	⅙ pie	17	384	40%
Blackberry cobbler-frozen (Stilwell)	4 oz	8	280	26%
Blueberry-frozen-(Banquet)	3.33 oz	11	270	37%
(Mrs. Smith's)-Old Fashioned	⅛ pie	17	460	33%
Ready to Bake	⅛ pie	17	380	40%
Thaw'N Serve-Lattice	⅛ pie	11	290	34%
homemade (9" dia)	⅙ pie	17	380	40%
Boston Cream-frozen				
(Mrs. Smith's)-Thaw'N Serve	⅛ pie	4	240	15%
(Weight Watchers)	3 oz	4	190	19%
Butterscotch-homemade (9" dia)	⅛ pie	12.5	304	37%
Cherry-frozen				
(Banquet)	3.33 oz	11	250	40%
(Mrs. Smith's)-Natural Juice	⅐ pie	18	410	40%
Old Fashioned	⅛ pie	19	460	37%
Ready To Bake	⅛ pie	16	400	36%
Thaw'N Serve-Lattice	⅛ pie	10	300	30%
homemade (9" dia)	⅙ pie	18	410	40%
Cherry Crumb-mix (Dromedary)	1 piece	6	231	23%
Cherry Streusel/frozen				
(Sara Lee) Free & Light	1 slice	2	160	11%
Chess/homemade(9" dia)	⅙ pie	24	485	45%
Chocolate-frozen-(Banquet)	2.33 oz	10	185	49%
–homemade (9" dia)	⅙ pie	22	433	46%
Chocolate Chiffon-homemade (9" dia)	⅛ pie	12	266	41%
Chocolate Cream-frozen				
(Mrs. Smith's)-Thaw'N Serve	⅛ pie	13	270	43%
Chocolate Meringue-homemade (9" dia)	⅙ pie	18	383	42%
Chocolate Mint-No Bake (Royal)	⅛ pie	15	260	52%
Chocolate Mocha-frozen				
(Weight Watchers)	2.75 oz	2	160	11%
Chocolate Mousse Pie-box mix				
(Jell-O)	⅛ pie	17	260	59%
(Royal)	⅛ pie	12	230	47%
frozen (Weight Watchers)	2.5 oz	6	170	32%
Chocolate Pecan-frozen				
(Mrs. Smith's)-Thaw'N Serve	⅛ pie	20	570	32%
Coconut-frozen-(Banquet)	2.33 oz	11	190	52%

Food and Description	Amount	Fat Grams	Total Calories	% Fat Calories
Coconut Cream-box mix				
(Jell-O)-No Bake frozen	1/8 pie	17	260	59%
(Mrs. Smith's)-Thaw'N Serve	1/8 pie	14	270	47%
Coconut Custard-frozen				
(Mrs. Smith's)-Ready To Bake	1/8 pie	15	330	41%
homemade (9" dia)	1/6 pie	19	357	48%
Cream-homemade (9" dia)	1/6 pie	23	455	46%
Custard-homemade (9" dia)	1/6 pie	17	330	46%
Egg Custard-frozen				
(Mrs. Smith's)-Ready To Bake	1/8 pie	9	300	27%
Fried-(Break Cake)-homemade	1	19	410	42%
apple	1	14	255	49%
cherry	1	14	250	50%
Grasshopper-homemade (9" dia)	1/6 pie	23	460	45%
Key Lime-homemade (9" dia)	1/6 pie	19	460	37%
Lemon-frozen-(Banquet)	2.33 oz	11	190	52%
Lemon Chiffon-homemade (9" dia)	1/6 pie	13.6	338	36%
Lemon Cream-frozen				
(Mrs. Smith's)- Thaw'N Serve	1/8 pie	12	245	44%
Lemon Meringue-frozen				
(Mrs. Smith's)-Thaw'N Serve	1/8 pie	6	290	19%
homemade (9" dia)	1/6 pie	14	355	36%
Mix-No Bake (Royal)	1/8 pie	11	310	32%
Mince-frozen				
(Mrs. Smith's) Ready To Bake	1/8 pie	19	470	36%
Mincemeat-frozen				
(Banquet)	3.33 oz	11	260	38%
homemade	1/6 pie	18	428	38%
Pastry Pockets-refigerated				
(Pillsbury)	1 Pocket	13	230	51%
Peach-frozen-(Banquet)	3.33 oz	11	245	40%
(Mrs. Smith's)-Old Fashioned	1/8 pie	16	365	40%
Thaw'N Serve-Lattice	1/8 pie	12	300	36%
homemade (9" dia)	1/6 pie	17	405	38%
Peach cobbler-frozen (Stilwell)	4 oz	5	270	17%
Pecan (little Debbie)	3 oz	3	280	10%
Pecan (little Debbie)	1.83 oz	2	170	11%
Pecan-frozen				
(Mrs. Smith's)-Thaw'N Serve	1/8 pie	16	480	30%
homemade (9" dia)	1/6 pie	32	575	50%
Pineapple-homemade (9" dia)	1/6 pie	17	400	38%
Pineapple Chiffon				
homemade-(9" dia)	1/6 pie	13	311	38%

Food and Description	Amount	Fat Grams	Total Calories	% Fat Calories
Pineapple Custard (9" dia)	1/6 pie	13	334	35%
Praline Pecan Mousse				
frozen-(Weight Watchers)	7 oz	7	190	33%
Pumpkin-frozen-(Banquet)	3.33 oz	8	200	36%
homemade (9" dia)	1/6 pie	17	320	48%
mix (Jell-O)-No Bake	1/8 pie	11	230	43%
mix-canned (Libby's)	1/6 pie	17	330	46%
Pumpkin Custard-frozen				
(Mrs. Smith's)-Ready To Serve	1/8 pie	11	310	32%
Thaw'N Serve	1/8 pie	8	300	24%
Raisin-homemade (9" dia)	1/6 pie	17	427	36%
Raisin Creme Pie (Little Debbie)	2.5 oz	10	290	31%
	1.17 oz	6	140	39%
Raspberry Mousse-frozen				
(Weight Watchers)	2.5 oz	2	150	12%
Red Raspberry-frozen				
(Mrs. Smith's)-Ready To Bake	1/8 pie	15	390	35%
Rhubarb-homemade (9" dia)	1/6 pie	17	400	38%
Shoo-fly-homemade (9" dia)	1/8 pie	13	395	30%
Snack-packaged-(Hostess)				
Apple	1	19	390	44%
Blackberry	1	15	380	36%
Blueberry	1	17	410	37%
Cherry	1	17	410	37%
Lemon	1	20	400	45%
Peach	1	15	380	36%
Strawberry	1	16	340	42%
(Hostess)-Pudding Pies				
Chocolate	1	19	490	35%
Vanilla	1	17	470	33%
(Little Debbie)-Marshmallow Pies				
Banana	3 oz	12	360	30%
	1.4 oz	6	170	32%
Chocolate	3 oz	13	370	32%
	1.38 oz	6	170	32%
Oatmeal Cream	1.33 oz	6	160	34%
	2.75 oz	14	350	36%
Pecan	3 oz	3	280	10%
Raisin Creme	2.5 oz	10	290	31%
(Sara Lee)-frozen				
Country Apple	1	7	230	32%
Fudge Brownie	1	14	280	45%
Southern Pecan	1	13	260	45%
Squash-homemade (9" dia)	1/6 pie	20	360	50%

Food and Description	Amount	Fat Grams	Total Calories	% Fat Calories
Strawberries'N Cream-frozen				
(Mrs. Smith's)-Thaw'N Serve	1/8 pie	16	330	44%
Strawberry-frozen				
(Banquet)	2.33 oz	9	170	48%
homemade (9" dia)	1/6 pie	10	246	37%
Strawberry-rhubarb-frozen				
(Mrs. Smith's)-Ready To Bake	1/8 pie	17	410	37%
homemade (9" dia)	1/8 pie	23	430	48%
Sweet Potato-homemade (9" dia)	1/6 pie	17	324	47%
PIE CRUST				
Mix	2 shells	93	1485	56%
Flako-9" dia	1/6 crust	15	250	54%
Krusteaz-baked	~ 1 oz	6	100	54%
Pillsbury Mix and Sticks	1/8 two crust			
	pie	17	270	57%
Mrs. Smith's-frozen	1/8 of 9 5/8"			
	shell	8	130	55%
Pepperidge Farm Patty shells	1 shell	15	210	64%
Petritz Deep Dish	1/6 shell	9	140	58%
Regular	1/6 shell	7	110	57%
Deep dish	1/6 shell	8	130	55%
Whole grain	1/6 shell	8	130	55%
9 5/8" dia	1/6 shell	11	170	58%
Ready Crust (Keebler)				
Butter flavored	1/8 crust	5	110	41%
Chocolate	1/8 crust	5	120	38%
Graham Cracker	1/8 crust	6	120	45%
Single Serve	1 tart	5	100	45%
Refrigerated (Pillsbury)	1/8 two crust			
	pie	15	240	56%
Standard Home Recipe (USDA) 9" dia	1 shell	60	900	60%
PIE CRUST-TYPE WEINER WRAP				
(Pillsbury)	1 wrap	2	60	30%
PIE FILLING				
PIE FILLING-CREAM-CANNED				
Comstock				
Banana	3.5 oz	2	110	16%
Chocolate	3.5 oz	3	130	21%
Coconut	3.5 oz	3	120	23%
Lemon	3.5 oz	1	140	13%
PIE FILLING-FRUIT				
Box				
Borden-mincemeat	2.5 oz	2	220	8%

Food and Description	Amount	Fat Grams	Total Calories	% Fat Calories
Canned				
Comstock				
Apricot	3.5 oz	–	110	–
Blueberry	3.5 oz	–	110	–
Cherry	3.5 oz	–	110	–
Mincemeat	3.5 oz	1	150	6%
Mountain fresh peach	3.5 oz	–	110	–
Pineapple	3.5 oz	–	100	–
Orchard fresh apple	3.5 oz	–	120	–
Pumpkin	3.5 oz	–	100	–
Raisin	3.5 oz	–	120	–
Strawberry	3.5 oz	–	100	–
Libby's				
Pumpkin	1 cup	–	210	–
Pumpkin-Solid pack	1 cup	1	80	11%
Pumpkin pie mix	1 cup	–	282	–
Baked	1/6 pie	17	330	46%
S&W-Mincemeat				
Old Fashioned				
mellowed w/brandy	3.5 oz	2	206	9%
Thank You				
Apple	3.5 oz	–	90	–
Cherry	3.5 oz	–	100	–
Jar-(None Such)				
Mincemeat				
plain	1/3 cup	1	200	5%
w/brandy & rum	1/3 cup	2	220	8%
PIE FILLING-INSTANT				
Mixes prepared w/whole milk (Jell-O)				
Banana cream	1/2 cup	4	160	23%
Butter pecan	1/2 cup	5	170	27%
Butterscotch	1/2 cup	4	140	26%
Chocolate	1/2 cup	4	130	28%
Chocolate fudge	1/2 cup	5	180	25%
Coconut cream	1/2 cup	6	180	30%
French vanilla	1/2 cup	4	160	23%
Lemon	1/2 cup	4	140	26%
Milk chocolate	1/2 cup	5	180	25%
Pineapple cream	1/2 cup	4	160	23%
Pistachio	1/2 cup	4	150	24%
Vanilla	1/2 cup	4	140	26%
PIE FILLING-INSTANT SUGAR-FREE				
Mixes prepared w/2% low-fat milk (Jell-O)				
Banana	1/2 cup	2	90	20%

Food and Description	Amount	Fat Grams	Total Calories	% Fat Calories
Butterscotch	½ cup	2	90	20%
Chocolate	½ cup	3	100	27%
Chocolate fudge	½ cup	3	100	27%
Pistachio	½ cup	3	100	27%
Vanilla	½ cup	2	90	20%
PIE FILLING-MICROWAVE				
Prepared as directed (Jell-O)				
Banana cream	½ cup	4	170	21%
Butterscotch	½ cup	4	170	21%
Chocolate	½ cup	5	170	27%
Milk chocolate	½ cup	6	160	34%
Mint chocolate	½ cup	5	160	28%
Vanilla	½ cup	4	160	23%
PIE FILLING-MIX				
Prepared w/whole milk				
(Jell-O)				
Banana cream (8" pie)				
excluding crust	⅙ pie	3	100	27%
Butterscotch	½ cup	4	170	21%
Chocolate	½ cup	5	180	25%
Chocolate fudge	½ cup	4	160	23%
Coconut cream (8" pie)				
excluding crust	⅙ pie	2	200	9%
Coconut Cream Pie Dessert				
(no crust)	⅛ pie	7	162	39%
Deluxe chocolate almond (no crust)	⅛ pie	7	162	39%
Deluxe chocolate mint (no crust)	⅛ pie	7	162	39%
Deluxe double chocolate				
(no crust)	⅛ pie	7	162	39%
French vanilla	½ cup	4	170	21%
Lemon (9" pie)-excluding crust	⅙ pie	2	200	9%
Milk chocolate	½ cup	4	140	26%
Vanilla	½ cup	4	160	23%
(Royal)				
Banana cream	½ cup	4	160	23%
Butterscotch	½ cup	4	160	23%
Chocolate	½ cup	4	180	20%
Custard	½ cup	5	150	30%
Dark'n sweet	½ cup	4	180	20%
Flan with caramel sauce	½ cup	5	150	30%
Key lime	½ cup	3	160	17%
Lemon	½ cup	3	160	17%
Vanilla	½ cup	4	160	23%
Vanilla tapioca	½ cup	4	160	23%
PIE FILLING-MIX-SUGAR-FREE				

Food and Description	Amount	Fat Grams	Total Calories	% Fat Calories
Prepared w/2% milk (JELL-O)				
Chocolate	½ cup	3	90	30%
Vanilla	½ cup	2	80	30%
PIGEONPEA				
fresh-cooked	½ cup	1	86	11%
raw	½ cup	1.5	350	4%
PIKE				
Northern				
cooked-dry heat	3 oz	.75	96	7%
raw	3 oz	1	75	12%
roe-raw	3 oz	1.7	110	14%
Walleye				
raw	3 oz	1	79	11%
PIMIENTO				
canned	1	–	11	–
	4 oz	–	30	–
diced or slices				
(Dromedary)	1 oz	–	10	–
(Dunbar's)	½ oz	–	4	–
PINA COLADA				
Nice & Natural	6 oz	–	80	–
PINE NUTS				
dried				
pignolia	1 oz	14	146	86%
pinyon	1 oz	17	161	95%
PINEAPPLE				
candied	4 oz	.5	357	1%
	1 oz	–	90	–
canned				
in water	1 slice	–	19	–
	1 cup		79	6%
in juice	1 slice	–	35	–
	1 cup		150	3%
in heavy syrup	1 slice	–	45	–
(Del Monte)				
chunks, crushed,tidbits, slices				
in juice	½ cup	–	70	–
chunks, crushed, slices				
in syrup	½ cup	–	90	–
spears in juice	2 spears	–	50	–
(Dole)				
all cuts in juice	½ cup	.5	70	6%
all cuts in syrup	½ cup	< 1	95	5%
(Nutradiet) sliced	½ cup	–	60	–

Food and Description	Amount	Fat Grams	Total Calories	% Fat Calories
	1 cup	.9	199	4%
(S&W)				
Hawaiian sliced				
in heavy syrup	2 slices	–	90	–
in pineapple juice	½ cup	–	70	–
fresh	1 slice	–	42	–
	1 cup	.66	77	8%
(Del Monte)	2 slices	–	90	–
	½ cup	–	52	–
frozen				
sweetened chunks	½ cup	–	104	–
unsweetened	3.5 oz	< 1	50	9%
PINEAPPLE-GRAPE DRINK	8 oz	–	117	–
PINEAPPLE-GRAPEFRUIT DRINK				
(Dole) w/pink grapefruit	6 oz	–	100	–
(Tropicana) single serve	10 oz	–	159	–
Twister	8 oz	–	112	–
PINEAPPLE-GRAPEFRUIT JUICE				
(Del Monte)	6 oz	–	90	–
(Dole)	6 oz	–	90	–
(Tropicana)	6 oz	–	90	–
PINEAPPLE-GRAPEFRUIT JUICE COCKTAIL				
(Ocean Spray)	6 oz	–	110	–
PINEAPPLE JUICE/canned	8 oz	–	139	–
(Del Monte)-unsweetened	6 oz	–	100	–
(Dole)-unsweetened	6 oz	–	103	–
(Mott's)	9.5 oz	–	169	–
(S&W)-unsweetened	6 oz	–	100	–
(Tree Top)	6 oz	–	100	–
frozen concentrate	8 oz	–	129	–
undiluted	6 oz	< 1	385	1%
Pineapple Nectar (Libby's)	6 oz	–	110	–
PINEAPPLE-ORANGE DRINK/canned	8 oz	–	125	–
PINEAPPLE-ORANGE JUICE				
(Del Monte)	6 oz	–	90	–
(Dole)	6 oz	–	100	–
PINEAPPLE-ORANGE-BANANA JUICE				
(Dole)	6 oz	< 1	90	5%
PINEAPPLE-ORANGE-GUAVA JUICE				
from frzn. conc.	6 oz	< 1	100	5%
PINEAPPLE-PINK GRAPEFRUIT JUICE				
(Del Monte)	6 oz	–	90	–
(Dole)	6 oz	–	101	–
PINEAPPLE SAUCE				

Food and Description	Amount	Fat Grams	Total Calories	% Fat Calories
(Dole)				
chunky	½ cup	–	90	–
smooth	½ cup	–	90	–
PINK BEANS				
boiled	½ cup	–	125	–
raw	½ cup	1	360	3%
PINTO BEAN				
boiled	½ cup	–	117	–
canned	½ cup	–	93	–
(Arrowhead Mills)	2 oz	1	200	5%
dry (Joan of Arc/Green Giant)	½ cup	1	90	10%
dry-picante style				
Joan of Arc	½ cup	1	100	9%
Green Giant	½ cup	1	100	9%
(Gebhardt)	7.5 oz	1	370	3%
(Progresso)	8 oz	1	165	6%
seasoned w/pork (Luck's)	7.25 oz	6	220	25%
w/Jalapeno (Ranch Style)	7.5 oz	2	180	10%
cooked from dry	½ cup	.5	133	3%
raw	½ cup	1	325	3%
sprouts-raw	½ cup	1	65	14%
PINTO BEAN DISHES				
canned w/onions seasoned w/pork				
(Luck's)	7.5 oz	6	220	25%
PISTACHIO NUT				
dried	1 oz	13.7	164	75%
	1 cup	61.9	739	75%
dry roasted	1 oz	15	172	79%
	1 cup	67.6	776	78%
(Dole)	1 oz	14	163	77%
(Planters)	1 oz	15	170	79%
in shell	1 oz	7	84	75%
natural (Planters)	1 oz	15	170	79%
red (Planters)	1 oz	15	170	79%
shelled	1 oz	15	168	80%
PITANGA				
fresh	1 lb	1.6	132	11%
	2	–	5	–
	1 cup	.7	57	11%
PIZZA & PIZZA SNACK (See also FAST FOOD)				
(CELENTANO)				
9-slice pizza	1 piece	5	160	28%
ThickCrust Pizza	⅓ pizza	7	240	26%

Food and Description	Amount	Fat Grams	Total Calories	% Fat Calories
(CELESTE)				
Cheese Pizza-For-One (6.5 oz)	1 pizza	24	500	43%
Deluxe Pizza-For-One				
(8.25 oz)	1 pizza	32	600	48%
Pepperoni Pizza-For-One				
(6.75 oz)	1 pizza	29	540	48%
Sausage Pizza-For-One				
(7.5 oz)	1 pizza	32	580	50%
Sausage & Mushroom Pizza-For-One				
(8.5 oz)	1 pizza	32	600	48%
Supreme Pizza-For-One (9 oz)	1 pizza	39	690	51%
Cheese Pizza	¼ pizza	17	330	46%
Deluxe Pizza	¼ pizza	22	390	51%
Pepperoni Pizza	¼ pizza	21	370	51%
Sausage Pizza	¼ pizza	22	390	51%
Supreme Pizza	¼ pizza	24	410	53%
(CHEF BOY-AR-DEE)				
Box Mix				
Cheese Pizza				
Complete 15⅜ oz	3.84 oz	6	230	24%
2 Complete 18⅞ oz	3.61 oz	5	210	21%
Pepperoni Pizza				
Complete 13.5 oz	3.38 oz	6	230	24%
Complete 15⅝ oz	4.16 oz	9	250	32%
2 complete 30 oz	3.75 oz	7	210	30%
Plain Pizza Mix 14 oz	3.5 oz	3	180	15%
Sausage Pizza				
Complete 16⅞ oz	4.22 oz	10	270	33%
(FOX) DELUXE PIZZA				
Golden Topping (6.8 oz)	½ pizza	11	240	41%
Hamburger (7.6 oz)	½ pizza	12	260	42%
Pepperoni (7 oz)	½ pizza	13	250	47%
Sausage (7.2 oz)	½ pizza	13	260	45%
Sausage & Pepperoni Combination				
(7.2 oz)	½ pizza	13	260	45%
(GRAINDANCE)				
Cheese w/whole wheat crust	¼ pizza	8	190	38%
(JENO'S)				
Crisp 'n Tasty Pizza				
Canadian Style Bacon (7.7 oz)	½ pizza	11	250	40%
Cheese(7.4 oz)	½ pizza	14	270	47%
Combination(7.8 oz)	½ pizza	16	300	48%
Hamburger (8.1 oz)	½ pizza	15	290	47%
Pepperoni (7.6 oz)	½ pizza	15	280	48%
Sausage (7.8 oz)	½ pizza	16	300	48%

Food and Description	Amount	Fat Grams	Total Calories	% Fat Calories
4-Pack Pizzas				
Cheese	1 pizza	8	160	45%
Combination	1 pizza	9	180	45%
Hamburger	1 pizza	9	180	45%
Pepperoni	1 pizza	9	170	48%
Sausage	1 pizza	9	180	45%
(JOHN'S) PIZZA				
Cheese 3-pack	1 pizza	12	300	36%
Deluxe Sausage	½ pizza	13	260	45%
Golden Topping	½ pizza	11	240	41%
Sausage	½ pizza	13	260	45%
Sausage 3-pack	1 pizza	12	300	36%
(LEAN CUISINE)				
French Bread Pizza				
Cheese	5⅛ oz	9	310	26%
Deluxe	6⅛ oz	12	340	32%
Pepperoni	5¼ oz	12	340	32%
Sausage	6 oz	10	330	27%
(LEAN POCKETS)				
Pizza Deluxe				
w/pepperoni & sausage	1 pocket	13	280	42%
(MICRO MAGIC)				
Deep Dish Combination Pizza	6.5 oz	34	605	51%
Deep Dish Pepperoni Pizza	6.5 oz	32	610	47%
Deep Dish Sausage Pizza	6.5 oz	31	590	47%
(MR. P'S PIZZA)				
Combination (7.2 oz)	½ pizza	13	260	45%
Golden Topping (6.8 oz)	½ pizza	11	240	41%
Hamburger (7.6 oz)	½ pizza	12	260	42%
Pepperoni (7 oz)	½ pizza	13	250	47%
Sausage (7.2 oz)	½ pizza	13	260	45%
(PAPPALO'S)				
French Bread Pizza				
Cheese (5.7 oz)	1 pizza	15	360	38%
Combination (6.5 oz)	1 pizza	21	430	44%
Pepperoni (6 oz)	1 pizza	20	410	44%
Sausage (6.3 oz)	1 pizza	18	410	40%
92% Fat Free				
Pepperoni (25.8 oz)	⅕ pizza	11	350	28%
Sausage and Pepperoni				
(16.6 oz)	⅕ pizza	12	360	30%
Supreme (22.6 oz)	¼ pizza	12	350	31%
Three Cheese (20.1 oz)	¼ pizza	7	310	20%
Pan Pizza				
Combination (26.5 oz)	⅙ pizza	15	340	40%

Food and Description	Amount	Fat Grams	Total Calories	% Fat Calories
Hamburger (26.3 oz)	⅙ pizza	12	310	35%
Pepperoni (25.2 oz)	⅙ pizza	14	330	38%
Sausage (26.3 oz)	⅙ pizza	18	360	45%
Thin Crust Pizza				
Combination (22 oz)	⅙ pizza	10	260	35%
Hamburger (22 oz)	⅙ pizza	8	240	30%
Pepperoni (22 oz)	⅙ pizza	11	270	37%
Sausage (22 oz)	⅙ pizza	9	250	32%
(PEPPERIDGE FARM) CROISSANT PASTRY PIZZA				
Cheese	1	27	490	50%
Deluxe	1	27	520	47%
Hamburger	1	27	510	48%
Pepperoni	1	25	490	50%
Sausage	1	29	540	48%
(PILLSBURY)				
Microwave French Bread Pizza				
Cheese (5.7 oz)	1 pizza	15	370	37%
Pepperoni (6 oz)	1 pizza	19	430	40%
Sausage (6.3 oz)	1 pizza	16	410	35%
Sausage & Pepperoni Combination (6.5 oz)	1 pizza	21	450	42%
Microwave Pizza				
Cheese (7.1 oz)	½ pizza	10	240	38%
Combination (9 oz)	½ pizza	15	310	44%
Pepperoni (8.5 oz)	½ pizza	15	300	45%
Sausage (8.75 oz)	½ pizza	13	280	42%
PIZZA ROLLS				
Cheese	3 oz/ ~ 6 rolls	12	240	45%
Hamburger	3 oz/ ~ 6 rolls	13	240	49%
Pepperoni & Cheese	3 oz/ ~6 rolls	13	230	51%
(Microwave)	3 oz/ ~6 rolls	13	240	49%
Sausage & Cheese (Microwave)	3 oz/ ~6 rolls	13	250	47%
Sausage & Pepperoni	3 oz/ ~6 rolls	13	230	51%
(RED BARON)				
Deep Dish Single Serve Pizza				
Cheese	5.5 oz	22.5	448.8	45%
Pepperoni	6 oz	26.9	479	51%
Sausage	6 oz	24.8	459.6	49%
Supreme	6 oz	25	466	48%

Food and Description	Amount	Fat Grams	Total Calories	% Fat Calories
12 Inch Pizza				
Canadian Bacon	22 oz	75	1446.5	47%
Cheese	21 oz	73.6	1429	46%
Hamburger	22 oz	65.6	1418.7	42%
Pepperoni	22 oz	93	1623.6	52%
Pepperoni Deluxe	22 oz	95	1875.7	46%
Sausage	22 oz	82.6	1525	49%
Sausage & Mushroom	24 oz	82	1541	48%
Sausage & Pepperoni	22.75 oz	94	1656.9	51%
Special Deluxe	23.6 oz	91	1858	44%
Supreme	24.5 oz	86	1581	49%
Microwave Pizza				
Hamburger	3.5 oz	13	290	40%
Pepperoni	3.5 oz	15	320	42%
Sausage	3.5 oz	14	300	42%
Sausage & Pepperoni	3.5 oz	16	310	47%
Supreme	3.5 oz	14	290	43%
SNACK TRAY PIZZAS				
Cheese (12)	4 pizzas	7	130	49%
Pepperoni (12)	4 pizzas	8	140	51%
Sausage (12)	4 pizzas	8	140	51%
(SCHWAN'S)/Home Delivery				
Deep Dish Single Serve Pizza				
Cheese	6 oz	25	550	41%
Pepperoni	6 oz	28	570	44%
Sausage	6 oz	27	570	43%
Supreme	6 oz	29	590	44%
7 ¼" Microwave Pizza				
Pepperoni	3.5 oz	17	310	49%
Supreme	3.5 oz	15	290	47%
Special Recipe Pizza				
Canadian Bacon	3.5 oz	15	280	48%
Cheese	3.5 oz	15	300	45%
Hamburger	3.5 oz	16	280	51%
Pepperoni	3.5 oz	18	330	49%
Sausage	3.5 oz	15	280	48%
Sausage & Pepperoni	3.5 oz	17	310	49%
Supreme	3.5 oz	16	290	50%
(STOUFFER'S) (See also LEAN CUISINE under FROZEN ENTREE/DINNER)				
French Bread Pizza				
Canadian Style Bacon-11⅝ oz	½ pizza	14	360	35%
Cheese-10⅜ oz	½ pizza	13	340	34%
Deluxe-12⅜ oz	½ pizza	21	430	44%
Double Cheese-11¾ oz	½ pizza	18	410	40%
Hamburger-12¼ oz	½ pizza	19	410	42%

Food and Description	Amount	Fat Grams	Total Calories	% Fat Calories
Pepperoni-11¼ oz	½ pizza	20	410	44%
Pepperoni & Mushroom-12¼ oz	½ pizza	22	430	46%
Sausage-12 oz	½ pizza	20	420	43%
Sausage & Mushroom-12.5 oz	½ pizza	19	410	42%
Sausage & Pepperoni-12.5 oz	½ pizza	23	450	46%
Vegetable Deluxe-12.75 oz	½ pizza	20	420	43%
(TOMBSTONE)				
12" pizza				
Canadian Style	¼ pizza/ 5.5 oz	13	340	34%
Cheese	¼ pizza/ 5.1 oz	13	330	36%
Cheese & Hamburger	¼ pizza/ 5.5 oz	16	360	40%
Cheese & Pepperoni	¼ pizza/ 5.4 oz	18	380	43%
Cheese & Sausage	¼ pizza/ 5.5 oz	14	350	36%
Cheese, Sausage, & Mushroom	¼ pizza/ 5.9 oz	15	360	38%
Combination Sausage	¼ pizza/ 5.6 oz	16	370	39%
Real Pepperoni	¼ pizza/ 5.8 oz	18	380	43%
Sausage Deluxe	¼ pizza/ 6 oz	14	350	36%
Smoked Sausage w/Pepperoni Seasoning	¼ pizza/ 5.5 oz	14	350	36%
Lite 93% Fat Free				
Sausage	4.1 oz	8	250	29%
Sausage and Pepperoni	4.1 oz	8	250	29%
Supreme	4.6 oz	8	250	29%
Vegetable	4.4 oz	8	250	29%
(TOTINO'S)				
Microwave (Small)				
Cheese	3.9 oz	8	250	29%
Pepperoni	4 oz	12	280	39%
Sausage	4.2 oz	16	320	45%
Sausage & Pepperoni	4.2 oz	15	310	44%
Party Pizza w/Leaner Meats (frozen)				
Canadian Bacon	½ pizza	10	290	31%
Combination	½ pizza	15	340	40%
Hamburger	½ pizza	13	320	37%
Pepperoni	½ pizza	14	330	38%

Food and Description	Amount	Fat Grams	Total Calories	% Fat Calories
Sausage	½ pizza	15	340	40%
My Classic Deluxe Pizza				
Combination (22.5 oz)	⅙ pizza	14	270	47%
Deluxe Cheese (18.7 oz)	⅙ pizza	9	210	39%
Pepperoni (21.1 oz)	⅙ pizza	13	260	45%
Pan Pizza				
Pepperoni (25.2 oz)	⅙ pizza	14	330	38%
Sausage (26.3 oz)	⅙ pizza	13	320	37%
Sausage & Pepperoni Combination				
(26.6 oz)	⅙ pizza	15	340	40%
Three Cheese (23.5 oz)	⅙ pizza	10	290	31%
Party Pizza				
Bacon (10 oz)	½ pizza	20	370	49%
Canadian Bacon (10.2 oz)	½ pizza	14	310	41%
Cheese (9.8 oz)	½ pizza	17	340	45%
Combination (10.5 oz)	½ pizza	21	380	50%
Hamburger (10.6 oz)	½ pizza	19	370	46%
Mexican Style (10.2 oz)	½ pizza	21	380	50%
Pepperoni (10.2 oz)	½ pizza	20	370	49%
Sausage (10.6 oz)	½ pizza	21	390	49%
Vegetable (10.7 oz)	½ pizza	13	300	39%
Pizza Slices				
Cheese	1	7	170	37%
Combination	1	10	200	45%
Pepperoni	1	9	190	43%
Sausage	1	10	200	45%
Temptin' Toppings				
Bacon (12.2 oz)	¼ pizza	11	220	45%
Canadian Style Bacon (12.4 oz)	¼ pizza	8	190	38%
Cheese (11.9 oz)	¼ pizza	10	210	43%
Hamburger (13 oz)	¼ pizza	10	210	43%
Mexican Style (12.3 oz)	¼ pizza	12	220	49%
Pepperoni (12.4 oz)	¼ pizza	11	220	45%
Sausage (12.3 oz)	¼ pizza	11	210	47%
Sausage & Pepperoni Comb.(13 oz)	¼ pizza	12	230	47%
Vegetable (12.9 oz)	¼ pizza	7	180	35%
(WEIGHT WATCHERS)				
French Bread Pizza				
Cheese	5.12 oz	12	310	35%
Deluxe	6.12 oz	13	310	38%
Pepperoni	5.25 oz	13	310	38%
Pizza				
Cheese	5.75 oz	8	310	23%
Deluxe Combination	6.75 oz	8	300	24%

Food and Description	Amount	Fat Grams	Total Calories	% Fat Calories
Pepperoni	5.87 oz	9	320	25%
Sausage	6.25 oz	8	310	23%
(ZAP)				
French Bread Pizza				
Cheese French Bread	4.5 oz	10	308	29%
Deluxe French Bread	4.8 oz	13	323	36%
Pepperoni French Bread	4.5 oz	16	347	42%
PIZZA CRUST				
(Chef Boyardee) mix				
Crust only	¼ pizza	2	150	12%
Quick & Easy	¼ mix	2	150	12%
(Ragu)-crust only-mix	¼ pizza	2	170	11%
Ready to Use				
Boboli-cheese	4" dia	6.5	301	19%
	8" dia	13	602	19%
	12" dia	26	1205	19%
Refrigerated-(Pillsbury)	⅛ crust	1	90	10%
Robin Hood/(Gold Medal)				
Pouch mix	⅙ mix	1	110	8%
PIZZA SAUCE (*See* SAUCE)				
PLANTAIN (*See* BANANA)				
PLUM				
canned				
in water	1 cup	–	102	–
in juice	1 cup	–	146	–
in heavy syrup	1 cup	–	230	–
fresh	1	< 1	36	13%
(Nutradiet)				
halves unpeeled	½ cup	–	52	–
whole unpeeled	½ cup	–	52	–
(S&W)				
halves unpeeled				
in heavy syrup	½ cup	–	135	–
whole fancy unpeeled				
in extra heavy syrup	½ cup	–	135	–
PLUM JUICE				
Plum Nectar (Kern's)	6 oz	–	110	–
POI	4 oz	–	134	–
POKEBERRY				
fresh-cooked	½ cup	–	16	–
raw	½ cup	–	20	–
POLLACK-or Pollock (*See also* SEAFOOD ENTREE/DINNER)				
Atlantic				
raw	3 oz	.83	78	10%

Food and Description	Amount	Fat Grams	Total Calories	% Fat Calories
Walleye				
raw	3 oz	.68	68	9%
cooked-dry heat	3 oz	.95	96	9%
POMEGRANATE/fresh	1	.5	104	4%
POMPANO/Florida				
breaded & fried	3 oz	16.8	271	56%
cooked-dry heat	3 oz	10	179	50%
raw	3 oz	8	140	51%
POP TART (See PASTRY, TOASTER)				
POPCORN				
(Act II)				
Frozen				
Butter Flavored	3 cups	10	190	47%
Real Butter	3 cups	8	140	51%
Lite				
Butter	3 cups	3	100	27%
50% less Salt	3 cups	3	100	27%
Natural	3 cups	3	100	27%
Natural	3 cups	8	140	51%
Sour Cream & Onion	3 cups	11	160	62%
Microwave				
Butter	3 cups	8	140	51%
Caramel	3 cups	14	280	45%
Airpopped-no butter added	1 cup	–	30	–
(Betty Crocker)				
Cheese	1 pouch	11	170	58%
Light-Butter	1 pouch	4	90	40%
Natural	1 pouch	8	140	51%
Salt Free Butter	1 pouch	9	140	58%
(Cape Cod)-Ready To Eat				
White Cheddar	1 oz	10	160	56%
Caramel Coated	1 oz	3	122	22%
w/peanuts	1.5 oz	5	180	25%
(Cracker Jacks)	1 oz	3	120	23%
(Deli Express)-Lite Pop				
Butter	3.2 cups	3	100	27%
Natural	3.2 cups	3	100	27%
(Eagle)-cheese/popped	.5 oz	6	80	68%
(Jiffy Pop)				
Butter	4 cups	6	130	42%
Light				
Butter flavored	3 cups	2	80	30%
Microwave				
Butter	3 cups	5	100	45%

Food and Description	Amount	Fat Grams	Total Calories	% Fat Calories
Natural	3 cups	5	100	45%
Regular	4 cups	6	130	42%
(Jolly Time)-Microwave				
Butter	3 cups	8	150	48%
Cheddar Cheese	3 cups	11	180	55%
Natural	3 cups	10	160	56%
Regular				
White-no butter	4 cups	1	75	12%
Yellow-no butter	4 cups	1	88	10%
(Keebler)-Ready to Eat-Pop Deluxe				
Honey Caramel Glazed	1 oz	3	120	23%
White Cheddar	1 oz	10	140	64%
Microwave-regular kernels	1 oz	5.7	100	51%
(Newman's Own-Butter)	3 cups	8	150	48%
Natural	3 cups	8	150	48%
(Old Vienna)				
Butter	1 oz	10	160	56%
Cheese	1 oz	10	160	56%
(Orville Redenbacher's)				
Air Popping Corn	4 cups	1	90	10%
Butter	3 cups	5	80	56%
Microwave	4 cups	6	110	49%
no salt	4 cups	7	110	57%
Butter Toffee-Microwave	2½ cups	12	210	51%
Caramel-Microwave	2½ cups	14	240	53%
Cheddar Cheese-Microwave	3 cups	10	150	40%
Light-Microwave				
Butter	3 cups	1	50	18%
Natural	3 cups	1	50	18%
Nacho Cheese-Microwave	3 cups	9	140	58%
Natural	3 cups	5	80	56%
Microwave	4 cups	7	110	57%
no salt	4 cups	8	120	60%
Popping Corn				
Plain	4 cups	1	90	10%
w/oil & salt	4 cups	8	160	45%
Ready-to-eat-Light	1 oz	5	100	45%
Sour Cream & Onion-Microwave	3 cups	10	150	60%
(Pillsbury)-Micro Wave				
Butter Flavor				
frozen	3 cups	13	210	56%
grocery shelf	3 cups	13	210	56%
Original				
frozen	3 cups	13	210	56%

Food and Description	Amount	Fat Grams	Total Calories	% Fat Calories
grocery shelf	3 cups	13	210	56%
Salt Free-frozen	3 cups	7	170	37%
(Planter's)-Microwave				
Butter	3 cups	8	140	51%
Natural	3 cups	9	140	58%
Popcorn Snack Cakes				
(Chico-San) Popcorn				
Butter	1 cake	–	40	–
Cheddar	1 cake	2	50	36%
Lightly Salted	1 cake	–	40	–
Plain	1 cake	–	35	–
(Quaker) PoppedCorn				
Butter	1 cake	–	35	–
Popped in oil-no butter added	1 cup	3	55	49%
(Pop-Secret)-Butter Flavor	3⅓ cups	9	150	54%
salt free	3 cups	9	140	58%
Cheese	2¼ cups	11	170	58%
Light-Butter	3 cups	3	70	39%
Natural	3 cups	4	90	40%
Natural Flavor	3⅓ cups	8	140	51%
Syrup-Coated	1 cup	1	135	7%
(Weight Watchers)-Microwave				
regular	1 oz pouch	1	100	9%
Ready-to-eat lightly salted	.66 oz	4	80	45%
Ready-to-eat White Cheddar	.66 oz	6	100	54%
(Wise)-Tender Eating Baby Popcorn	.5 oz	6	70	77%
W/real White Cheddar Cheese	.5 oz	5	70	64%
POPPY SEED	1 tsp	1	15	60%
POPSICLES (See FRUIT ICES)				
PORGY				
breaded & fried	3 oz	13	246	48%
cooked-dry heat	3 oz	8.7	172	46%
PORK (See also BACON, HAM, LUNCHEON MEAT, SAUSAGE)				

(NOTE: Lean = meat trimmed of all separable fat before cooking.
Lean & fat = untrimmed and cooked or eaten as purchased.)

Food and Description	Amount	Fat Grams	Total Calories	% Fat Calories
Arm Picnic				
fresh				
lean & fat-braised	3 oz	22	296	67%
lean & fat-roasted	3 oz	22	284	70%
lean-braised	3 oz	12	213	51%
lean-roasted	3 oz	11	195	51%
Arm Picnic				
cured				
lean & fat-roasted	3 oz	18	240	68%

Food and Description	Amount	Fat Grams	Total Calories	% Fat Calories
lean-roasted	3 oz	6	146	37%
Backfat				
raw	1 oz	25	230	100%
	1 lb	402	3685	100%
Blade, Boston				
braised-lean & fat	3 oz	24	316	68%
	1 steak/			
	~ 5.6 oz	45.88	594	70%
broiled-lean & fat	3 oz	24	297	73%
	1 steak/			
	~ 6.5 oz	52.6	647	73%
roasted-lean & fat	3 oz	21	273	69%
	1 steak/			
	~ 6.5 oz	46.76	594	71%
Blade, Boston				
braised-lean only	3 oz	14.95	250	54%
	1 steak/			
	~ 4.5 oz	22.86	382	54%
broiled-lean only	3 oz	15.67	233	61%
	1 steak/			
	~ 5 oz	27.8	413	61%
roasted-lean only	3 oz	14	218	58%
	1 steak/			
	~5.5 oz	26.6	404	59%
Brains				
braised	3 oz	8	117	62%
Chitterlings				
cooked-simmered	3 oz	24	258	84%
	1 lb	73	923	71%
Ears				
cooked-simmered	1 Ear	11.88	183	58%
Feet				
cooked-simmered	2.5 oz	8.8	138	57%
Feet				
Cured, Pickled	1 oz	4.58	58	71%
Simmered	3 oz	10.6	166	57%
Heart				
braised	1 Heart	6.5	191	31%
Jowl				
raw	4 oz	78.66	740	96%
	1 oz	19.7	186	95%
Kidney				
braised	3 oz	4	128	28%

Food and Description	Amount	Fat Grams	Total Calories	% Fat Calories
Leg				
lean & fat-roasted	3 oz	18	252	64%
lean-roasted	3 oz	10	189	48%
Liver				
braised	3 oz	3.7	141	24%
Loin, Blade				
braised-lean & fat	3 oz	28.98	348	75%
broiled-lean & fat	3 oz	28.77	334	78%
pan-fried-lean & fat	3 oz	31	352	79%
roasted-lean & fat	3 oz	25.88	310	75%
Loin, Blade				
braised-lean only	3 oz	17.5	266	59%
broiled-lean only	3 oz	18	255	64%
pan-fried-lean only	3 oz	16.86	240	63%
roasted-lean only	3 oz	16	238	60%
Loin, Center				
braised-lean & fat	3 oz	21.5	301	64%
broiled-lean & fat	3 oz	18.78	269	63%
pan-fried-lean & fat	3 oz	25.9	318	73%
roasted-lean & fat	3 oz	18	268	60%
Loin, Center				
braised-lean only	3 oz	11.65	231	45%
broiled-lean only	3 oz	8.9	196	41%
pan-fried-lean only	3 oz	13.5	226	54%
roasted-lean only	3 oz	11	204	49%
Loin, Center Rib				
braised-lean & fat	3 oz	23	312	66%
broiled-lean & fat	3 oz	22	291	68%
pan-fried-lean & fat	3 oz	28	331	76%
roasted-lean & fat	3 oz	20	271	66%
Loin, Center Rib				
braised-lean only	3 oz	12	236	46%
broiled-lean only	3 oz	12.7	219	52%
pan-fried-lean only	3 oz	13	219	53%
roasted-lean only	3 oz	11.7	208	51%
Loin, Whole				
braised-lean & fat	3 oz	23.7	312	68%
broiled-lean & fat	3 oz	23	294	70%
roasted-lean & fat	3 oz	20.65	271	69%
Loin, whole				
braised-lean only	3 oz	12	232	47%
broiled-lean only	3 oz	13	218	54%
roasted-lean only	3 oz	11.8	204	52%

Food and Description	Amount	Fat Grams	Total Calories	% Fat Calories
Lungs				
braised	3 oz	2.65	85	28%
Shank				
lean & fat-roasted	3 oz	19	260	66%
lean-roasted	3 oz	9	184	44%
Shoulder, Whole				
roasted-lean & fat	3 oz	21.8	277	71%
Shoulder, Whole				
roasted-lean only	3 oz	12.74	207	55%
Sirloin				
braised-lean & fat	3 oz	21.8	299	66%
broiled-lean & fat	3 oz	21	281	67%
roasted-lean & fat	3 oz	17	247	62%
Sirloin				
braised-lean only	3 oz	11	221	45%
broiled-lean only	3 oz	11.5	207	50%
roasted-lean only	3 oz	11	201	49%
Spareribs				
braised-lean & fat	3 oz	25.75	338	69%
braised from 1 lb raw	~ 6 oz	53.6	703	69%
Spleen				
braised	3 oz	2.7	128	19%
Stomach				
raw	3 oz	8	135	53%
Tail				
cooked-simmered	3 oz	30	336	80%
Tenderloin				
roasted-lean only	3 oz	4	141	26%
Tongue				
braised	3 oz	14.8	215	62%
cured-canned (Hormel) 8 lb	3 oz	13	190	62%
Top Loin				
braised-lean & fat	3 oz	24.78	324	69%
broiled-lean & fat	3 oz	24	306	71%
pan-fried-lean & fat	3 oz	28	333	76%
roasted-lean & fat	3 oz	21	280	68%
Top Loin				
braised-lean only	3 oz	12	236	46%
broiled-lean only	3 oz	12.7	219	52%
pan-fried-lean only	3 oz	13	219	53%
roasted-lean only	3 oz	11.7	208	51%
PORK ENTREE/DINNER (*See also* FROZEN ENTREE/DINNER)				
Breaded Pork Steaks/frozen (Hormel)	3 oz	15	220	61%

Food and Description	Amount	Fat Grams	Total Calories	% Fat Calories
Cajun Pork/Hunt's Minute Gourmet				
box	6.6 oz	23	460	45%
Great Beginnings (Hormel) Box				
prepared	5 oz	8	140	51%
Ham & Swiss Cheese Croissant/frozen -				
(Sara Lee)	1	18	340	48%
Ham Croquette/homemade	1/~2 oz	9.8	163	54%
Pork Loin-sliced w/gravy/homemade	4 oz	9	162	50%
Scalloped Potatoes & Ham/frozen	9 oz	16	340	42%
(Schwan's)/frozen - Center Cut Pork Loin				
Chops	7 oz	14	300	42%
Chopped pork fritter	2.66 oz	9	200	41%
Ham Steak Patties	2 oz	16	180	80%
Pork Dinner Loin	4 oz	4	230	16%
POT PIE (*See* individual listings, i.e., BEEF, CHICKEN, TURKEY)				
POTATO				
White				
raw/no skin	1 medium	–	88	–
raw/with skin	1 medium	–	110	–
baked/no skin	~ 5.5 oz	–	145	–
baked/with skin	~ 7 oz	–	220	–
baked-skin only	1 medium	–	115	–
boiled/no skin	½ cup	–	67	–
	~ 4.75 oz	–	116	–
boiled/with skin	½ cup	–	68	–
canned/no skin	½ cup	–	54	–
small whole new (S&W)	½ cup	–	45	–
whole new potatoes (Del Monte)	½ cup	–	45	–
flakes/dry	1 cup	–	164	–
flakes-(Arrowhead Mills)	2 oz	–	140	–
Country Store				
(Borden)/dry	⅓ cup	–	70	–
frozen/cottage cut				
cooked in oven	10 pcs	4	109	33%
frozen-fried in veg. oil	10 pcs	8	158	46%
french-fried/frozen-heated	10 pieces	4	109	33%
french fries/from restaurant	10 pieces	8	158	46%
granules/dry	1 cup	1	704	1%
microwaved/no skin	1 large	–	156	–
microwaved/with skin	1 large	–	212	–
POTATO CHIPS				
(Cottage Fries)-no salt added	1 oz	11	160	62%
Eagle)-Crispy Cut	1 oz	10	150	60%
Barbeque Flavored	1 oz	8	150	48%

Food and Description	Amount	Fat Grams	Total Calories	% Fat Calories
Extra Crunchy	1 oz	8	150	48%
Hawaiian	1 oz	8	150	48%
Lattice Cut	1 oz	10	150	60%
Mesquite Barbecue	1 oz	10	150	60%
Onion Ridged	1 oz	10	150	60%
Plain	1 oz	10	150	60%
Ridged-plain	1 oz	10	150	60%
Russet	1 oz	8	150	48%
Sour Cream & Onion	1 oz	10	150	60%
Thins	1 oz	10	150	60%
Barbeque Flavored	1 oz	10	150	60%
(Health Valley)-Country	1 oz	10	160	56%
no salt	1 oz	10	160	56%
Country Ripples	1 oz	10	160	56%
Dip-no salt	1 oz	10	160	56%
Plain	1 oz	10	160	56%
(Keebler)-Ripplin's-all flavors	1 oz	9	150	54%
(Laura Scudder)-Bar-B-Q	1 oz	9	150	54%
For Dips	1 oz	10	150	60%
Hawaiian	1 oz	9	150	54%
Natural Style	1 oz	10	150	60%
Plain	1 oz	10	150	60%
Sour Cream & Onion	1 oz	9	150	54%
(Lay's)				
Crunch Tators				
Hoppin Jalapeno	1 oz	7	140	45%
Mighty Mesquite	1 oz	7	140	45%
Original	1 oz	8	140	51%
Regular Chips				
Bar B Q	1 oz	9	150	54%
Cheddar Cheese	1 oz	10	150	60%
Italian Cheese	1 oz	9	150	54%
Jalapen'N Cheddar	1 oz	9	150	54%
Plain	1 oz	10	150	60%
Salt & Vinegar	1 oz	9	150	54%
Sour Cream & Onion	1 oz	10	160	56%
Unsalted	1 oz	10	150	60%
(New York Deli)	1 oz	11	160	62%
(O'Boises)-Original	1 oz	9	150	54%
Sour Cream & Onion	1 oz	9	150	54%
(O'Grady's)-Au Gratin	1 oz	8	150	48%
Hearty Seasoning	1 oz	8	140	51%
Plain	1 oz	9	150	54%
(Old Vienna)-Plain	1 oz	9	150	54%

Food and Description	Amount	Fat Grams	Total Calories	% Fat Calories
(Poore Brothers)				
Bar-B-Que	1 oz	10	150	60%
Cajun	1 oz	10	150	60%
Chili & Lemon	1 oz	10	150	60%
Dill Pickle	1 oz	10	150	60%
Jalapeno	1 oz	10	150	60%
Regular	1 oz	10	150	60%
no salt	1 oz	10	150	60%
Sour Cream & Onion	1 oz	10	150	60%
(Pringle's)				
B-B-Q-Light	1 oz	8	150	48%
Cheez-ums	1 oz	13	170	69%
Idaho Rippled				
French Onion	1 oz	12	170	64%
Original	1 oz	12	170	64%
Taco'n Cheddar	1 oz	12	170	64%
Light	1 oz	8	150	48%
Light Ranch	1 oz	8	150	48%
Regular	1 oz	13	170	69%
Sour Cream'N Onion	1 oz	12	170	64%
(Ruffles)				
Bacon & Sour Cream	1 oz	9	150	54%
Bar-B-Q	1 oz	9	150	54%
Cajun Spice	1 oz	10	150	60%
Cheddar & Sour Cream	1 oz	9	150	54%
Light				
plain	1 oz	6	130	62%
sour cream & onion	1 oz	6	120	30%
Mesquite Grille B-B-Q	1 oz	10	160	56%
Original	1 oz	10	150	60%
Ranch	1 oz	10	160	56%
Sour Cream & Onions	1 oz	9	150	54%
Tato Skins (*See* POTATO SNACKS)				
(Wise)-Natural	1 oz	11	160	62%
Ridges-Barbecue	1 oz	10	150	60%
POTATO DISHES				
Au Gratin				
box mix	1 cup	10	230	39%
frozen (Banquet)	½ cup	2	98	18%
homemade w/butter	½ cup	9	160	51%
microwaveable				
(Green Giant) Pantry Express	½ cup	5	120	38%
Baked w/broccoli & cheese				
frozen (Weight Watchers)	10.5 oz	7	280	23%

Food and Description	Amount	Fat Grams	Total Calories	% Fat Calories
Baked w/sour cream & chives				
frozen (Pillsbury)	5 oz	10	230	39%
Baked w/Cheddar Cheese				
frozen (Oh Boy!)	6 oz	4	142	25%
Baked w/Real Bacon				
frozen (Oh Boy!)	6 oz	3	116	23%
Baked w/Sour Cream, Onion, & Chives				
frozen (Oh Boy!)	6 oz	5	129	35%
Baked w/Cheese flavored topping				
frozen (Pillsbury)	5 oz	6	200	27%
(Betty Crocker) box mixes				
prepared				
Au Gratin	1 Serving	6	150	24%
Cheddar & bacon	1 Serving	6	150	24%
Hash browns w/onions	1 Serving	6	160	34%
Julienne	1 Serving	6	140	39%
Homestyle Skin-On Potatoes				
American Cheese				
Prepared	⅙ box	5	140	32%
Unprepared	⅙ box	1	190	5%
Cheddar Cheese				
Prepared	⅙ box	5	140	32%
Unprepared	⅙ box	2	100	17%
Microwave				
Au Gratin	1 Serving	5	140	32%
Cheese Please (Idahoan)	½ cup	5	150	30%
creamy scalloped	1 Serving	6	150	36%
mild cheddar cheese	1 Serving	5	150	30%
Rich sour cream	1 Serving	5	150	30%
Potato Medleys-box mixes-prepared				
Broccoli Au Gratin	1 Serving	4	140	26%
Scalloped				
w/Broccoli	1 Serving	5	150	30%
w/green beans & mushrooms	1 Serving	5	140	32%
w/cheddar cheese & mushroom	1 Serving	4	140	26%
Scalloped	1 Serving	5	140	32%
Smokey Cheddar	1 Serving	6	150	36%
Sour Cream & Chive	1 Serving	7	160	39%
Twice Baked				
Bacon & Cheddar	1 Serving	11	210	47%
Herbed Butter	1 Serving	13	220	53%
Mild Cheddar w/onion	1 Serving	11	190	52%
Sour Cream & Chive	1 Serving	11	200	50%

Food and Description	Amount	Fat Grams	Total Calories	% Fat Calories
Escalloped Potatoes/Vegetable Clasics				
(Del Monte) microwave	4.5 oz	9	140	58%
(French's)				
Box Mixes-prepared				
Cheddar and Bacon Casserole	1 Serving	5	130	35%
Creamy Italian Scalloped	1 Serving	3	120	23%
Creamy Stroganoff	1 Serving	4	130	28%
Crispy Top Scalloped w/Savory				
Onion	1 Serving	5	140	32%
Real Cheese Scalloped	1 Serving	5	140	32%
Real Sour Cream & Chives	1 Serving	7	150	42%
Tangy Au-Gratin	1 Serving	5	130	35%
Hash Browns				
homemade w/veg oil	½ cup	10.85	163	60%
frozen/plain	½ cup	8.97	170	48%
frozen/butter sauce	3.5 oz	8.9	178	45%
refrigerated				
(Simply Potatoes)	4 oz	< 1	100	5%
(Kraft) Box Mixes-prepared				
Broccoli Au Gratin	⅙ box	5	140	32%
Potatoes & Cheese-Two Cheese	⅙ box	4	140	26%
Scalloped Potatoes	⅙ box	5	140	32%
Mashed				
w/whole milk	½ cup	.6	81	7%
w/whole milk and margarine	½ cup	4	94	38%
from dehydrated flakes				
w/milk & butter added	½ cup	6	165	33%
Instant				
(Instamash)				
microwave-box mix	½ cup	1	80	11%
French's				
box mix/prepared	½ cup	6	130	42%
Hungry Jack box mix/prepared	½ cup	7	140	45%
Potato Buds (Betty Crocker)				
Box Mix/dry	½ cup	–	70	–
Box Mix/prepared	½ cup	6	130	42%
Spuds (French's)				
Mix-prepared	½ cup	7	140	45%
(Micromagic)				
frozen				
french fries	3 oz	13	290	40%
Skinny fries	3.5 oz	15	350	39%
Tater Sticks	4 oz	22	390	51%

Food and Description	Amount	Fat Grams	Total Calories	% Fat Calories
Microwave				
(Del Monte) Vegetable Classics				
Potatoes Au Gratin in Tangy				
Chili Sauce	½ cup	11	190	52%
(Ore Ida) frozen				
Cheddar browns	3 oz	2	80	23%
Cottage Fries	3 oz	5	120	38%
Crinkle Cuts, Lites	3 oz	2	90	20%
Crinkle Cuts, Microwave	3.5 oz	8	180	40%
Crispers!	3 oz	15	230	59%
Crispy Crowns	3 oz	10	170	53%
Deep Fries-for the oven				
Crinkle Cuts	3 oz	6	160	34%
Regular Cuts	3 oz	7	160	39%
French Fries-Golden Crinkles	3 oz	4	120	30%
French Fries-Golden Fries	3 oz	4	120	30%
French Fries-Pixie Crinkles	3 oz	5	140	32%
French Fries-Shoestrings	3 oz	6	150	36%
Fries Country Style Dinner	3 oz	3	110	25%
Golden Patties	2.5 oz	8	140	51%
Golden Twirls	3 oz	7	160	39%
Hash Browns-Microwave	2 oz	7	120	60%
Hash Browns-Shredded	3 oz	–	70	–
Hash Browns-Southern Style	3 oz	–	70	–
Potatoes O'Brien	3 oz	–	60	–
Small Whole Potatoes	3 oz	–	70	–
Tater Tots	3 oz	7	150	42%
Tater Tots-Microwave	2 oz	9	200	41%
Tater Tots-bacon flavored	3 oz	6	150	36%
Tater Tots w/onion	3 oz	6	150	36%
Toaster Hash Browns	1.75 oz	6	100	54%
Topped Baked				
Broccoli & Cheese	5⅞ oz	4	160	23%
Vegetable Primavera	6⅛ oz	7	160	39%
Twice Baked				
butter flavor	5 oz	9	210	39%
cheddar cheese	5 oz	11	230	43%
sour cream & chives	5 oz	9	210	39%
Wedges Home Style	3 oz	3	110	25%
Whole Small	3 oz	–	70	–
Zesties!	3 oz	8	160	45%
Pierogi (dumpling)/frozen				
(Mrs. T's)				
Potato Cheese	1	1	70	13%

Food and Description	Amount	Fat Grams	Total Calories	% Fat Calories
Potato Onion	1	–	50	–
(Pillsbury) box mixes/prepared				
cheddar & bacon	1 Serving	5	130	35%
creamy Italian style	1 Serving	3	120	23%
potato pancake	3 pancakes	2	90	20%
scalloped w/cheese	1 Serving	5	140	32%
scalloped w/creamy white sauce	1 Serving	5	140	32%
sour cream & chives	1 Serving	7	150	42%
Tangy Au Gratin	1 Serving	5	130	35%
Potato Fillets/frozen				
(Gorton's)	2 fillets	20	310	58%
Potato Pancakes				
(French's) box mix				
homemade				
w/butter & milk	1 pancake	12.6	495	23%
Dinner Pancakes	3-3" pancakes	2	90	20%
Potato Puffs/frozen	1 puff	.8	16	45%
	½ cup	6.7	138	44%
Potato Salad w/mayonnaise				
canned German Style				
(Read)	½ cup	3	120	23%
canned Home Style				
(Read)	1 cup	22	340	58%
homemade	½ cup	10	179	50%
Potato Sticks/frozen				
(Gorton's)	4 sticks	16	260	55%
Potatoes O'Brien w/bread crumbs & butter				
homemade	½ cup	1	79	11%
Scalloped/homemade				
w/butter	½ cup	4.5	105	39%
w/cheese	½ cup	9.5	175	49%
Scalloped flavored w/ham				
(Lunch Bucket)	8.5 oz	12	250	43%
frozen/plain	½ cup	6	123	44%
frozen w/cheese	½ cup	9.6	177	49%
Scalloped potatoes & ham/frozen				
(Swanson's)	9 oz	16	340	42%
POTATO SNACKS (See also POTATO CHIPS)				
(Keebler)-Tato Skins-all flavors	1 oz	8	150	48%
(Planter's)-Potato Crunchies	1.25 oz	11	190	52%
Potato Sticks	1 cup	12	190	57%
	1 oz	9	148	55%
(Durkee) O&C-plain	1.5 oz	15	231	58%
POTATO SOUP (See SOUP)				

Food and Description	Amount	Fat Grams	Total Calories	% Fat Calories
POTATO STARCH (Manischewitz)	½ cup	–	385	–
POULTRY SEASONING	1 tsp	–	5	–
POUT-OCEAN/raw	3 oz	1	70	13%
PRESERVES (See JAM/JELLY/PRESERVES)				
PRETZELS				
(Eagle)-Beer	1 oz	2	110	16%
plain	1 oz	2	110	16%
(Estee)-unsalted	5 pieces	< 1	25	18%
(Featherweight)-unsalted pretzels	1 oz	1	110	8%
(Laura Scudder's)-Bavarian	1 oz	1	110	8%
unsalted	1 oz	1	120	8%
Sticks	1 oz	1	110	8%
Twists	1 oz	1	110	8%
(Nabisco)-Mister Salty				
Butter Flavored	1 oz	1	110	8%
Dutch Pretzels	1 oz	1	110	8%
Fat Free	1 oz	0	100	–
Junior Pretzels	1 oz	2	110	16%
Mini	1 oz	1	110	8%
Pretzel Rings	1 oz	2	110	16%
Pretzel Sticks	1 oz	1	90	10%
Pretzel Twists	1 oz	2	110	16%
Very Thin Pretzel Sticks	1 oz	1	110	8%
(Planter's)-Pretzels	1 oz	1	110	8%
(Pocket Pretzels) Peanut Butter				
Filled	1 oz	4	126	29%
(Rokeach)-Dutch	1 oz	< 1	110	5%
no salt	1 oz	< 1	110	5%
(Rold Gold)				
Rods	1 oz	2	110	16%
Sticks	1 oz	1	110	8%
Twists	1 oz	1	110	8%
Tiny Tims	1 oz	2	110	16%
(Snyder's) Hard Pretzels				
Old Fashioned	1 oz	–	110	–
Sour Dough	1 oz	–	110	–
(Super Pretzel)-frozen-baked soft	2.25 oz	–	190	–
oat bran	2.25 oz	–	178	–
(Syfert's)-Butter-rods	1 oz	1	110	8%
PRICKLY PEAR	1	.5	42	11%
PRUNE				
canned in heavy syrup	5	–	90	–
	1 cup	< 1	240	2%

Food and Description	Amount	Fat Grams	Total Calories	% Fat Calories
dried				
cooked				
no sugar	1 cup	< 1	225	2%
w/sugar	1 cup	< 1	294	2%
moist pack (Del Monte)	2 oz	–	120	–
uncooked	10 Pitted	< 1	201	2%
(Del Monte)				
w/pits	2 oz	–	120	–
w/o pits	2 oz	–	140	–
dried				
(Mariani)				
large	¼ cup	1	140	6%
pitted	¼ cup	1	140	6%
(Sunsweet)				
bite size				
pitted	2 oz	–	140	–
large	2 oz	–	120	–
medium	2 oz	–	120	–
Xtra large	2 oz	–	120	–
PRUNE JUICE				
canned	4 oz	–	90	–
(Del Monte)-unsweetened	6 oz	–	120	–
(Mott's)				
country style	6 oz	–	129	–
unsweetened	6 oz	–	130	–
(S&W)-unsweetened	6 oz	–	120	–
(Sunsweet)	6 oz	–	130	–
w/prune pulp	6 oz	–	130	–
PUDDING & MOUSSE (*See also* CUSTARD)				
Apple Brown Betty				
homemade	1 cup	7.6	325	21%
Bread				
homemade with raisins	1 cup	16	495	29%
Canned				
banana	½ cup	4	150	24%
butterscotch	½ cup	4	150	24%
chocolate	½ cup	4	190	19%
egg custard	½ cup	6	140	39%
fudge	½ cup	4	190	10%
lemon	½ cup	2	170	11%
rice	½ cup	3	150	18%
tapioca	½ cup	4	140	26%
vanilla	½ cup	4	150	24%

Food and Description	Amount	Fat Grams	Total Calories	% Fat Calories
Corn				
homemade	1 cup	9.8	255	35%
(Del Monte)-Pudding Cups				
banana	5 oz	5	180	25%
butterscotch	5 oz	5	180	25%
chocolate	5 oz	6	190	28%
chocolate fudge	5 oz	6	190	28%
tapioca	5 oz	4	180	20%
vanilla	5 oz	5	180	25%
(Featherweight)-Sweet Pretenders/canned				
butterscotch	½ cup	1	100	9%
chocolate	½ cup	1	100	9%
vanilla	½ cup	2	100	18%
Indian Pudding/homemade-baked	½ cup	4.5	120	34%
Mix				
(D-Zera)-Reduced Calorie-prepared w/skim milk				
butterscotch	½ cup	–	70	–
chocolate	½ cup	–	60	–
vanilla	½ cup	–	70	–
(Estee)				
butterscotch	½ cup	.5	70	6%
chocolate	½ cup	.5	70	6%
lemon	½ cup	.5	70	6%
vanilla	½ cup	.5	70	6%
(Jell-O)-Deluxe Chocolate Collection				
chocolate almond & chocolate creme dessert/				
prepared as directed	½ cup	8	220	33%
(Jell-O)-instant - prepared w/whole milk				
banana cream	½ cup	4	160	23%
butter pecan	½ cup	5	170	27%
butterscotch	½ cup	4	140	26%
chocolate	½ cup	4	130	28%
chocolate fudge	½ cup	5	180	25%
coconut cream	½ cup	6	180	30%
french vanilla	½ cup	4	160	23%
lemon	½ cup	4	140	26%
milk chocolate	½ cup	5	180	25%
pineapple cream	½ cup	4	160	23%
pistachio	½ cup	4	150	24%
vanilla	½ cup	4	140	26%
(Jell-O)-instant-sugar free-prepared with 2% low-fat milk				
banana	½ cup	2	90	20%
butterscotch	½ cup	2	90	20%
chocolate	½ cup	3	100	27%

Food and Description	Amount	Fat Grams	Total Calories	% Fat Calories
chocolate fudge	½ cup	3	100	27%
pistachio	½ cup	3	100	27%
vanilla	½ cup	2	90	20%
(Jell-O)-Microwave puddings-prepared w/whole milk				
banana cream	½ cup	4	170	21%
butterscotch	½ cup	4	170	21%
chocolate	½ cup	5	170	27%
milk chocolate	½ cup	6	160	34%
mint chocolate-	½ cup	5	160	28%
vanilla	½ cup	4	160	23%
(Jell-O)-regular puddings-prepared w/whole milk				
banana cream	½ cup	3	100	27%
butterscotch	½ cup	4	170	21%
chocolate	½ cup	5	180	25%
chocolate fudge	½ cup	4	160	23%
coconut cream	½ cup	6	170	32%
french vanilla	½ cup	4	170	21%
lemon	½ cup	2	200	9%
milk chocolate	½ cup	4	160	23%
vanilla	½ cup	4	140	26%
(Jell-O)-regular sugar-free puddings-prepared with 2% milk				
chocolate	½ cup	3	90	30%
vanilla	½ cup	2	80	23%
(Jell-O)-Mousse-Rich & Luscious-prepared w/whole milk				
chocolate	½ cup	6	150	36%
chocolate fudge	½ cup	6	150	36%
(Jell-O)-Rice Pudding				
Americana prep w/whole milk	½ cup	4	170	21%
(Jell-O)-Whip'N Chill Deluxe Dessert Mix				
chocolate	½ cup	2	70	26%
lemon	½ cup	2	70	26%
mint	½ cup	2	70	26%
strawberry	½ cup	2	70	26%
vanilla	½ cup	2	70	26%
(Royal)-Instant Pudding				
banana cream/ prepared w/whole milk	½ cup	5	180	25%
butterscotch/ prepared w/whole milk	½ cup	5	180	25%
chocolate/ prepared w/whole milk	½ cup	4	190	19%
chocolate almond/ prepared w/2% milk	½ cup	3	180	15%

Food and Description	Amount	Fat Grams	Total Calories	% Fat Calories
chocolate chocolate chip/				
prep w/whole milk	½ cup	4	190	19%
chocolate mint/				
prepared w/whole milk	½ cup	4	190	19%
dark'n sweet/				
prepared w/whole milk	½ cup	4	190	19%
lemon/prepared w/whole milk	½ cup	5	180	25%
pistachio nut/				
prepared w/whole milk	½ cup	4	170	21%
toasted butter almond/				
prep w/whole milk	½ cup	4	170	21%
toasted coconut/				
prepared w/whole milk	½ cup	4	170	21%
vanilla/				
prepared w/whole milk	½ cup	5	180	25%
(Royal)-Instant-sugar-free/prepared w/2% milk				
butterscotch	½ cup	2	100	18%
chocolate	½ cup	3	110	25%
vanilla	½ cup	2	100	18%
(Royal)-regular (cooked)/prepared w/whole milk				
banana cream	½ cup	4	160	23%
butterscotch	½ cup	4	160	23%
chocolate	½ cup	4	180	20%
custard	½ cup	4	150	24%
dark'n sweet	½ cup	5	180	25%
flan w/caramel sauce	½ cup	5	150	30%
vanilla	½ cup	4	160	23%
vanilla tapioca	½ cup	4	160	23%
(Weight Watchers)-Instant/prepared w/skim milk				
butterscotch	½ cup	–	90	–
chocolate	½ cup	1	90	10%
vanilla	½ cup	–	90	–
(Weight Watchers)-Mousse-frozen				
chocolate	2.5 oz	6	170	32%
praline pecan	2. oz	7	190	33%
(Weight Watchers)-Mousse-instant/ prepared w/skim milk				
cheesecake	½ cup	2	60	30%
chocolate	½ cup	3	60	45%
raspberry	½ cup	3	60	45%
strawberry	½ cup	3	60	45%
white chocolate almond	½ cup	3	60	45%

Food and Description	Amount	Fat Grams	Total Calories	% Fat Calories
Rice-homemade-with raisins	½ cup	6	245	22%
Snack				
(Hunt's)/Snack Pack				
banana	4.25 oz	9	180	45%
butterscotch	4.25 oz	8	180	40%
chocolate	4.25 oz	7	180	35%
chocolate fudge	4.25 oz	9	170	48%
chocolate marshmallow	4.25 oz	7	170	37%
german chocolate	4.25 oz	8	190	38%
lemon	4.25 oz	3	150	18%
rice	4.25 oz	10	190	47%
tapioca	4.25 oz	5	120	38%
vanilla	4.25 oz	7	180	35%
(Hershey's) Chocolate Bar Flavor - in the dairy case				
chocolate	4 oz	6	180	30%
chocolate & almond	4 oz	6	180	30%
kisses-chocolate & vanilla	4 oz	6	180	30%
york peppermint pattie	4 oz	6	180	30%
(Hunt's) Snack Pack-Light				
chocolate	4 oz	2	100	18%
tapioca	4 oz	1	199	8%
(Jell-O)-in the dairy case				
chocolate	4 oz	6	170	32%
choc caramel swirls	4 oz	6	170	32%
choc vanilla swirls	4 oz	6	170	32%
double chocolate swirls	4 oz	6	170	32%
vanilla	4 oz	7	180	35%
vanilla chocolate swirls	4 oz	6	180	32%
(Jell-O) Free				
chocolate	4 oz	–	100	–
chocolate vanilla swirls	4 oz	–	100	–
(Jell-O)-Light-Pudding Snacks				
chocolate	4 oz	2	100	18%
chocolate fudge	4 oz	1	100	9%
chocolate vanilla combo	4 oz	2	100	18%
vanilla	4 oz	2	100	17%
(Swiss Miss)-in the dairy case				
chocolate	4 oz	6	180	30%
chocolate fudge	4 oz	7	170	37%
tapioca	4 oz	4	150	24%
vanilla w/fudge topping	4 oz	7	180	35%
(Swiss Miss)-Light-Pudding Snacks				
chocolate	4 oz	1	100	9%
chocolate fudge	4 oz	1	100	9%

Food and Description	Amount	Fat Grams	Total Calories	% Fat Calories
vanilla	4 oz	1	100	9%
vanilla/chocolate parfait	4 oz	1	100	9%
(Yoplait) Pudding Snacks				
double chocolate	4 oz	4	150	24%
milk chocolate	4 oz	4	170	21%
vanilla	4 oz	4	150	24%
Tapioca				
canned	5 oz	5	160	28%
homemade	1 cup	8	221	33%
apple	1 cup	–	293	–
(Jell-O)-Americana prepared w/whole milk				
chocolate	½ cup	5	170	27%
vanilla	½ cup	4	160	23%
1-Minute	1 Tbs	–	35	
PUDDING POPS				
(Jell-O) - Pudding Pops				
chocolate	1	2	80	23%
chocolate caramel swirl	1	2	80	23%
chocolate-covered chocolate	1	7	130	49%
chocolate-covered vanilla	1	7	130	49%
chocolate vanilla swirl	1	2	70	26%
chocolate w/chocolate chips	1	3	80	34%
vanilla	1	2	70	26%
vanilla w/chocolate chips	1	3	80	34%
PUMMELO/raw	1	–	228	–
	1 cup	–	71	–
PUMPKIN				
canned				
(Del Monte)	½ cup	–	35	–
(Festal)	½ cup	1	40	23%
solid pack (Libby's)	1 cup	1	80	11%
fresh-boiled-mashed	1 cup	–	48	–
raw-cubed	1 cup	–	30	–
PUMPKIN FLOWERS				
cooked	½ cup	< 1	10	45%
raw	½ cup	< 1	5	90%
PUMPKIN LEAVES/cooked	½ cup	< 1	7	64%
PUMPKIN PIE MIX/canned (Libby's)	1 cup	–	210	–
PUMPKIN PIE SPICE	1 tsp	–	6	–
PUMPKIN SEEDS (and SQUASH SEEDS)				
dried	1 oz	13	154	76%
	1 cup	63	747	76%
kernels-roasted	1 oz	11.96	148	73%
	1 cup	95.6	1184	73%

Food and Description	Amount	Fat Grams	Total Calories	% Fat Calories
whole-roasted	1 oz	5.5	127	39%
	1 cup	12	285	38%
PUNCH				
Dietetic or low-calorie:				
Kool-Aid Soft Drink Mix				
sugar-free	8 oz	–	4	–
Sweetened:				
Cherry Kool-Aid/sweetened	8 oz	–	90	–
Grape Kool-Aid/sweetened	8 oz	–	90	–
Orange Kool-Aid/sweetened	8 oz	–	90	–
Tropical Punch Kool-Aid				
sweetened	8 oz	–	100	–
PURSLANE				
boiled	½ cup	–	10	–
raw	1 cup	–	7	–

Q

Food and Description	Amount	Fat Grams	Total Calories	% Fat Calories
QUAIL				
breast meat only-raw	~ 2 oz	1.67	69	22%
meat & skin-raw	~ 4 oz	13	210	56%
meat only-raw	~ 3 oz	4	123	29%
QUICHE (See EGG MEALS)				
QUINCE	1	–	53	–

R

Food and Description	Amount	Fat Grams	Total Calories	% Fat Calories
RABBIT				
Domestic				
breaded & fried/boneless	3 oz	8.8	199	40%
chopped/diced	1 cup	14	302	42%

Food and Description	Amount	Fat Grams	Total Calories	% Fat Calories
ground	1 cup	11	238	42%
stewed	4 oz	11.5	245	42%
	1 lb	45.8	980	42%
Wild/raw-boneless	3 oz	8.5	182	42%
RADISH/raw	10 pieces	–	7	–
Chinese	½ cup	–	13	–
Oriental				
raw	½ cup	–	8	–
dried	¼ cup	–	75	–
White Icicle	1 piece	–	14	–
RAISIN				
Golden				
seedless	1 cup	.75	453	2%
(Del Monte)	3 oz	–	260	–
(Dole)	½ cup	–	262	–
(Sun Maid)	½ cup	–	260	–
Muscat (Sun Maid)	½ cup	1	270	3%
natural (Del Monte)	3 oz	–	250	–
seedless	1 cup	.68	434	1%
	1 pack-½ oz	–	40	–
cooked w/sugar	1 cup	–	628	–
(Sun Maid)	1 oz	–	96	–
uncooked ground				
packed	1 cup	< 1	780	1%
unpacked	1 cup	–	578	–
sun-dried				
(Dole)	½ cup	–	250	–
(Sun Maid)	½ cup	–	250	–
with seeds	1 cup	.8	428	2%
RASPBERRY				
Black				
canned in water	1 cup	2	110	16%
fresh	1 cup	2	100	18%
Red				
fresh	1 cup	.66	61	10%
	1 pint	1.7	154	10%
canned in hvy syrup	1 cup	< 1	234	2%
frozen-lite syrup (Birds Eye)	5 oz	< 1	90	5%
frozen				
sweetened	1 cup	< 1	256	2%
unsweetened	3.5 oz	< 1	50	9%
RASBERRY-CRANBERRY JUICE COCKTAIL				
(Seneca)	6 oz	–	110	–
RASPBERRY JUICE	1 cup	–	100	–

Food and Description	Amount	Fat Grams	Total Calories	% Fat Calories
Black				
Raspberry/fresh	4 oz	–	49	–
Raspberry,Country				
from frozen conc	6 oz	–	90	–
Raspberry (Dole) Pure & Light	6 oz	–	87	–
Red				
Red Raspberry (Smucker's)	8 oz	–	120	–
Red Raspberry Delight/bottled	6 oz	–	90	–
RAVIOLI-BEEF				
Canned				
(Chef Boyardee)	7 oz	5	180	25%
(Estee)	7.5 oz	11	230	43%
(Franco-American)	7.5 oz	4.7	223	19%
Hearty Beef	7.5 oz	11	290	34%
Hearty Pasta	7.5 oz	11	280	35%
W/Meat Sauce	7.5 oz	10.8	284	34%
RAVIOLIO'S-BEEF				
Canned (Franco-American)	7.5 oz	8	250	29%
RED BEAN				
canned	½ cup	–	100	–
(Van Camp's)	1 cup	1	190	5%
dry				
(Joan of Arc/Green Giant)	½ cup	1	90	10%
RED BEAN SOUP (See SOUP)				
REFRIED BEANS (See MEXICAN FOOD)				
RELISH				
(Claussen)	1 Tbs	–	14	–
(Heinz)				
Hamburger relish	1 oz	–	30	–
Hot Dog relish	1 oz	–	35	–
India relish	1 oz	–	35	–
Sweet relish	1 oz	–	30	–
Pickle Relish	1Tbs	–	12	–
(Vlasic)				
Dill relish	1 oz	–	2	–
Green tomato piccalilli	1 oz	–	35	–
Hamburger relish	1 oz	–	40	–
Hot Dog relish	1 oz	1	40	–
Hot piccalilli relish	1 oz	–	35	–
India relish	1 oz	–	30	–
Sweet relish	1 oz	–	30	–
RHUBARB				
cooked-sweetened	1 cup	–	280	–
frozen-cooked w/sugar	1 cup	–	278	–

Food and Description	Amount	Fat Grams	Total Calories	% Fat Calories
raw-diced	½ cup	–	13	–
RICE				
(Arrowhead Mills)				
brown rice				
quick	2 oz	1	200	5%
Brown				
cooked				
long grain				
cold	1 cup	.9	173	5%
hot	1 cup	1	232	4%
raw				
long grain	1 cup	3.5	666	5%
short grain	1 cup	3.8	720	5%
Long grain				
cooked	½ cup	–	90	–
Long Grain & Wild Rices				
Brown & Wild				
dry	½ cup	1	130	7%
prepared w/butter	½ cup	4	150	24%
Chicken Stock Sauce				
dry	½ cup	2	140	13%
prepared w/butter	½ cup	5	160	28%
Original				
dry	½ cup	< 1	100	5%
prepared w/butter	½ cup	2	120	15%
Original Fast Cooking Recipe				
dry	½ cup	< 1	100	5%
prepared w/butter	½ cup	4	130	28%
Rice In An Instant				
dry	⅔ cup	< 1	120	4%
prepared w/butte	⅔ cup	2	130	14%
Whole Grain Brown				
dry	⅔ cup	1	130	7%
prepared w/butter	⅔ cup	3	150	18%
(MJB) brown rice				
Quick/cooked	½ cup	1	110	8%
(Mahatma)				
Brown/dry	1 oz	–	110	–
Instant/dry	1 oz	–	110	–
cooked/no butter	½ cup	–	110	–
White/dry	1 oz	–	100	–
(Minute Rice)				
Boil In Bag/prepared	½ cup	–	90	–
Brown/instant/prepared	½ cup	1	120	8%

Food and Description	Amount	Fat Grams	Total Calories	% Fat Calories
Premium Long Grain/prepared	⅔ cup	–	120	–
White/prepared	⅔ cup	< 1	120	4%
(New Frontier)				
Standard				
Brown Rice				
cooked	1 Serving	.9	111	7%
dry	3.5 oz	1.9	354	5%
Wild Rice				
cooked	1 Serving	< 1	147	3%
dry	3.5 oz	.7	353	2%
Ultra Roast				
Brown Rice				
cooked	1 Serving	.9	111	7%
dry	3.5 oz	3	395	7%
Wild Rice				
cooked	1 Serving	.9	147	3%
dry	3.5 oz	1	394	2%
(Pritikin)				
Pilaf Brown	½ cup	< 1	90	5%
Spanish Brown	½ cup	< 1	100	5%
(Success)				
Brown				
Boil In Bag/prepared	½ cup	–	103	–
10 Minute/prepared	½ cup	–	103	–
Natural Long Grain				
pre-cooked/prepared	½ cup	< 1	90	5%
(Texmati)				
Brown	½ cup	–	85	–
Lite Bran	½ cup	–	84	–
White Long Grain	½ cup	–	82	–
(Uncle Ben's)				
Boil In Bag/as packaged	½ cup	< 1	90	5%
Aromatica/prepared	½ cup	–	100	–
Converted				
dry	⅔ cup	< 1	120	4%
prepared w/butter	⅔ cup	2	140	13%
Microwave				
(Vita Fiber)				
Rice Grain	1 oz	6	100	54%
White				
cooked/long grain				
cold	1 cup	< 1	158	3%
hot	1 cup	< 1	223	2%

Food and Description	Amount	Fat Grams	Total Calories	% Fat Calories
parboiled/long grain				
cooked/cold	1 cup	–	154	–
cooked/hot	1 cup	–	186	–
dry	1 cup	.6	683	1%
raw				
long grain	1 cup	.7	672	1%
medium grain	1 cup	.8	708	1%
short grain	1 cup	.8	726	1%
Wild Rice/raw	4 oz	< 1	400	1%
RICE AND SAUCE				
(Lipton)-box				
Beef flavored	½ cup	4	160	23%
RICE BRAN	4 oz	18	315	51%
RICE CAKES				
Rice Cakes, Mini				
(Chico San) all flavors	5 pieces	–	50	–
(Hain)				
Apple Cinnamon	5 pieces	< 1	60	8%
Barbque	5 pieces	3	70	39%
Cheese	5 pieces	2	60	30%
Honey Nut	5 pieces	< 1	60	8%
Teriyaki	5 pieces	< 1	50	9%
(Hollywood)				
Apple Cinnamon & Plain	½ oz	< 1	50	9%
Cheese	½ oz	2	60	30%
Honey Nut	½ oz	1	60	15%
Rice Cakes, regular size/most brands				
(ie Chico San, Pritikin, Quaker, etc)				
all flavors	1 cake	–	35	–
Crispy Cakes (Pacific Rice Products)				
all flavors	1	–	20	–
Rice, Carob				
(El Molino)				
mint	1⅞ oz	6	125	43%
plain	1⅞ oz	6	125	43%
RICE DISHES				
(Birds Eye) International Rice Recipes				
frozen				
French Style	3.3 oz	–	110	–
Italian Style	3.3 oz	1	120	8%
Spanish Style	3.3 oz	–	110	–
(Casbah)				
Couscoous Pilaf				
prepared	½ cup	–	100	–

Food and Description	Amount	Fat Grams	Total Calories	% Fat Calories
Pilaf-dry	2 oz	–	90	–
Pilaf nutted-prepared	½ cup	2	160	11%
Spanish Pilaf-dry	1 oz	–	90	–
Tabouly Mix (*See* TABOULI)				
(Chun King) mix-dry	.25 oz	–	20	–
(Country Inn) as packaged without butter				
Broccoli Rice Au Gratin	½ cup	3	130	21%
Chicken Rice Royale	½ cup	1	120	8%
Chicken Stock Rice	½ cup	1	130	7%
Herbed Rice Au Gratin	½ cup	3	140	19%
Rice Alfredo	½ cup	4	140	26%
Rice Florentine	½ cup	3	140	19%
Vegetable Pilaf	½ cup	1	120	8%
Vegetable Rice Medley	½ cup	1	140	6%
(Country Inn) 10 Minute Recipes as packaged without butter				
Asparagus Au Gratin	½ cup	3	130	21%
Broccoli Almondine	½ cup	2	130	14%
Cauliflower Au Gratin	½ cup	3	130	21%
Creamy Chicken & Mushroom	½ cup	3	140	19%
Creamy Mushroom & Wild Rice	½ cup	3	140	19%
Green Bean & Almondine Casserole	½ cup	2	120	15%
Homestyle Chicken & Vegetables	½ cup	3	140	19%
Chicken & Cheese Risotto	½ cup	2	120	15%
(Featherweight)				
Spanish Rice	7.5 oz	–	140	–
(Golden Grain) Rice-A-Roni				
Beef Flavor				
dry	1.33 oz	1	130	7%
prepared	½ cup	5	170	27%
Chicken Flavor				
dry	1.33 oz	1	140	6%
prepared	½ cup	5	170	27%
Chicken & Broccoli				
dry	1.23 oz	1	120	8%
repared	½ cup	3	130	21%
Chicken & Mushroom				
dry	1.33 oz	1	130	7%
prepared	½ cup	7	180	35%
Chicken & Vegetables				
dry	1.20 oz	1	120	8%
prepared	½ cup	4	150	24%
Fried Rice w/Almonds				
dry	1.04 oz	1	110	8%

Food and Description	Amount	Fat Grams	Total Calories	% Fat Calories
prepared	½ cup	5	140	32%
Herb & Butter				
dry	1.04 oz	1	110	8%
prepared	½ cup	4	140	26%
Long Grain & Wild				
Chicken w/almonds				
dry	1.20 oz	1	120	8%
prepared	½ cup	4	140	26%
Rice Pilaf				
dry	1.45 oz	1	150	6%
prepared	½ cup	6	190	28%
Risotto				
dry	1.5 oz	1	160	6%
prepared	½ cup	6	200	27%
Spanish				
dry	1.07 oz	1	110	8%
prepared	½ cup	4	150	24%
Stroganoff				
dry	1.35 oz	3	150	18%
prepared	½ cup	8	190	38%
Wild Rice Pilaf				
dry	1.06 oz	1	100	9%
prepared	½ cup	3	130	21%
Yellow				
dry	1.35 oz	3	150	18%
prepared	½ cup	8	190	38%
(Golden Grain) Rice-A-Roni				
Savory Classics				
Almond Chicken & Wild Rice				
dry	1.3 oz	1	110	8%
prepared	½ cup	4	140	26%
Broccoli Au Gratin				
dry	1.12 oz	3	130	21%
prepared	½ cup	9	180	45%
Cauliflower Au Gratin				
dry	1.2 oz	4	140	26%
prepared	½ cup	7	170	37%
Chicken & Broccoli Dijon				
prepared	1 Serving	5	160	28%
Chicken Florentine				
dry	1.12 oz	1	110	8%
prepared	½ cup	4	130	28%
Creamy Parmesan & Herbs				
dry	1.22 oz	4	140	26%

Food and Description	Amount	Fat Grams	Total Calories	% Fat Calories
prepared	½ cup	7	170	37%
Garden Pilaf				
dry	1.12 oz	1	110	8%
prepared	½ cup	4	140	26%
Green Bean Salad Almondine				
dry	1.25 oz	5	150	30%
prepared	½ cup	11	210	45%
Oriental Stir Fry				
dry	1.08 oz	1	100	9%
prepared	½ cup	6	150	34%
Spring Vegetables & Cheese				
dry	1.22 oz	4	140	26%
prepared	½ cup	7	170	37%
Zesty Cheddar				
dry	1.30 oz	4	150	24%
prepared	½ cup	7	180	40%
(Green Giant)				
One Serving Vegetables/frozen				
Rice Medley	4.5 oz	4	130	28%
Rice'n Broccoli in Cheese Sauce	4.5 oz	5	140	32%
Rice Originals/frozen				
Italian Blend White Rice & Spinach in a Cheese Sauce	½ cup	4	120	30%
Rice Jubilee	½ cup	6	150	36%
Rice Medley	½ cup	3	120	23%
Rice'n Broccoli in Flavored Cheese Sauce	½ cup	4	120	30%
Rice Pilaf	½ cup	2	120	15%
Rice W/Herb Butter Sauce	½ cup	5	150	30%
White & Wild Rice	½ cup	2	120	15%
(Hain)				
3-Gain Side Dishes				
Chicken Meatless Style	½ cup	1	100	9%
Herb	½ cup	1	80	11%
Rice Almondine	½ cup	5	130	35%
Rice Oriental 3-Grain Goodness	½ cup	5	120	38%
(Health Valley)				
Amaranth Pilaf	7.5 oz	3	176	15%
Zesty Lentil Pilaf	4 oz	2.75	110	23%
(Heinz)				
Beef Flavored				
dry	1 oz	–	100	–
Chicken Flavored				
dry	1 oz	1	100	9%

Food and Description	Amount	Fat Grams	Total Calories	% Fat Calories
Long Grain Wild-prepared	½ cup	1	100	9%
Rice Pilaf-dry	1 oz	–	100	–
Spanish-canned	7.25 oz	5	150	30%
Spanish Pilaf-dry	1 oz	–	100	–
(Kashhi)				
7 Whole Grain & Sesame Pilaf-dry	2 oz	1	177	5%
(Konriko)				
Wild Pecan Rice	½ cup	1	89	10%
(Kraft)				
Rice & Cheese-prepared				
3-Cheese & Herbs	½ cup	4	150	24%
Cheddar Pilaf	½ cup	4	150	24%
Cheddar Broccoli	½ cup	5	150	30%
Cheddar & Chicken	½ cup	4	150	24%
(La Choy)				
Chinese Fried Rice-canned	¾ cup	1	190	5%
(Lipton)				
Rice & Beans				
dry	¼ pkg	< 1	130	4%
prepared	½ cup	3	160	17%
Rice & Sauce				
Beef				
dry	¼ pkg	< 1	120	4%
prepared	½ cup	4	160	23%
Broccoli & Cheddar				
dry	¼ pkg	2	130	14%
prepared	½ cup	7	180	35%
Chicken				
dry	¼ pkg	1	125	7%
prepared	½ cup	4	150	24%
Herb & Butter				
dry	¼ pkg	2	125	14%
prepared	½ cup	5	160	28%
Long Grain & Wild				
dry	¼ pkg	–	120	–
prepared	½ cup	3	150	18%
Mushroom				
dry	¼ pkg	< 1	123	4%
prepared	½ cup	3	150	18%
Pilaf				
dry	¼ pkg	< 1	120	4%
prepared	½ cup	6	170	32%
Rice Asparagus w/Hollandaise Sauce				
dry	¼ pkg	1	123	7%

Food and Description	Amount	Fat Grams	Total Calories	% Fat Calories
Spanish				
dry	¼ pkg	< 1	120	4%
prepared	½ cup	3	140	19%
(MJB)				
Fried Rice Oriental/cooked	½ cup	1	110	8%
Herb & Butter/cooked	½ cup	1	100	9%
Mexican Style/cooked	½ cup	–	120	–
Rice Pilaf/cooked	½ cup	1	110	8%
Savory Beef/cooked	½ cup	1	100	9%
Savory Chicken/cooked	½ cup	1	100	9%
(Minute MicroWave)				
Rice Dishes				
Beef Flavored				
family	½ cup	3	160	17%
single	½ cup	2	150	12%
Cheddar Cheese & Broccoli				
family	½ cup	5	160	28%
single	½ cup	4	160	23%
Chicken Flavored				
family	½ cup	4	160	23%
single	½ cup	3	150	18%
French Style Pilaf				
family	½ cup	3	130	15%
single	½ cup	2	120	15%
(Minute Rice)				
Drumstick-prepared w/butter	½ cup	4	150	24%
Fried-prepared w/oil	½ cup	5	160	28%
Long Grain & Wild-prepared w/butter	½ cup	4	150	24%
Rib Roast-prepared w/butter	½ cup	4	150	24%
(Near East)				
Chicken Flavored Pilaf				
dry	1 oz	–	100	–
prepared	½ cup	4	140	26%
Rice Pilaf Mix				
dry	1 oz	–	100	–
Spanish				
dry	1½ oz	–	110	–
prepared	½ cup	4	160	23%
Taboule (See TABOULI)				
Spanish Rice				
(Van Camp's)-canned	1 cup	3	150	18%
(Suzi Wan)				
Honey Lemon Chicken mix	1 Serving	1	200	5%
w/added ingredients	7.5 oz	11	370	27%

Food and Description	Amount	Fat Grams	Total Calories	% Fat Calories
Stir Fry Broccoli mix	1 Serving	3	200	14%
w/added ingredients	7.5 oz	15	370	37%
Sweet'n Sour mix	1 Serving	1	220	4%
w/added ingredients	7.5 oz	5	340	13%
Teriyaki mix	1 Serving	1	180	5%
w/added ingredients	7.5 oz	12	360	30%
As packaged without butter				
Chicken & Broccoli	½ cup	1	120	8%
Chicken & Vegetables	½ cup	1	120	8%
Sweet'n SourRice	½ cup	1	130	7%
Teriyaki Rice	½ cup	1	120	8%
Three Flavor Rice	½ cup	1	120	8%
(Weight Watchers)				
Spanish Rice				
dry	½ cup	1	100	9%
prepared	½ cup	3	120	23%
(Wick Fowler's)				
Rice Kits				
dry				
Cajun	1 serving	1	120	8%
Jalapeno	1 serving	1	130	7%
Ranchero	1 serving	1	110	8%
RICE DRINK				
(Don Jose) Hor chata				
Non dairy rice drink	6 oz	4	120	30%
RICE NOODLES				
canned	½ cup	5	130	35%
RICE POLISH				
stirred and spooned into cup	1 cup	13	278	42%
RICE PUDDING (See PUDDING)				
RICE TOPPINGS				
(Mayacamas)				
Mix prepared				
Calcutta	2 oz	1	22	41%
Chicken Herb	2 oz	1	23	39%
Creole	2 oz	1	23	39%
Garden Pea	2 oz	1	22	41%
Mediterranean	2 oz	1	22	41%
Mexicali	2 oz	1	23	39%
ROAST BEEF (See BEEF, LUNCHEON MEAT)				
ROAST BEEF HASH				
Canned (Mary Kitchen)	7.5 oz	22	350	57%
ROAST BEEF SPREAD (See LUNCHEON MEAT)				

Food and Description	Amount	Fat Grams	Total Calories	% Fat Calories
ROCKFISH				
Pacific				
cooked	3 oz	1.7	103	15%
raw	3 oz	1	80	11%
ROLL				
Brown & Serve				
(Pepperidge Farm)-frozen				
Club Enriched	1	1	100	9%
French Enriched (3 per pkg)	½	1	120	8%
French Enriched (2 per pkg)	½	2	180	10%
Hearth Enriched	1	1	50	18%
(Roman Meal)	1	2	77	23%
(Wonder)				
Gem Style	1	2	80	23%
W/Buttermilk	1	2	80	23%
Crusty Italian Rolls du Jour	1	1	80	11%
Petite French Rolls du Jour	1	2	230	8%
Butterflake-refrigerated (Pillsbury)	1	5	140	32%
Cloverleaf				
commercial				
ready to serve	1	1.6	83	17%
brown & serve	1	1.9	84	20%
homemade (2½" dia)	1	3	119	23%
Colonial Wheat (Rainbo)	1	19	300	57%
Corn Twists-refrigerated-(Pillsbury)	1	4	70	51%
Cracked Wheat	1	.8	95	8%
Crescent-frozen-(Pillsbury)	1	5.5	100	50%
Dinner				
(Pepperidge Farm)	1	2	60	30%
(Roman Meal)	1	1	45	20%
(Wonder)	1	1	80	11%
Finger w/Poppy Seeds				
(Pepperidge Farm)	1	2	60	30%
Finger w/Sesame Seeds				
(Pepperidge Farm)	1	2	60	30%
French Roll	1	1	130	7%
(Earth Grains)	1	1	100	9%
(Pepperidge Farm) 9 per pkg	1	1	110	8%
4 per pkg	½	2	120	15%
Garlic Rolls/frozen (Cole's)	1	5	100	45%
Health Nut Rolls (Oroweat)	1	3	160	17%
Hot Roll Mix (Pillsbury)	2	4	240	15%
Kaiser (Earth Grains)	1	2	190	10%
Old Fashioned (Pepperdge Farm)	1	2	50	36%

Food and Description	Amount	Fat Grams	Total Calories	% Fat Calories
Onion (Earth Grains)	1	2	190	10%
Pan (Wonder)	1	1	80	11%
Parkerhouse/from frozen dough (Pepperidge Farm)	1	1	75	12%
Butter Crescent	1	6	110	49%
French Twist	1	1	110	8%
Golden Twist	1	6	110	49%
Golden Twist-frozen dough	1	6	120	45%
Parker House Rolls	1	1	60	15%
Party Enriched	1	1	30	30%
Sourdough French	1	1	100	9%
Popover				
homemade	1	3.7	90	37%
mix	1	5	170	27%
Potato Roll	1	2	130	14%
Rye	1	–	87	–
Sandwich Quartet (Pepperidge Farm)				
Croissant	1	9	180	25%
Dijon		1	4	180
Golden Egg	1	6	200	27%
Rye	1	4	170	21%
Sandwich Rolls (Pepperidge Farm)				
Dijon Frankfurter	1	3	130	21%
Frankfurter Enriched side sliced	1	3	140	19%
Frankfurter Enriched top sliced	1	3	140	19%
Onion Buns w/poppy seeds	1	3	150	18%
Sandwich Buns w/sesame seeds	1	3	160	17%
Sliced Hamburger Enriched	1	2	130	14%
Soft Family Enriched	1	2	110	16%
(Weight Watchers)				
Hamburger Buns	1	< 1	80	6%
Hot Dog	1	< 1	80	6%
Reduced Calorie Wheat Buns	1	< 1	80	6%
(Wonder)				
Hamburger Buns	1	2	120	15%
Light	1	1	80	11%
Hoagie Rolls	1	7	400	16%
Hot Dog Buns-Light	1	1	80	11%
Hot Dog Rolls	1	1	80	11%
Country Grain Hot	1	1	100	9%

Food and Description	Amount	Fat Grams	Total Calories	% Fat Calories
Scone				
homemade	1.5 oz	6.5	140	42%
(Krusteaz)	2 oz	10	210	43%
Sour dough	1	1	130	7%
Submarine (Earth Grains)	½ roll	1	180	5%
Sub, Hoagie	1/~3.5 oz	7	400	45%
Wheat Dinner Rolls (Home Pride)	1	1	70	13%
White-hard	1	1.6	156	9%
White-soft dinner	1	2	85	21%
frozen homestyle (Rich's)	1	1	75	12%
homemade	1/~1 oz	3	120	23%
(Home Pride)	1	2	80	23%
White-soft				
hamburger and/or hotdog	1	2	150	12%
hamburger (Holsum)	1	2	120	15%
hambruger (Roman Meal)	1	2	113	16%
hotdog (Roman Meal)	1	2	104	17%
hotdog (Wonder)	1	1	80	11%
Whole Wheat	1	1	93	10%
ROMAN BEAN				
canned (Progresso)	8 oz	1	210	4%
ROSEMARY/dried	1 tsp	–	4	–
ROUGHY				
Orange				
raw	3 oz	5.95	107	49%
RUM (*See* DISTILLED LIQUOR)				
RUTABAGA				
fresh-boiled	½ cup	–	39	–
raw	½ cup	–	25	–
RYE (*See* DISTILLED LIQUOR)				

S

Food and Description	Amount	Fat Grams	Total Calories	% Fat Calories
SABLEFISH				
raw	3 oz	13	165	71%
smoked	3 oz	17	220	70%
SAFFRON	1 tsp	–	2	–
SAGE/ground	1 tsp	–	2	–

Food and Description	Amount	Fat Grams	Total Calories	% Fat Calories
SALAD DRESSING				
MIXES (& STANDARD HOME RECIPE [USDA])				
(NOTE: Mixes were prepared as directed on package.)				
Bleu Cheese (Estee)	1 Tbs	< 1	8	56%
Bleu Cheese & herbs (Good Seasons)				
Prepared	1 Tbs	8	70	100%
Unprepared	1 packet	–	4	–
Blue Cheese				
Hidden Valley	1 Tbs	6	58	93%
Thick 'n Creamy	1 Tbs	9	100	81%
Chunky	1 Tbs	8	75	96%
Buttermilk farm style (Good Seasons)				
Prepared	1 Tbs	6	60	90%
Unprepared	1 packet	–	4	–
Cheese Garlic (Good Seasons)				
Prepared	1 Tbs	8	70	100%
Unprepared	1 packet	–	4	–
Cheese Italian (Good Seasons)				
Lite				
Prepared	1 Tbs	3	25	100%
Unprepared	1 packet	–	4	–
Regular				
Prepared	1 Tbs	8	70	100%
Unprepared	1 packet	–	4	–
Classic Herb (Good Seasons)				
Prepared	1 Tbs	8	70	100%
Unprepared	1 packet	–	2	–
Cooked/Standard Home Recipe (USDA)				
W/regular margarine	1 Tbs	2	25	72%
Creamy Style (Good Seasons)				
Prepared	1 Tbs	5	50	90%
Unprepared	1 packet	–	2	–
French/Standard Home				
Recipe (USDA)	1 Tbs	9.8	88	100%
French, Creamy (Estee)	1 Tbs	–	16	–
French, Old Fashion	1 Tbs	9	85	95%
French, Thick 'n Creamy	1 Tbs	9	100	81%
Garlic			1 Tbs	9
Garlic, Creamy (Estee)	1 Tbs	–	2	–
Garlic & Herbs (Good Seasons)				
Prepared	1 Tbs	8	70	100%
Unprepared	1 packet	–	4	–
(Hain)-No Oil				
Bleu Cheese	1 Tbs	1	14	64%

Food and Description	Amount	Fat Grams	Total Calories	% Fat Calories
Buttermilk	1 Tbs	–	12	–
Caesar	1 Tbs	–	4	–
French	1 Tbs	–	12	–
Garlakes/dry	1 Tbs	< 1	228	2%
prepared w/water	1 cup	< 1	242	2%
/boiled-no skin-mashed	½ cup	.5	172	3%
/canned-mashed	1 cup	.5	258	2%
pieces	1 cup	< 1	183	3%
w/syrup	1 cup	< 1	212	2%
/fresh-baked-mashed	½ cup	< 1	103	4%
(Hidden Valley)				
Original Buttermilk				
Regular	1 Tbs	5.7	58	88%
Reduced calorie	1 Tbs	3	33	82%
Ranch Style	1 Tbs	5.7	58	88%
Italian (Good Seasons)				
Prepared	1 Tbs	8	70	100%
Unprepared	1 packet	–	2	–
Italian-Lite (Good Seasons)				
Prepared	1 Tbs	3	25	100%
Unprepared	1 packet	–	4	–
Italian-Mild (Good Seasons)				
Prepared	1 Tbs	8	70	100%
Unprepared	1 packet	–	4	–
Italian-No Oil (Good Seasons)	1 Tbs	–	6	–
Italian-Style (Weight Watchers)				
Individual packets	1 packet	–	9	–
Italian-Zesty				
Estee	1 Tbs	–	4	–
Good Seasons				
Lite				
Prepared	1 Tbs	3	25	100%
Unprepared	1 packet	–	4	–
Regular				
Prepared	1 Tbs	8	70	100%
Unprepared	1 packet	–	2	–
Lemon & Herbs (Good Seasons)				
Prepared	1 Tbs	8	70	100%
Unprepared	1 pkt	–	2	–
(Macayamas)				
Blue Cheese	1 Tbs	5	47	96%
Buttermilk & Herb	1 Tbs	4	45	80%
Cheese Garlic	1 Tbs	9	86	94%
Garlic-Lemon-Dill	1 Tbs	5	45	100%

Food and Description	Amount	Fat Grams	Total Calories	% Fat Calories
Honey Herb	1 Tbs	9	82	98%
Italian Supreme	1 Tbs	9	82	98%
Ranch (Good Seasons)				
Lite				
Prepared	1 Tbs	2	30	60%
Unprepared	1 packet	–	4	–
Regular				
Prepared	1 Tbs	6	60	90%
Unprepared	1 packet	–	4	–
Thousand Island (Estee)	1 Tbs	–	8	–
Vinegar and Oil/Standard Home				
Recipe (USDA)	1 Tbs	8	70	100%
READY TO USE				
Bacon & Buttermilk	1 Tbs	8	80	90%
Bacon & Tomato				
Estee	1 Tbs	< 1	8	56%
Kraft				
Reduced calorie	1 Tbs	2	30	60%
Regular	1 Tbs	7	70	90%
Bacon, Creamy				
Kraft-reduced calorie	1 Tbs	2	30	60%
(Bama)	1 Tbs	4	50	72%
(Bernstein)				
Caesar	1 Tbs	5	48	94%
Cheese Fantastico	1 Tbs	5	50	95%
French Vinaigrette	1 Tbs	5	48	94%
Italian				
Low-cal	1 Tbs	< 1	4	100%
Restaurant Recipe	1 Tbs	7	60	100%
W/cheese-low-cal	1 Tbs	3	45	60%
W/cheese & garlic	1 Tbs	5	45	100%
Light Fantastico				
Cheese Fantastico	1 Tbs	1	15	60%
Classico Italian	1 Tbs	–	20	–
Creamy Dijon	1 Tbs	1	25	36%
Parmesan Garlic Ranch	1 Tbs	2	35	51%
Restaurant Ranch	1 Tbs	1	25	36%
Roquefort	1 Tbs	7	65	96%
Thousand Island	1 Tbs	6	62	87%
Vinaigrette-Low-cal	1 Tbs	< 1	2	100%
(Bertolli)				
Creamy Olive Oil	1 Tbs	6	60	90%
Original Olive Oil	1 Tbs	8	80	90%
Zesty Olive Oil	1 Tbs	7	70	90%

Food and Description	Amount	Fat Grams	Total Calories	% Fat Calories
Blue Cheese/generic	1 Tbs	8	75	96%
Estee	1 Tbs	< 1	8	56%
Nutradiet	1 Tbs	2	25	72%
Blue Cheese Chunky				
Kraft				
Reduced calorie	1 Tbs	2	30	60%
Regular	1 Tbs	6	60	90%
Lite	1 Tbs	4	40	90%
Nutradiet	1 Tbs	2	25	72%
Wish Bone				
Lite	1 Tbs	4	40	90%
Regular	1 Tbs	8	70	100%
Buttermilk, Creamy				
Estee	1 Tbs	–	6	–
Kraft				
Reduced calorie	1 Tbs	3	30	90%
Regular	1 Tbs	8	80	90%
Buttermilk & Chives, Creamy	1 Tbs	8	80	90%
Buttermilk Ranch (Nutradiet)	1 Tbs	2	25	100%
Buttermilk Recipe (Seven Seas)				
Light	1 Tbs	1	50	18%
Regular	1 Tbs	8	80	90%
Caesar				
(Weight Watchers)				
Bottled	1 Tbs	–	4	–
Individual packets	1 packet	–	6	–
(Wish Bone)	1 Tbs	8	78	92%
Catalina French (Kraft)				
Reduced calorie	1 Tbs	1	18	50%
Regular	1 Tbs	5	60	75%
Coleslaw Dressing (Kraft)	1 Tbs	6	70	77%
(Cook's Classic)-Cook's Caesar	1 Tbs	5	50	90%
Cucumber, Creamy				
(Kraft)				
Reduced calorie	1 Tbs	2	25	72%
Regular	1 Tbs	8	70	100%
(Nutradiet)	1 Tbs	2	20	72%
Dijon, Creamy (Estee)	1 Tbs		8	56%
Dijon Vinaigrette-Classic (Wish Bone)				
Lite	1 Tbs	2	25	72%
Regular	1 Tbs	6	61	89%
(Dorothy Lynch) Homestyle				
Reduced calorie	1 Tbs	< 1	30	15%

Food and Description	Amount	Fat Grams	Total Calories	% Fat Calories
(El Molino)-Herbal Secrets No-Oil				
Bleu Cheese	1 Tbs	< 1	12	38%
Creamy Italian	1 Tbs	< 1	7	64%
French	1 Tbs	< 1	10	45%
Herb & Spice	1 Tbs	< 1	6	75%
Italian	1 Tbs	< 1	5	90%
Vinaigrette	1 Tbs	< 1	5	90%
(Featherweight)				
Caesar	1 Tbs	1	14	64%
Creamy Cucumber	1 Tbs	–	4	–
French	1 Tbs	–	14	–
Herb	1 Tbs	–	6	–
Italian	1 Tbs	–	4	–
New Bleu	1 Tbs	–	4	–
Red Wine Vinegar	1 Tbs	–	6	–
Russian	1 Tbs	–	6	–
Thousand Island	1 Tbs	–	18	–
Zesty Tomato	1 Tbs	–	2	–
French				
Kraft				
Reduced calorie	1 Tbs	2	25	72%
Regular	1 Tbs	6	60	90%
Nutradiet	1 Tbs	–	18	–
Pritikin-no oil	1 Tbs	–	10	–
Weight Watchers	1 Tbs	–	10	–
Wish Bone-Lite	1 Tbs	2.5	30	75%
French, Deluxe (Wish Bone)	1 Tbs	5.5	60	83%
French, Garlic (Wish Bone)				
Lite	1 Tbs	2.5	30	75%
Regular	1 Tbs	5	55	82%
French, Sweet 'N Spicy (Wish Bone)				
Lite	1 Tbs	< 1	18	25%
Regular	1 Tbs	5	60	75%
Garlic, Creamy				
Estee	1 Tbs	–	2	–
Kraft	1 Tbs	5	50	90%
Wish Bone	1 Tbs	8	74	97%
Golden Caesar (Kraft)	1 Tbs	7	70	90%
(Hain)				
Creamy Caesar	1 Tbs	6	60	90%
Low salt	1 Tbs	6	60	90%
Creamy French	1 Tbs	6	60	90%
Creamy Italian	1 Tbs	8	80	90%
No salt	1 Tbs	8	80	90%

Food and Description	Amount	Fat Grams	Total Calories	% Fat Calories
Cucumber Dill	1 Tbs	8	80	90%
Dijon	1 Tbs	5	50	90%
Garlic & Sour Cream	1 Tbs	7	70	90%
Honey Sesame	1 Tbs	5	60	75%
Italian Cheese	1 Tbs	6	55	98%
Old Fashioned Buttermilk	1 Tbs	7	70	90%
Poppy Seed Ranchers	1 Tbs	7	60	100%
Savory Herb	1 Tbs	10	90	100%
Swiss Cheese	1 Tbs	7	60	100%
Thousand Island	1 Tbs	5	50	90%
Traditional Italian	1 Tbs	8	80	90%
No salt	1 Tbs	6	60	90%
(Henri's)				
Chef's Ranch House	1 Tbs	7	70	90%
Hearty French	1 Tbs	6	70	77%
Original French	1 Tbs	6	60	90%
Sweet & Saucy French	1 Tbs	6	70	77%
Tas-Tee Dressing	1 Tbs	4	50	72%
(Herb Magic)				
Creamy Cucumber	1 Tbs	–	8	–
Italian	1 Tbs	–	4	–
Sweet & Sour	1 Tbs	–	18	–
Vinaigrette	1 Tbs	–	6	–
Zesty Tomato	1 Tbs	–	14	–
(Hidden Valley)				
Original-reduced calorie	1 Tbs	4	40	90%
Original Creamy	1 Tbs	8	80	90%
Original Ranch-reduced calorie	1 Tbs	4	40	90%
Original w/bacon	1 Tbs	8	80	90%
Ranch Italian-reduced calorie	1 Tbs	3	30	90%
Take Heart-Nonfat				
Blue Cheese	1 Tbs	–	12	–
French	1 Tbs	–	20	–
Italian	1 Tbs	–	14	–
Original	1 Tbs	1	20	45%
Ranch	1 Tbs	1	20	45%
Thousand Island	1 Tbs	–	25	–
Italian				
Generic				
Low cal	1 Tbs	1.5	16	84%
Regular	1 Tbs	7	69	91%

Food and Description	Amount	Fat Grams	Total Calories	% Fat Calories
(Kraft)				
House				
Reduced calorie	1 Tbs	3	30	90%
Regular	1 Tbs	6	60	90%
Oil-free	1 Tbs	–	4	–
Presto	1 Tbs	7	70	90%
(Nutrdiet)/no oil	1 Tbs	–	2	–
(Pritikin)/no oil	1 Tbs	–	6	–
(Weight Watchers)				
Bottled	1 Tbs	–	6	–
Individual packets	1 packet	–	9	–
(Wish Bone)				
Lite	1 Tbs	–	6	–
Regular	1 Tbs	4	45	80%
Italian, Creamy				
(Estee)	1 Tbs	–	4	–
(Kraft)				
Reduced calorie	1 Tbs	2	25	72%
w/real sour cream	1 Tbs	5	50	90%
Lite	1 Tbs	2	25	72%
(Nutradiet)	1 Tbs	1	10	90%
(Wish Bone)				
Lite	1 Tbs	–	7	–
Regular	1 Tbs	5	56	80%
Italian, Dijon (Nutradiet)	1 Tbs	1	8	100%
Italian French (Estee)	1 Tbs	–	4	–
Italian, Herbal (Wish Bone)	1 Tbs	7	70	90%
Italian, Robusto (Wish Bone)	1 Tbs	7	70	90%
Italian, Zesty (Kraft)				
Reduced calorie	1 Tbs	2	20	90%
Regular	1 Tbs	5	50	90%
Italian W/Cheese/low-cal	1 Tbs	1	12	75%
(Kraft) Free-Nonfat				
Blue Cheese	1 Tbs	–	16	–
Catalina	1 Tbs	–	16	–
French	1 Tbs	–	20	–
Italian	1 Tbs	–	6	–
Ranch	1 Tbs	–	16	–
Thousand Island	1 Tbs	–	20	–
(Kraft) Regular				
Peppercorn	1 Tbs	9	90	90%
(Life All Natural)				
Avocado w/tofu	1 Tbs	7	70	90%
Creamy salad egg free	1 Tbs	4	39	92%

Food and Description	Amount	Fat Grams	Total Calories	% Fat Calories
Garlic w/tofu	1 Tbs	7	70	90%
Tofu	1 Tbs	7	75	84%
(Marzetti) Slaw Dressing-Light	1 Tbs	3	50	54%
Miracle French (Kraft)	1 Tbs	6	70	77%
Miracle Whip				
Cholesterol-free	1 Tbs	7	70	90%
Free	1 Tbs	–	20	–
Light	1 Tbs	4	45	80%
Regular	1 Tbs	7	70	90%
(Naturally Fresh)-Refrigerated				
Bleu Cheese	1 Tbs	8	90	80%
Honey Mustard	1 Tbs	6	80	68%
Italian Herb Vinaigrette	1 Tbs	6	60	90%
Poppy Seed	1 Tbs	4	80	45%
Ranch-Lite	1 Tbs	3	30	90%
Slaw Dressing	1 Tbs	5	70	64%
Thousand Island	1 Tbs	5	50	90%
Oil & Vinegar (Kraft)	1 Tbs	8	70	100%
Olive Oil Vinaigrette				
(Wish Bone)-Lite	1 Tbs	.9	16	51%
Onion & Chive				
(Wish Bone)-Lite	1 Tbs	3	35	77%
Onion & Chives, Creamy (Kraft)	1 Tbs	7	70	90%
(Oriental Chef)				
Honey Orange	1 Tbs	3	40	68%
Original French	1 Tbs	3	40	68%
Snappy Ginger	1 Tbs	4	40	90%
Tangy Soy	1 Tbs	4	35	100%
(Ott's)				
Italian	1 Tbs	9	80	100%
Original	1 Tbs	3	40	90%
Reduced calorie	1 Tbs	1	25	36%
(Peggy Jane's)				
Garden Herb	1 Tbs	4	45	80%
Honey Mustard	1 Tbs	6	60	90%
Honey Sesame	1 Tbs	5	60	75%
Pepper Cream	1 Tbs	8	80	90%
Poppy Seed	1 Tbs	4	60	60%
Ranch				
(Pritikin)/No Oil	1 Tbs	–	18	–
(Weight Watchers)-creamy				
Bottled	1 Tbs	–	25	–
Individual packets	1 packet	–	35	–
(Wish Bone)-Lite	1 Tbs	4	45	80%

Food and Description	Amount	Fat Grams	Total Calories	% Fat Calories
Rancher's Choice, creamy (Kraft)				
Reduced calorie	1 Tbs	3	30	90%
Regular	1 Tbs	10	90	100%
Red Wine Vinaigrette				
(Wish Bone)	1 Tbs	3.6	50	65%
Red Wine Vinegar (Estee)	1 Tbs	–	2	–
Red Wine, Vinegar and Oil (Kraft)	1 Tbs	4	60	60%
(Richard Simmons) Salad Spray				
Dijon Vinaigrette	1 spray	–	1	–
	18 sprays	1	14	64%
French	1 spray	–	1	–
	18 sprays	1	14	64%
Italian	1 spray	–	1	–
	18 sprays	1	14	64%
Roma Cheese	1 spray	–	1	–
	18 sprays	1	14	64%
Roka Blue Cheese (Kraft)				
Reduced calorie	1 Tbs	1	16	56%
Regular	1 Tbs	6	60	90%
Roquefort	1 Tbs	8	77	94%
Russian				
Kraft				
Reduced calorie	1 Tbs	1	30	30%
Regular	1 Tbs	5	60	75%
Nutradiet	1 Tbs	1	25	36%
Wish Bone				
Lite	1 Tbs	< 1	25	18%
Regular	1 Tbs	2.5	47	48%
Russian, Creamy (Kraft)	1 Tbs	5	60	75%
Sesame Seed/generic	1 Tbs	6.9	68	91%
(Seven Seas)				
Buttermilk Recipe				
Light	1 Tbs	5	50	90%
Regular	1 Tbs	8	80	90%
Free				
Italian	1 Tbs	–	4	–
Ranch	1 Tbs	–	16	–
Red Wine Vinegar	1 Tbs	–	6	–
French-Light	1 Tbs	3	35	77%
French, Creamy	1 Tbs	6	60	90%
Thousand Island-Light	1 Tbs	2	30	60%
Thousand Island, Creamy	1 Tbs	5	50	90%
Thousand Island				
(Bob's) Famous Thousand Island	1 Tbs	6	66	82%

Food and Description	Amount	Fat Grams	Total Calories	% Fat Calories
(Estee)	1 Tbs	–	8	–
(Kraft)				
Reduced calorie	1 Tbs	2	30	60%
Regular	1 Tbs	5	60	75%
(Nutradiet)	1 Tbs	2	25	72%
(Wish Bone)				
Lite	1 Tbs	3	40	68%
Regular	1 Tbs	5.6	61	83%
Thousand Island & Bacon (Kraft)	1 Tbs	5	60	75%
Thousand Island Lite-Less Oil	1 Tbs	3	40	68%
Tomato Vinaigrette				
(Weight Watchers)	1 Tbs	–	8	–
Tomato Zesty-No Oil (Pritikin)	1 Tbs	–	18	–
Vinaigrette, No Oil (Pritikin)	1 Tbs	–	10	–
Viva				
Herbs & Spices				
Light	1 Tbs	3	30	90%
Regular	1 Tbs	6	60	90%
Italian				
Creamy				
Light	1 Tbs	4	45	80%
Regular	1 Tbs	7	70	90%
Light-Reduced calorie	1 Tbs	4	40	90%
Regular	1 Tbs	8	70	100%
Ranch				
Light	1 Tbs	5	50	90%
Regular	1 Tbs	8	80	90%
Red Wine Vinegar & Oil				
Light	1 Tbs	4	45	80%
Regular	1 Tbs	7	60	100%
Western (Richelieu)				
Reduced calorie	1 Tbs	1	35	26%
Regular	1 Tbs	5	70	64%
(Western) 98% Fat Free				
French	1 Tbs	1	35	26%
SALAD TOPPINGS				
(McCormick/Schilling)				
Cheese	1 Tbs	.7	31	20%
Garden Veg	1 Tbs	.7	34	19%
Regular	1 Tbs	.8	32	23%
SALAMI (*See also* LUNCHEON MEAT)				
Beerwurst/Beer Salami				
4" dia-⅛"thick	1 slice	6.76	75	81%
Salami/cooked	1oz	5.9	7	42%

Food and Description	Amount	Fat Grams	Total Calories	% Fat Calories
SALMON (*See also* SEAFOOD ENTREE/DINNER)				
Atlantic				
canned	3 oz	2.8	173	15%
canned solids & liquid	8 oz	6	268	20%
	15 oz	11.9	502	21%
cooked-dry heat	3 oz	6	155	35%
raw	3 oz	5	121	37%
Blueback-fancy				
(Nutradiet)	½ cup	11	188	53%
Chinook				
raw	3 oz	8.88	153	52%
smoked	3 oz	3.67	99	33%
Chum				
raw	3 oz	3	102	27%
canned	3 oz	4.68	120	35%
Coho				
raw	3 oz	5	124	36%
cooked-moist heat	3 oz	6	157	34%
Pink				
raw	3 oz	2.9	99	26%
canned	3 oz	5	118	38%
(Bumble Bee)	3.5 oz	8	160	45%
(Chicken Of The Sea)/spring water	3.5 oz	2	97	19%
(Del Monte)	½ cup	7	160	39%
(Featherweight)	2 oz	3	70	39%
(Libby's)	7¾ oz	13	310	38%
Red				
canned	3 oz	8	154	47%
(Bumble Bee)	3.5 oz	10	180	50%
(Del Monte)	½ cup	9	180	45%
(Nutradiet)	½ cup	11	188	53%
(S&W)-Fancy	½ cup	10	190	47%
cooked-dry heat	3 oz	5	140	32%
Smoked	3 oz	8	150	48%
SALSIFY/cooked/sliced	½ cup	–	46	–
SALT	Any amount	–	–	–
unseasoned	1 tsp	–	–	–
SALT SUBSTITUTE				
(Health Valley) Instead of Salt				
All Purpose	1 tsp	< 1	11	41%
Chicken Flavor	1 tsp	< 1	8	56%
Fish	1 tsp	< 1	11	41%
Steak & Ham	1 tsp	< 1	6	75%
Vegetable	1 tsp	< 1	13	35%

Food and Description	Amount	Fat Grams	Total Calories	% Fat Calories
seasoned	1 tsp	–	2	–
seasoned No-Salt	1 tsp	–	4	–
unseasoned	1 tsp	–	–	–
SANDWICH SPREAD				
(Best Foods)	1 Tbs	5	50	90%
(Hellman's)	1 Tbs	5	50	90%
(Kraft)	1 Tbs	5	50	90%
SAPODILLO				
Tropical American	1	1.9	140	12%
	1 cup	2	178	10%
SARDINES				
Atlantic				
canned in Olive Oil				
(Crown Prince)-Brisling				
includes oil	3.75 oz	42	460	82%
canned in Olive Oil				
(S&W) Norwegian Brisling				
drained	2 oz	10	130	69%
canned in sardine oil				
(Crown Prince)				
includes oil	3.75 oz	42	460	82%
canned in soya oil	2 pieces	2.75	50	50%
canned in tobasco sauce				
(Underwood)				
drained	1 can/			
	~ 3 oz	18	30	70%
canned in tomato sauce				
(Crown Prince)				
incudes sauce	3.75 oz	18	240	68%
(Del Monte)	½ cup	12	360	30%
Pacific				
canned in mustard sauce				
(Underwood)				
includes sauce	3.75 oz	16	220	66%
canned in tomato sauce	1	4.5	68	60%
(includes bone)	1 can/			
	~ 13 oz	44	658	60%
(Underwood)				
includes sauce	3.75 oz	16	220	66%
SAUCE (*See also* GRAVY)				
DEHYDRATED				
(NOTE: Prepared as directed. Pkg servings are unprepared.)				
A la King/(Durkee)	1 cup	8	133	54%
Alfredo/(Knorr)	2 oz	2	30	60%

Food and Description	Amount	Fat Grams	Total Calories	% Fat Calories
Alfredo/(Mayacamas)	2 oz	19	198	86%
Bearnaise/(Knorr)	2 oz	1	16	56%
/(Mayacamas)	1 Tbs	3	32	84%
/with milk and butter	1 cup	68	701	87%
Bolognese/(Fresh Chef)	4 oz	7	130	49%
Cheddar Cheese/(Mayacamas)	1 Tbs	3	31	87%
Cheese				
dry	1 Pkg	8.9	158	51%
(Durkee)	1 pkg	8	157	46%
	1 cup	16.9	316	48%
(French's)	¼ pkg	2	40	45%
prepared	¼ cup	4	80	45%
with milk	1 cup	17	307	50%
Clam Spaghetti/(Mayacamas)	4 oz	21	250	76%
Curry				
dry	1 oz	6.5	121	48%
(Knorr)	2 oz	2	35	51%
(Mayacamas)	1 Tbs	3	32	84%
with milk	1 cup	14.7	270	49%
Dill Sauce, Creamy for Fish/(Durkee)				
Roastin' Bag	1 pkg	14	153	82%
(Escoffier)/Diable Sauce	1 Tbs	–	20	–
/Robert Sauce	1 Tbs	–	20	–
Green Pepper/(Knorr)	2 oz	1	20	45%
Hollandaise/(Durkee)	¾ cup	14	173	73%
/(Mayacamas)	1 Tbs	3	32	84%
Hollandaise W/Butter & with water	1 cup	19.74	237	75%
Hollandaise W/Veg. Oil, milk & butter	1 cup	68	703	87%
Honey Mustard				
(Mayacamas)	1 Tbs	3	32	84%
Lemon Dill				
(Knorr)	2 oz	1	30	30%
Lyonnaise				
(Knorr)	2 oz	1	25	36%
Marinara				
(Mayacamas)	4 oz	11	147	67%
Mushroom	1 pkg/1 oz	3	99	27%
with milk	1 cup	10	228	40%
Newburg				
(Knorr)	2 oz	1	20	45%
Pesto				
(Fresh Chef)	4 oz	60	630	86%
(Knorr)	2 oz	1	18	50%
(Mayacamas)	1 Tbs	7	64	98%

Food and Description	Amount	Fat Grams	Total Calories	% Fat Calories
Red Clam				
(Fresh Chef)	4 oz	4	90	40%
Sour Cream				
	1 pkg/1.2 oz	11	180	55%
with milk	1 cup	30	509	53%
Spaghetti				
(Durkee)				
extra thick & rich	1 pkg	.68	72	9%
w/tomato paste	2¼ cups	1	212	4%
regular	1 pkg	–	85	–
w/tomato paste	2½ cups	1	224	4%
with mushrooms	1 pkg	–	69	–
w/tomato paste	2⅔ cups	.8	208	4%
(French's)				
Italian Style	¼ pkg	–	35	–
prepared	⅝ cup	4	100	36%
Mushrooms	¼ pkg	1	30	30%
prepared	⅝ cup	4	100	36%
(Knorr)	2 oz	1	12	75%
(Mayacamas)				
w/mushrooms	4 oz	11	149	66%
(Prego)-Extra Chunky				
mushroom & green pepper	4 oz	6	110	49%
mushroom & tomato	4 oz	5	110	41%
tomato, onion, & garlic	4 oz	6	110	49%
(Ragu)-Slow Cooked Homestyle				
tomato & herbs	4 oz	5	110	33%
W/meat	4 oz	4	110	33%
W/mushrooms & meat	4 oz	5	110	33%
Sparerib				
(Durkee)				
Roastin'Bag	1 pkg	2	162	11%
Stroganof	1 pkg/1.6 oz	4	161	22%
with milk and water	1 cup	10.7	271	36%
(Durkee)	1 pkg	.7	90	7%
w/beef, oil, & sour cream	4 cups	285	3280	78%
	1 cup	71	820	78%
Sweet and Sour	1 cup	–	294	–
(Kikkoman)	2⅛ oz pkg	–	228	–
Sweet and Sour Sauce				
Glaze Entree Mix				
(Chun King)	3.8 oz	–	370	–
(Tabasco)	½ tsp	–	2	–
Taco (Old El Paso)	1 pkg	1	100	9%

Food and Description	Amount	Fat Grams	Total Calories	% Fat Calories
Teriyaki Sauce	1 pkg	1	30	30%
	1 Tbs	–	8	–
	1 cup	.9	131	6%
White (Durkee)	1 pkg	11	155	64%
	1 cup	19.7	317	56%
White Clam (Fresh Chef)	4 oz	10	130	69%
White-Onion (Mayacamas)	1 Tbs	3	32	84%
READY-TO-SERVE & HOMEMADE				
BY BRAND:				
(Bull's Eye)	2 Tbs	–	50	–
(Chris' & Pitt's)	1 Tbs	–	15	–
(Estee)	1 Tbs	–	18	–
(Featherweight)	1 Tbs	–	14	–
(Hain)				
Honey	1 Tbs	1	14	64%
(Heinz)				
Chunky	1 Tbs	–	20	–
Hickory Smoke	1 Tbs	–	20	–
Hot	1 Tbs	–	20	–
Mushroom	1 Tbs	–	20	–
Onion	1 Tbs	–	20	–
Regular	1 Tbs	–	20	–
(Hunt's)				
Hickory	1 Tbs	–	20	–
Original	1 Tbs	–	25	–
(Kingsford)				
Masterpiece Mesquite	1 Tbs	–	30	–
Masterpiece Original	1 Tbs	–	30	–
(Kraft)				
Garlic	2 Tbs	1	40	23%
Hot	2 Tbs	1	40	23%
Hickory Smoke	2 Tbs	1	40	23%
Hot Hickory Smoke	2 Tbs	1	40	23%
Misquite Smoke	2 Tbs	1	40	23%
Original				
(Kraft)				
Hickory Smoke Onion Bits	2 Tbs	1	50	18%
Italian Seasonings	2 Tbs	1	50	18%
Kansas City Style	2 Tbs	1	50	18%
Onion Blts	2 Tbs	1	50	18%
Thick'n Spicy	2 Tbs	1	50	18%
Thick'n Spicy Hickory Smoke	2 Tbs	1	50	18%
Thick'n Spicy Original	2 Tbs	1	50	18%

Food and Description	Amount	Fat Grams	Total Calories	% Fat Calories
(Kraft)				
Thick'n Spicy Chunky	2 Tbs	1	60	15%
Thick'n Spicy w/Honey	2 Tbs	1	60	15%
Thick 'n Spicy Kansas City Style	2 Tbs	1	60	15%
(Maul's)	3.5 oz	2	123	15%
Smoky	3.5 oz	–	124	–
Sweet & Mild	3.5 oz	2	167	11%
Sweet & Smoky	3.5 oz	–	160	–
With Onion Bits	3.5 oz	2	126	14%
(Open Pit)				
Hickory Smoke	1 Tbs	–	25	–
Hickory thick'n tangy	1 Tbs	–	25	–
Hot'n Tangy	1 Tbs	–	25	–
Mesquite'n Tangy	1 Tbs	–	25	–
Original	1 Tbs	–	25	–
Original w/onions	1 Tbs	–	25	–
Sweet'n Tangy	1 Tbs	–	25	–
BY KIND:				
Alfredo, Fetticini (Prego)	5 oz	12.6	251	45%
Barbecue (most commercial types)	1 cup	4.5	188	22%
Cattleman's (French's)				
mild	1 Tbs	–	25	–
smoky	1 Tbs	–	25	–
Chili	1 Tbs	–	17	–
(Del Monte)	¼ cup	–	70	–
(Featherweight)	1 Tbs	–	8	–
(Heinz)	1 Tbs	–	17	–
Chili Hot Dog Sauce	1.25 oz	2	44	41%
(Chef Boyardee)-w/beef	1 oz	1	30	30%
(Gebhardt)	2 Tbs	1	20	45%
(Wolf)	⅙ cup	2	40	45%
Clam Sauce				
homemade	½ cup	22	275	72%
red	2 oz	1.6	41	35%
white	2 oz	4.8	61	71%
Cocktail Sauce				
(Del Monte)-Seafood	¼ cup	–	70	–
(Estee)	1 Tbs	–	10	–
(Heinz)-Seafood	1 Tbs	–	20	–
(Sauceworks)	1 Tbs	–	12	–
(Durkee) Famous Sauce	1 Tbs	7	69	91%
Enchilada (See also MEXICAN FOOD)				
(Del Monte)				
hot	½ cup	–	45	–

Food and Description	Amount	Fat Grams	Total Calories	% Fat Calories
mild	½ cup	–	45	–
(La Victoria)	1 cup	5	80	56%
Green Chili (Old El Paso)	¼ cup	1	30	30%
Hot (Old El Paso)	¼ cup	1	25	36%
Plain (Old El Paso)	¼ cup	–	18	–
Heinz 57	1 Tbs	–	15	–
Horseradish				
(Heinz)	1 Tbs	7	75	84%
(Sauceworks)	1 Tbs	5	50	90%
Horseradish, creamy style & prepared	1 Tbs	1	10	90%
Horseradish Mustard				
(Kraft)	1 Tbs	1	14	64%
Manwich				
(Hunt's)				
sauce only	2.5 oz	1	35	26%
w/ground beef on hamburger roll	5.8 oz	13	310	38%
sauce only				
Extra Thick & Chunky	2.5 oz	.5	60	8%
Marinara (tomato)	4 oz	4	86	42%
Mustard Sauce-Hot (Sauceworks)	1 Tbs	2	35	51%
Newberg Sauce w/sherry (Snow's)	⅓ cup	8	120	60%
Picante Salsa (*See also* MEXICAN FOOD)				
(Del Monte)				
Hot	¼ cup	–	20	–
Hot & Chunky	¼ cup	–	15	–
(Old El Paso)	2 Tbs	–	10	–
Picante Sauce (*See also* MEXICAN FOOD)				
(Azteca)				
Medium	1 Tbs	–	4	–
Mild	1 Tbs	–	4	–
(Del Monte)				
Burrito	¼ cup	–	20	–
Green Chili Mild	¼ cup	–	20	–
Rojo Mild	¼ cup	–	20	–
(Estee)	2 Tbs	–	8	–
(Old El Paso)	2 Tbs	–	8	–
Pizza				
canned				
(Chef Boyardee)w/cheese	2.6 oz	4	70	51%
	3.88 oz	6	90	60%
(Contadina)				
quick & easy	¼ cup	1	30	30%
w/Italian cheese	¼ cup	1	30	30%
w/pepperoni	¼ cup	2	40	45%

Food and Description	Amount	Fat Grams	Total Calories	% Fat Calories
w/tomato chunks	¼ cup	1	25	36%
canned				
(Ragu) Extra Tomatoes	3 Tbs	1	25	36%
canned w/cheese				
(Chef Boyardee)	2.6 oz	3	50	54%
Pizza Quick Sauce				
(Ragu)				
chunky style	3 Tbs	2	45	40%
garlic & basil	3 Tbs	2	40	45%
pepperoni	3 Tbs	3	50	54%
traditional	3 Tbs	2	40	45%
with cheese	3 Tbs	2	40	45%
Rib Sauce (Gold's)	1 oz	–	60	–
Salsa				
Thick 'N Chunky (Old El Paso)	2 Tbs	–	6	–
Sloppy Joe Barbecue Sauce (Libby's)				
w/beef	⅓ cup	7	110	57%
w/pork	⅓ cup	8	120	60%
Soy	1 Tbs	–	11	–
	1 oz	–	23	–
	¼ cup	–	30	–
(Chun King)	1 tsp	–	6	–
(Kikkoman)				
Lite	1 Tbs	–	12	–
Regular	1 Tbs	–	18	–
(La Choy)	1 Tbs	< 1	8	56%
Spaghetti				
canned	1 cup	11.9	272	39%
canned (Chef Boyardee)				
Original w/meat	3.75 oz	6	120	45%
Original w/mushrooms	3.75 oz	3	80	34%
With Meat	3.75 oz	3	80	34%
With Mushrooms	3.75 oz	1	60	15%
canned (Hunt's)				
Chunky Style	4 oz		50	9%
Homestyle	4 oz	2	60	30%
Meat	4 oz	2	70	26%
Mushroom	4 oz	2	70	26%
Traditional	4 oz	2	70	26%
Spaghetti Sauce from Jars				
(Chef Boyardee)				
Meatless	4 oz	1	60	15%
with ground beef	4 oz	3	90	30%
	4.14 oz	3	100	27%

Food and Description	Amount	Fat Grams	Total Calories	% Fat Calories
with mushrooms	4 oz	2	70	26%
(Enrico's) All Natural				
no salt	4 oz	1	60	15%
plain	4 oz	1	60	15%
(Estee)	4 oz	2	60	30%
(Featherweight) Healthy Recipes	4 oz	1	60	15%
(Prego)				
Al Fresco Garden Tomato				
w/Mushrooms	4 oz	5	100	45%
Al Fresco Garden Tomato				
w/Peppers	4 oz	6	100	54%
flavored with meat	4 oz	6	150	36%
extra chunky mushrooms				
& grn pepper	4 oz	6	110	33%
extra chunky mushrooms				
& onion	4 oz	5	110	41%
extra chunky mushrooms				
& tomato	4 oz	6	110	33%
extra chunky sausage				
& green pepper	4 oz	9	170	48%
extra chunky tomato & onion	4 oz	6	110	33%
marinara	4 oz	5	100	45%
no salt added	4 oz	6	100	54%
plain	4 oz	6	140	39%
with mushrooms	4 oz	5	140	32%
with mushrooms & chunk tomatoes	4 oz	4.7	121	35%
(Pritikin)				
plain	4 oz	–	60	–
with mushrooms	4 oz	–	60	–
(Ragu)				
Chunky Garden Style				
Green Peppers & Mushrooms	4 oz	2	80	23%
Italian Garden Combination	4 oz	2	80	23%
Mushrooms and Onions	4 oz	2	80	23%
Sweet Green & Red Bell Peppers	4 oz	2	80	23%
Xtra tomatoes, garlic & onions	4 oz	2	80	23%
(Ragu)				
Extra Thick & Zesty				
flavored w/meat	4 oz	4	100	36%
plain	4 oz	4	100	36%
with mushrooms	4 oz	5	110	41%
(Ragu)				
Fresh Italian				
Garden Medley	4 oz	3	80	34%

Food and Description	Amount	Fat Grams	Total Calories	% Fat Calories
Garlic & Basil	4 oz	3	80	34%
Hot & Spicy	4 oz	3	70	39%
Parmesan	4 oz	4	90	40%
Sliced Mushrooms	4 oz	3	70	39%
Tomatoes & Herbs	4 oz	3	80	34%
(Ragu)				
Homestyle				
flavored w/meat	4 oz	2	70	26%
plain	4 oz	2	70	26%
with mushrooms	4 oz	2	70	26%
(Ragu/Old World Style)				
marinara sauce	4 oz	4	90	40%
plain	4 oz	3	80	34%
with meat	4 oz	2	80	23%
with mushrooms	4 oz	4	80	45%
with xtra cheese	4 oz	3	80	34%
with xtra garlic	4 oz	3	80	34%
(Ragu)				
Thick & Hearty				
flavored w/meat	4 oz	4	120	30%
plain	4 oz	4	110	33%
with leaner ground beef	4 oz	4	120	30%
with mushrooms	4 oz	4	110	33%
(Weight Watchers)				
flavored with meat	⅓ cup	1	50	18%
with mushrooms	4 oz	–	40	–
Steak Sauce				
(A-1)	1 Tbs	–	14	–
(Estee)	½ oz	–	15	–
(French's)	1 Tbs	–	16	–
Stir Fry				
(Kikkoman)	1 Tbs	–	18	–
Sweet'n Sour Sauce				
(Chun King)	1.8 oz	–	60	–
(Contadina)	4 oz	3	150	18%
(Kikkoman)	1 Tbs	–	18	–
(LaChoy)	1 Tbs	–	30	–
(Sauceworks)	1 Tbs	–	20	–
Taco (See also MEXICAN FOOD)				
(Del Monte)				
Hot	¼ cup	–	15	–
Mild	¼ cup	–	15	–
(Estee)	2 Tbs	–	14	–

Food and Description	Amount	Fat Grams	Total Calories	% Fat Calories
(Heinz)				
Mild	1 Tbs	–	6	–
Medium	1 Tbs	–	6	–
(Old El Paso)	2 Tbs	–	10	–
Tartar				
(Hellman's & Kraft)	1 Tbs	8	72	100%
(Sauceworks)				
Natural Lemon & Herb	1 Tbs	8	72	100%
(Weight Watchers)	1 Tbs	3	35	77%
Teriyaki	1 Tbs	–	15	–
	1 oz	–	30	–
(Kikkoman)	1 Tbs	–	18	–
Teriyaki Baste and Glaze				
(Kikkoman)	1 Tbs	–	27	–
Tomato				
canned	4 oz	–	37	–
(Hidden Valley)	7.5 oz	.5	58	8%
Herb (Hunt's)	4 oz	4	80	45%
Italian (Hunt's)	4 oz	2	60	30%
plain (Del Monte)	1 cup	1	70	13%
Special (Hunt's)	4 oz	–	35	–
with bits (Hunt's)	4 oz	–	30	–
with cheese (Hunt's)	4 oz	1	45	20%
with herbs & cheese	4 oz	2	72	25%
with mushrooms (Hunt's)	4 oz	–	25	–
with onions				
(Del Monte)	1 cup	1	100	9%
(Hunt's)	4 oz	–	40	–
with onions, green peppers, & celery	4 oz	.9	50	6%
with tomato tidbits	4 oz	.5	39	12%
Welsh Rarebit Cheese Sauce				
(Snow's)	½ cup	11	170	58%
White Cream Sauce				
canned	4 oz	9	118	69%
homemade				
thin	1 cup	21.8	303	65%
medium	1 cup	31	405	69%
thick	1 cup	39	495	71%
Worcestershire				
(French's)				
regular	1 Tbs	–	10	–
smoky	1 Tbs	–	10	–
(Heinz)	1 Tbs	–	10	–
(Lea & Perrin)	1 oz	–	30	–

Food and Description	Amount	Fat Grams	Total Calories	% Fat Calories
SAUERKRAUT/canned	½ cup	–	22	–
canned-(Del Monte)	½ cup	–	25	–
canned (S&W)	5 oz	–	14	–
(Vlasic)-Old Fashioned	1 oz	–	4	–
SAUERKRAUT DISHES				
Pierogi (dumpling)-frozen (Mrs. T's)	1	–	60	–
SAUERKRAUT JUICE/canned	10 oz	–	28	–
SAUSAGE (*See also* LUNCHEON MEAT)	1.5 oz	11.6	134	78%
Beef Breakfast Strips (Sizzlean)	2 strips	5	70	64%
Cooked-smoked	1 oz	7.6	89	77%
(Eckrich)/Brown 'N Serve-beef	1 link	12	120	90%
Pork Sausage				
brown & serve	1 link/			
	~ 1 oz	5	50	90%
country style/raw	1 patty/			
	2 oz	22.97	238	87%
	1 link/			
	1 oz	11	118	84%
cooked	1 patty/			
	1 oz	8	100	72%
	1 link/			
	.5 oz	8	96	75%
fresh-link-cooked	1 oz	11	118	84%
fresh-patty-cooked	1 oz	8	100	72%
(Jimmy Dean)-16 oz pkg-all flavors	1 patty	13	140	84%
light-turkey & pork	1 oz	6	80	67%
skinless links	2 Links	17	180	85%
square patties	1 patty	13	140	84%
Links/frozen (Schwan's)	1 oz	10	110	82%
Little Sizzlers (Hormel)-cooked	2 sausages	9	103	79%
Midget Links (Hormel)-cooked	2 sausages	7	143	44%
Patties/frozen (Schwan's)	2 oz	23	240	86%
Smoked Rope/frozen (Schwan's)	3.5 oz	30	330	82%
(Swift)				
Premium brown'n serve smoke-flavored	1 Link	11	120	83%
Premium brown'n serve microwave links	1 Link	12	120	90%
Lite	1 Link	6	90	60%
Premium brown'n serve country recipe links	1 Link	12	130	83%
Lite	2 Links	11	120	83%
Premium brown'n serve country recipe patties	1 pattie	12	130	83%

Food and Description	Amount	Fat Grams	Total Calories	% Fat Calories
Premium brown'n serve links w/bacon	1 Link	11	120	83%
Premium brown'n serve links w/ham	1 Link	13	130	90%
Premium brown'n serve maple-flavored links	1 Link	12	120	90%
Lite	1 Link	5	60	75%
Premium brown'n serve original Lite Links	1 link	5	60	75%
Premium brown'n serve original patties	1 pattie	12	120	90%
Smoked Link/4" long-1⅛" dia	1 link	21.59	265	73%
/2" long-¾" dia	1 link	5	62	73%
SAVORY/ground	1 tsp	–	4	–
SCALLION	5-5" pieces	–	45	
SCALLOP (See also SEAFOOD ENTREE/DINNER)				
Mixed				
breaded & fried	2 large/ ~ 1 oz	3	67	40%
imitation	3 oz	< 1	85	5%
raw	3 oz	.6	75	7%
SCOTCH (See DISTILLED LIQUOR)				
SCOTCH BROTH (See SOUP)				
SCROD (See SEAFOOD ENTREE/DINNER)				
SCUP/raw	3 oz	2	90	20%
SEA BASS				
breaded & fried	3 oz	7	176	36%
cooked-dry heat	3 oz	2	105	17%
raw	3 oz	1.7	82	19%
SEA SALT	1 tsp	–	–	–
SEA TROUT/raw	3 oz	3	88	31%
SEAFOOD CHOWDER (See SOUP)				
SEAFOOOD ENTREE/DINNER (See also FROZEN ENTREE/DINNER)				

(NOTE: Serving sizes for box dishes are for prepared portions. The homemade dishes included here are not made with low-fat substitutes. The data listed can vary, pending the type and amount of certain ingredients used. These data are to be used as a viable guide for the same dish you might make in your home. The same goes for the commercial box mixes—the data may vary slightly, pending on the fat and calorie content of the seafood used in preparation.)

(Booth) frozen				
Block				
Atlantic Flounder	4 oz	1	90	10%
Atlantic Sole	4 oz	1	90	10%
Cod	4 oz	1	89	10%

Food and Description	Amount	Fat Grams	Total Calories	% Fat Calories
Ocean Catfish	4 oz	3	115	24%
Ocean Perch	4 oz	1	100	9%
Whiting	4 oz	1	100	9%
Fisherboy				
fish nuggets	2 oz	10	160	56%
fish portions	2 oz	7	130	49%
fish sticks	2.4 oz	11	190	52%
Individually Wrapped Fillets				
Cod	4 oz	1	90	10%
Flounder	4 oz	–	90	–
Haddock	4 oz	–	90	–
Perch	4 oz	1	100	9%
Whiting	4 oz	1	80	11%
Fishburgers	3 oz	9	170	48%
Clam Fritter				
homemade	1/~1.5 oz	6	124	44%
Clams				
frozen-breaded & fried				
(Mrs. Paul's)	2.5 oz	13	240	49%
Clams, Crunchy Strips-frozen (Gorton's)	3.5 oz	22	330	60%
Cod				
Baked Scrod				
Microwave with toasted bread crumbs				
frozen (Gorton's)	6 oz	18	320	51%
Cod, Fillet of				
frozen				
(Booth Light Entree)				
Au Gratin	9.5 oz	11	280	35%
Mushroom	9.5 oz	11	280	35%
Cod Fillets				
Microwave/crunchy-frozen	1 fillet	22	330	60%
Crab				
cakes				
fried in margarine-homemade	1/~4 oz	10.8	203	48%
Deviled				
canned	4.5 oz	13	252	46%
homemade	½ cup	12	185	58%
Stuffed				
homemade	½ cup	4	86	42%
Fillet Almondine				
frozen (Gorton's)	5.5 oz	25	350	64%
Fish Cakes				
frozen	1 reg size or 5 bite size	10.7	162	59%

Food and Description	Amount	Fat Grams	Total Calories	% Fat Calories
homemade-fried	1 reg size or 5 bite size	4.8	103	42%
Fish Fillets in Buttery Herb Sauce				
frozen-microwave (Gorton's)	6.25 oz	8	190	38%
Fish Kabobs-frozen (Van de Kamp's)	4 oz	15	240	56%
Fish Loaf-homemade	~ 5 oz	5.6	186	27%
Fish'N Chips-frozen (Swanson)	6.5 oz	18	370	44%
Fish'N Fries-frozen (Swanson)	6.5 oz	17	350	44%
Fish Nuggets-frozen (Swanson)	9.5 oz	19	410	42%
Fish Sticks-frozen (4"x2"x½")	1 stick	3	76	36%
(Frionor) frozen - uncooked unless otherwise noted				
Batter Fried Deep Fry				
2 oz Cod Wedge	4 oz	–	210	–
fried	4 oz	13	250	47%
Batter Fried Oven Ready				
2 oz Cod Wedge	4 oz	11	220	45%
3 oz Cod Wedge	3 oz	8	160	45%
4 oz Cod Long	4 oz	10	210	43%
4 oz Cod Rectangle	4 oz	10	210	43%
3 oz Pollock Wedge	3 oz	8	170	42%
4 oz Pollock Wedge	4 oz	11	220	45%
2 oz Whiting Wedge	4 oz	11	230	43%
3 oz Whiting Wedge	3 oz	8	170	42%
4 oz Whiting Rectangle	4 oz	7	160	39%
Breaded Precooked				
1 oz Cod Stick, Grade A	4 oz	9	210	39%
3 oz Cod Rectangle, Grade A	3 oz	7	150	42%
3 oz Cod Rectangle	3 oz	8	180	40%
3.2 oz Cod Rectangle, Grade A	3.2 oz	6	140	39%
3.6 oz Cod Rectangle, Grade A	3.6 oz	7	160	39%
4 oz Cod Rectangle, Grade A	4 oz	9	200	41%
1 oz Minced Cod Stick	4 oz	9	210	39%
3 oz Minced Cod Rectangle	3 oz	7	160	39%
1 oz Haddock Stick, Grade A	4 oz	9	210	39%
3 oz Haddock Rectangle, Grade A	3 oz	8	180	40%
3 oz Haddock Rectangle	3 oz	7	130	49%
3 oz Pollock Rectangle	3 oz	8	180	40%
4 oz Pollock Rectangle, Grade A	4 oz	10	230	39%
3 oz Whiting Rectangle, Grade A	3 oz	7	160	39%
3.6 oz Whiting Rectangle, Grade A	3.6 oz	7	160	39%
3 oz Great Silver Smelt Rectangle	3 oz	6	150	36%
Fancy Stuffed Flounder				
9 oz stuffed w/broccoli, cheese & lobster	9 oz	13	270	43%

Food and Description	Amount	Fat Grams	Total Calories	% Fat Calories
9 oz stuffed w/crabmeat	9 oz	16	230	63%
Fishfries				
1.25 oz Country Style Alaska Pollock	3.75 oz	–	130	–
1.25 oz Country Style Cod	3.75 oz	–	130	–
1.25 oz Santa Fe Style Alaska Pollock	3.75 oz	–	120	–
1.25 oz Santa Fe Style Cod	3.75 oz	–	120	–
1.25 oz Southern Cornmeal Style Alaska Pollock	3.75 oz	–	120	–
Fishfries, Golden Broil				
5 oz Cod Fillet Shape	5 oz	8	170	42%
3 oz Cod Tail-r-Cut	3 oz	5	110	41%
4.5 oz Cod Tail-r-Cut	4.5 oz	7	160	39%
Fishfries, Gourmet Raw Breaded				
3 oz Cod Fillet Shape	3 oz	–	110	–
fried	3 oz	9	190	43%
Fishfries, Honey Granola Crunch				
1 oz Alaska Pollock Nugget	4 oz	20	340	53%
3 oz Alaska Pollock Rectangle	3 oz	11	200	50%
1 oz Cod Nugget	4 oz	21	340	56%
3 oz Cod Rectangle	3 oz	16	260	55%
1 oz Whiting Nugget	4 oz	20	340	53%
3 oz Whiting Rectangle	3 oz	14	240	53%
Fishfries, Microwavable				
fully cooked				
Fish Sandwich w/chese	5 oz	17	330	46%
2.5 oz	2.5 oz	5	130	35%
3 oz	3 oz	6	150	36%
Fishfries, Norwegian Fish Fillets				
Cod Fillets	4 oz	–	70	–
Salmon Sides	4 oz	10	180	50%
Fishfries, Oven Crispy				
1 oz Cod Triangle Nugget	4 oz	11	220	45%
2 oz Cod Wedge	4 oz	9	210	39%
3 oz Cod Wedge	3 oz	7	160	39%
3 oz Great Silver Smelt Wedge	3 oz	7	160	39%
2 oz Whiting Wedge	4 oz	9	210	39%
3 oz Whiting Wedge	3 oz	7	170	37%
3.6 oz Whiting Wedge	3.6 oz	9	190	43%
3.6 oz Whiting Rectangle	3.6 oz	9	190	43%
Fishfries, Oven Crispy Crunchy				
.5 oz Bunch O'Crunch minced Cod Nugget	2.5 oz	13	200	59%

Food and Description	Amount	Fat Grams	Total Calories	% Fat Calories
.67 oz Bunch O'Crunch minced				
Cod Stick	2.7 oz	15	230	59%
1 oz Cod Nugget	4 oz	11	240	41%
1 oz Cod Select Nugget	4 oz	13	240	49%
1 oz Great Silver Smelt Nugget	4 oz	11	220	45%
1 oz Whiting Nugget	4 oz	11	210	47%
1 oz Whiting Select Nugget	4 oz	14	250	50%
Fishfries, Oven Crispy Fish & Cheese				
3.6 oz Cod'N Cheese Rectangle	3.6 oz	15	250	54%
Fishfries, Raw Breaded				
3 oz Cod Rectangle, Grade A	3 oz	–	120	–
fried	3 oz	11	200	50%
4 oz Cod Tail-r-Cut	4 oz	–	160	–
fried	4 oz	12	240	45%
5⅓ Cod Tail-r-Cut	5⅓ oz	–	210	–
fried	5⅓ oz	18	350	46%
Fishfries, Raw Unbreaded				
4 oz Cod English Cut, Glazed,				
Grade A	4 oz	–	70	–
4 oz Cod Rectangle	4 oz	–	70	–
12.66 Cod Nordic Cut	4 oz	–	70	–
25.6 oz Cod Shim	4 oz	–	70	–
4 oz Haddock English Cut, Glazed	4 oz	–	70	–
12.66 oz Haddock Nordic Cut	4 oz	–	70	–
Fishfries, Shellfish				
Norwegian Shrimp	4 oz	1	100	9%
Fishfries, Tender Crisp				
3 oz Cod Fillet Shape	3 oz	–	110	–
fried	3 oz	12	200	54%
(Gorton's)				
frozen				
Crispy Batter Sticks	4 sticks	14	210	60%
Crispy Batter Fillets	2 fillets	20	300	60%
Crunchy Fish Sticks	4 sticks	15	220	61%
Crunchy Fish Fillets	2 fillets	20	320	56%
Fishmarket Fresh				
cod	5 oz	1	110	8%
flounder	5 oz	1	110	8%
haddock	5 oz	1	110	8%
ocean perch	5 oz	3	140	19%
sole	5 oz	1	110	8%
Light Recipe				
Lightly Breaded Fillets	1 fillet	7	170	37%
Tempura Fish Fillets	1 fillet	12	190	57%

Food and Description	Amount	Fat Grams	Total Calories	% Fat Calories
Microwave				
Crunch Whole Shrimp	5 oz	20	380	47%
Fillets-2 larger cut	1 fillet	22	330	60%
Fish Sticks	6 sticks	22	340	58%
Fish Fillets	2 fillets	26	350	67%
Haddock in Lemon Butter	1 pkg	19	320	53%
Shrimp Scampi	1 pkg	24	350	62%
Stuffed Flounder	1 pkg	15	300	45%
Sole in Lemon Butter	1 pkg	19	320	53%
Value Pack				
Fish Portion	1 fillet	11	180	55%
Fish Sticks	4 sticks	11	210	47%
Jambalaya				
homemade	1 cup	6.7	250	24%
(Kibun & Kibun Gold)/frozen				
Dill Sauce & Fish	10 oz	5	280	16%
Mediterranean Fish	10 oz	1	230	4%
Piccata	10 oz	25	470	48%
Primavera	10 oz	19	360	48%
Sea Pasta Pacific Fish & Shrimp				
w/o dressing	½ pkg.	1	140	6%
with dressing	½ pkg	9	210	39%
Sea Stix	4 oz	< 1	110	4%
Sea Tails	4 oz	< 1	110	4%
Seafood Fettucini Alfredo	10 oz	11	330	30%
Seafood Linguini	10 oz	6	260	21%
Seafood Marinara	11 oz	2	240	8%
Seafood Newburg	10 oz	7	300	21%
Seafood Piccata	1 serving	21	450	42%
Seafood Primivera	1 serving	7	300	21%
(Lean Cuisine)/frozen entrees				
Filet of Fish Divan	12⅜ oz	8	260	28%
Tuna Lasagna	9.75 oz	10	270	33%
Lobster Newburg-homemade	~ 6.5 oz	35	455	69%
(Mrs. Paul's) frozen				
Au Natural				
Cod Fillets	5 oz	2	110	16%
Flounder Fillets	5 oz	2	110	16%
Haddock Fillets	5 oz	2	110	16%
Perch Fillets	5 oz	2	110	16%
Sole Fillets	5 oz	2	110	16%
Light Fillets				
Catfish	1 fillet	10	250	36%
Cod	1 fillet	7	220	29%

Food and Description	Amount	Fat Grams	Total Calories	% Fat Calories
Flounder	1 fillet	11	260	38%
Haddock	1 fillet	5	220	21%
Ocean Perch	1 fillet	13	270	43%
Pollock	1 fillet	11	240	41%
Sole	1 fillet	11	260	38%
Light Seafood Entrees				
Fish Au Gratin	9 oz	9	270	30%
Fish and Pasta Florentine	9 oz	8	230	31%
Fish Dijon	8¾ oz	9	210	39%
Fish Florentine	8 oz	6	200	32%
Fish Mornay	9 oz	10	250	36%
Shrimp Cajun Style	9 oz	3	200	14%
Shrimp and Clams w/Linguini	10 oz	9	280	29%
Shrimp Primivera	9½ oz	4	190	19%
Tuna Pasta Casserole	10 oz	7	270	23%
Prepared Seafoods				
Batter Dipped Fish Fillets	2 fillets	13	320	37%
Buttered Fish Fillets	2 fillets	9	170	48%
Catfish Fillet Strips	4 oz	13	240	49%
Combination Seafood Platter	9 oz	31	590	47%
Crispy Crunchy Fish Fillets	2 fillets	16	280	51%
Crispy Crunchy Fish Sticks	4 sticks	10	200	45%
Crispy Crunchy Flounder	2 fillets	15	270	50%
Crispy Crunchy Haddock	2 fillets	13	280	42%
Crispy Crunchy Ocean Perch	2 fillets	19	320	53%
Crunchy Fish Sticks-Minced	4 oz	10	200	45%
Crunchy Light Batter Fish Fillets	2 fillets	17	310	49%
Crunchy Light Batter Fish Sticks	4 sticks	13	240	49%
Crunchy Light Batter Flounder	2 fillets	16	310	47%
Crunchy Light Batter Haddock	2 fillets	17	330	46%
Deviled Crabs	1 cake	7	170	37%
Deviled Crab Miniatures	3½ oz	12	250	43%
Fish Cakes	2 cakes	11	250	40%
Fish Cake Thins	2 cakes	13	290	40%
Fried Scallops	3½ oz	9	230	35%
Fried Shrimp	3 oz	11	200	50%
Light Batter Fried Clams	2½ oz	13	240	49%
Supreme Light Batter Fish Fillet	1 fillet	12	210	51%
Oyster Stew				
homemade	1 cup	15	233	58%
Oysters Rockefeller-homemade	4 oysters	2.7	90	27%
Paella				
homemade-including saffron rice, seafood & vegtables	~ 8 oz	11	350	28%

Food and Description	Amount	Fat Grams	Total Calories	% Fat Calories
Pollack				
Alaskan Batter dipped fillets				
frozen (Mrs. Paul's)	2 fillets	13	320	37%
crispy crunchy breaded				
frozen (Mrs. Paul's)	2 fillets	18	290	56%
crunchy batter				
frozen (Mrs. Paul's)	3 oz	17	310	49%
Salmon Cake				
homemade	3.5 oz	15	248	54%
Salmon Casserole				
homemade	1 cup	35	555	57%
Salmon Patty				
homemade	3.5 oz	12	239	45%
Salmon Rice Loaf				
homemade	6 oz	8	212	34%
(Schwan's)				
home delivery				
frozen				
Batter Crisp	2 oz	8	150	48%
Blue Lake Loins	3.5 oz	1	90	10%
Breaded Clam Strips	3.5 oz	11	220	45%
Breaded Fantail Shrimp	3.5 oz	2	210	9%
Breaded Halibut Fillets	4 oz	2	230	8%
Breaded Round Shrimp	3.5 oz	2	210	9%
Breaded Shrimp Pieces	3.5 oz	2	210	9%
Cajun Style Catfish	3.5 oz	12	180	60%
Catfish Fingers	3.5 oz	13	230	51%
Cod Fillets	3.5 oz	1	80	11%
Cod Fish Nuggets	3.5 oz/ 7 nuggets	10	200	45%
Fish 'N Batter	2 oz	8	140	51%
Fancy Seafood Legs	3.5 oz	.5	100	5%
Flounder Fillets	3.5 oz	1	90	10%
Haddock Fillets	3.5 oz	1	90	10%
Haddock Squares	4 oz	8	210	34%
Haddock Sticks	1 oz	2	48	38%
Halibut Steaks	3.5 oz	2	110	16%
Lobster Tails	3.5 oz	2	110	16%
New England Style Scrod	5 oz	17	280	55%
Ocean Perch	3.5 oz	2	100	18%
Orange Roughy	3.5 oz	7	120	53%
Oven-ready Breaded Shrimp	3.5 oz	1	210	4%
Peeled & De-veined Shrimp	3.5 oz	2	100	18%
Pollock Fillets	3.5 oz	1	90	10%

Food and Description	Amount	Fat Grams	Total Calories	% Fat Calories
Red Snapper Steaks	3.5 oz	1	100	0%
Salmon Fillets	5 oz	8	210	34%
Scallops	3.5 oz	1	90	10%
Shell On Shrimp	3.5 oz	1	90	10%
Slipper Lobster	3.5 oz	1	90	10%
Stuffed Shrimp	2 oz/1 piece	4	100	36%
Stuffed Scrod				
-w/Broccoli & Mozzarella	5 oz	7	150	42%
Stuffed Sole Monterey	6 oz	8	200	36%
Unbreaded Shrimp	3.5 oz	2	120	15%
Walleye Fillets	3.5 oz	2	90	20%
Seafood Creole				
w/rice				
frozen				
(Swanson)	9 oz	6	240	23%
(Seafood Elites)				
Sole Fillet				
frozen				
with broccoli & mozzarella	1	7	150	42%
with lemon & wild rice	1	7	150	42%
with spinach & cheddar	1	6	130	42%
Seafood Gumbo				
homemade	5 oz	1	48	19%
Seafood Linguini				
frozen				
(Weight Watchers)	9 oz	7	220	29%
Shrimp				
frozen				
(Booth Light Entree)				
Fettucine Alfredo	10 oz	8	260	28%
New Orleans	10 oz	5	230	20%
(Brilliant)				
cooked	2 oz	–	30	–
Shrimp Creole				
homemade w/rice	1 cup	8.7	301	26%
Shrimp Curried				
homemade	¾ cup	11.5	232	45%
Sole				
frozen				
with Wine Sauce				
(Gorton's)	6.5 oz	7	180	35%
Sole, Fillet of				
frozen				
(Le Menu)	10 oz	14	360	35%

Food and Description	Amount	Fat Grams	Total Calories	% Fat Calories
Tuna Fillets				
(Gorton's Natural Cut)				
25% less fat				
breaded 6 cruncy fillets	2 fillets	14	260	48%
(Tuna Helper)				
box - prepared:				
Buttery Rice 'n Tuna	1 Serving	11	280	35%
Creamy Mushroom	1 Serving	6	220	25%
Creamy Noodles 'n Tuna	1 Serving	7	250	25%
Cheesy Noodles'n Tuna	1 Serving	9	250	32%
Tuna Au Gratin	1 Serving	11	280	35%
Tuna Pot Pie	1 Serving	27	420	58%
Tuna Salad	1 Serving	30	440	61%
Tuna Tetrazzini	1 Serving	8	240	30%
Tuna Loaf, Smoked				
(Neptune) Tunables	1 oz	1.8	40	41%
Tuna Meat Pie				
frozen				
(Banquet)	7 oz	33	540	55%
Tuna Noodle Casserole				
frozen				
(Swanson's)	9 oz	11	250	40%
Tuna Pattie				
homemade	3 oz	3	80	34%
(Van de Kamp's)				
frozen				
battered				
Fish fillets	1 fillet	10	200	45%
Fish Sticks	4 sticks	9	170	48%
Haddock Fillets	2 fillets	13	250	47%
Halibut Fillets	2 fillets	9	180	45%
Ocean Perch Fillets	2 fillets	14	260	49%
breaded				
Fish Fillets				
crispy-microwave	1 fillet	7	130	49%
crispy-oven	2 fillets	15	260	52%
large	1 fillet	16	300	48%
Fish Sticks-crispy-microwave	3 sticks	8	150	48%
Fish Sticks-oven	4 sticks	10	190	47%
Haddock Fillets-oven	2 fillets	15	260	52%
lightly breaded-microwave				
Cod	9 oz	19	300	57%
Flounder	9 oz	18	300	54%
Haddock	9 oz	17	300	51%

Food and Description	Amount	Fat Grams	Total Calories	% Fat Calories
Ocean Perch	9 oz	19	310	55%
Sole	9 oz	18	300	54%
Today's Catch				
Cod	4 oz	1	100	9%
Flounder	4 oz	1	100	9%
Haddock	4 oz	1	100	9%
Ocean Perch	4 oz	2	110	16%
Sole	4 oz	1	100	9%
SEAFOOD SALAD	3.5 oz	10	160	56%
SEASONINGS (See individual listings such as PAPRIKA, SAGE, etc. and ORIENTAL FOOD SEASONINGS)				
SEAWEED				
agar				
dried	3 oz	< 1	260	2%
raw	3 oz	< 1	23	20%
kelp/raw	3 oz	.6	37	15%
laver	3 oz	< 1	31	15%
spirulina				
dried	3 oz	6.6	249	24%
raw	3 oz	< 1	22	21%
wakame/raw	3 oz	< 1	40	11%
SELTZER WATER (See SODA)				
SESAME BUTTER	1 oz	15	169	80%
Tahini	2 Tbs	16	180	80%
Toasted	2 Tbs	20	200	90%
SESAME FLOUR				
high fat	4 oz	42	595	64%
low fat	4 oz	2	380	5%
partially defatted	4 oz	14	440	29%
SESAME NUT MIX/(Planters)				
dry roasted	1 oz	12	160	68%
oil roasted	1 oz	13	160	73%
SESAME SEEDS				
dried				
kernels	1 Tbs	4	47	77%
whole	1 Tbs	4.5	52	78%
kernels-toasted	1 oz	13.6	161	76%
	1 cup	80	873	83%
Whole roasted & toasted	1 oz	13.6	161	76%
SHAD/American				
cooked-dry heat	3 oz	9.6	171	51%
raw	3 oz	11.7	167	63%
roe-raw	3 oz	1.7	111	14%
SHALLOT/raw	1 Tbs	–	7	–

Food and Description	Amount	Fat Grams	Total Calories	% Fat Calories
SHARK				
batter dipped & fried	3 oz	11.75	194	55%
raw	3 oz	3.8	111	31%
SHEEPSHEAD				
cooked-dry heat	3 oz	1	107	8%
raw	3 oz	2	92	20%
SHELLIE BEAN/canned	½ cup	–	37	–
sprouts/canned (La Choy)	⅔ cup	–	8	–
SHERBET	1 cup	4	270	13%
(Borden)-orange	½ cup	1	110	8%
(Dreyer's)/all flavors-data averaged	½ cup	1	110	8%
(Pet)/orange	½ cup	1	130	7%
(Sealtest)				
Orange	½ cup	1	130	7%
Rainbow	½ cup	1	130	7%
Strawberry	½ cup	1	130	7%
(Thrifty)				
Apricot Mango	½ cup	1	130	7%
Rainbow	½ cup	1	120	8%
SHORTENING (*See* FAT)				
SHRIMP (*See also* SEAFOOD ENTREE/DINNER)				
breaded & fried	3 oz	10	206	44%
	4 Large/ ~ 1 oz	3.68	73	45%
canned	4 Large/ 1 cup	1.67	102	15%
	1 cup	3	155	17%
canned-deveined-medium/whole (S&W)	2 oz	–	65	–
cooked-moist heat	3 oz	.9	84	10%
	4 Large/ ~ 1 oz	–	22	–
dried	1 oz	.8	82	9%
imitation (from surimi)	3 oz	1	86	10%
paste	3 oz	8	155	47%
raw	3 oz	1	90	10%
SHRIMP SALAD/homemade	¾ cup	11.9	210	51%
SHRIMP SOUP, CREAM OF (*See* SOUP)				
SLOPPY JOE SAUCE (*See* SAUCE)				
SMELT/Rainbow				
breaded & fried	3 oz	10.6	214	45%
cooked-dry heat	3 oz	2.6	106	22%
raw	3 oz	2	83	22%
SNACK CAKES				
(Break Cake)				
Apple Sandwich Cakes	1-1.83 oz	3	90	30%

Food and Description	Amount	Fat Grams	Total Calories	% Fat Calories
Banana Creme	1-2 oz	9	240	34%
Blueberry Sandwich Cakes	1-1.83 oz	4	100	36%
Devil's Food Creme	1-2 oz	9	230	35%
Oatmeal Creme	1-2 oz	9	240	34%
100's				
Chocolate cup cakes	1	2	100	18%
Cinnamon Streusel	1	2	100	18%
Peanut Butter Creme	1-2 oz	9	240	34%
Raisin Creme	1-2 oz	9	240	34%
Raspberry Sandwich Cakes	1-1.83 oz	3	100	27%
Cupcakes				
chocolate				
(Break Cake)	2 cakes	10	350	26%
homemade-plain	1	5	103	44%
homemade-choc frosting	1	8	175	41%
white				
homemade-plain	1	5	114	35%
homemade-choc frosting	1	8	186	39%
homemade-white frosting	1	6	165	33%
yellow				
homemade-plain	1	5	125	36%
homemade-choc frosting	1	8	195	37%
devil's food w/creme filling	1 cake	4	105	34%
(Dolly Madison)				
Blue Ribbon Creme Filled	1 cake	3	90	30%
Creme Zinger	1 cake	3	90	30%
Pecan Roller	1 roll	5	120	38%
White Zinters	1 cake	4	140	26%
Yellow Zingers	1 cake	4	140	26%
Zinger Raspberry	1 cake	5	130	35%
(Hostess) packaged				
Big Wheels	1 cake	10	173	52%
Choco Bliss	1 cake	7	200	32%
Choco Diles	1 cake	11	240	41%
Chocolate Cupcakes	1 cake	8	170	42%
Crumb Cake	1 cake	4	160	23%
Devil's Food Cupcakes	1 cake	4	136	27%
Ding Dongs	1 cake	9	170	48%
Fruit Loaf	1	9	400	20%
Ho Hos	1 cake	6	120	45%
Hostess O's	1 cake	8	220	33%
Lights				
Apple Spice	1.5 oz	1	130	7%
Chocolate-w/chocolatey frosting	1.25 oz	1	110	8%

Food and Description	Amount	Fat Grams	Total Calories	% Fat Calories
	1.5 oz	1	130	7%
w/vanilla pudding	1.25 oz	1	110	8%
	1.5 oz	1	140	6%
Raspberry Filled	1.5 oz	1	130	7%
Twinkies	1.25 oz	2	110	17%
Lil' Angels	1 cake	1	90	10%
Orange Cupcakes	1 cake	5	150	30%
Pudding Cakes	1 cake	4	170	21%
Snoball	1 cake	2	140	13%
Suzy Q's				
-Banana	1 cake	8	240	30%
-Chocolate	1 cake	8	250	29%
Tiger Tail	1 cake	2	140	13%
Twinkie	1 cake	2	140	13%
(Little Debbie) packaged				
Apple Delights	1 pkg	4	140	26%
Apple Spice Snack	1 pkg	11	270	37%
Banana Slices	1 pkg	12	340	32%
Banana Twins	1 pkg	9	250	32%
Be My Valentine	1 pkg	17	330	46%
Caravella	1 pkg	9	200	41%
Cherry Cordials	1 pkg	8	170	42%
Choco-Cakes	1 pkg/			
	2.17 oz	13	270	43%
	1 pkg/			
	2.7 oz	15	330	41%
Choc-O-Jel	1 pkg	7	150	42%
Chocolate Chip Snack	1 pkg	16	320	45%
Chocolate Slices	1 pkg	9	320	25%
Chocolate Twins	1 pkg	7	240	26%
Christmas Treecakes	1 pkg	11	220	45%
Coffee Cake	1 pkg	9	250	32%
Coconut Crunch	1 pkg	19	320	53%
Coconut Rounds	1 pkg	7	150	42%
Debbie Doodle Dandies	1 pkg	16	320	45%
Dessert Cups	1 pkg	1	80	1%
Devil Cremes	1 pkg/1.3 oz	7	160	39%
	1 pkg/2.5 oz	13	300	39%
Devil Slices	1 pkg	9	320	25%
Devil Squares	1 pkg	11	270	37%
Dutch Apple	1 pkg	8	230	31%
Easter Bunny Cakes	1 pkg	15	320	42%
Fancy Cakes	1 pkg	16	340	42%
Figaroos	1 pkg	4	160	23%

Food and Description	Amount	Fat Grams	Total Calories	% Fat Calories
Fudge Crispy	1 pkg	7	260	25%
Fudge Rounds	1 pkg/			
	1.19 oz	6	150	36%
	1 pkg/			
	2.75 oz	12	330	33%
Golden Cremes	1 pkg/1.4 oz	6	150	36%
	1 pkg/2.5 oz	11	270	37%
Holiday Cakes, chocolate	1 pkg	14	310	41%
Holiday Cakes, vanilla	1 pkg	16	320	45%
Lemon Stix	1 pkg	10	220	41%
Marshmallow Supremes	1 pkg	5	130	35%
Mint Sprints	1 pkg	10	200	45%
Nutty Bar	1 pkg/2 oz	20	310	58%
	1 pkg/2.5 oz	23	390	53%
Peanut Butter & Jelly Sdw	1 pkg	6	150	36%
Peanut Butter Bars	1 pkg/2.5 oz	18	370	44%
	1 pkg/1.8 oz	13	260	45%
Peanut Cluster	1 pkg	12	230	47%
Pecan Twins	1 pkg	10	220	41%
Pumpkin Delights	1 pkg	6	140	39%
Snack Cakes-Chocolate	1 pkg/3 oz	19	390	44%
	1 pkg/2.5 oz	14	320	40%
Snack Cakes-Vanilla	1 pkg/3 oz	19	390	44%
	1 pkg/2.6 oz	16	330	44%
Spice	1 pkg	11	270	37%
Star Crunch	1 pkg	6	150	36%
Swiss Cake Rolls	1 pkg	12	270	40%
Swiss Rolls	1 pkg	12	280	39%
(Sara Lee)				
All Butter Pound	1 cake	11	200	50%
Choc Fudge	1 cake	10	190	47%
Classic Cheesecake	1 cake	14	200	63%
Deluxe Carrot Cake	1 cake	7	180	35%
(Tastykake)				
Banana Treats	1	4	147	25%
Cupcake				
Chocolate	1	3.5	113	28%
Vanilla	1	3	116	23%
Juniors				
chocolate	1	8	365	20%
coconut	1	4	317	11%
Koffee Kakes	1	12	317	34%
Kandy Kake				
chocolate	1	4	95	38%

Food and Description	Amount	Fat Grams	Total Calories	% Fat Calories
peanut butter	1	5	103	44%
Koffee Kakes-cream filled	1	6	145	37%
Krimpets				
butterscotch	1	2	118	15%
chocolate cream filled	1	4	142	25%
jelly	1		96	8%
vanilla cream filled	1	4	139	26%
Spice-w/brown sugar frosting				
homemade (9"dia)	1/10 cake	16	411	35%
Sponge-tube-no icing				
homemade (9¾" dia)	1/12 cake	3.8	196	17%
Strawberry Cream-frozen				
(Pepperidge Farm)	2 oz	7	190	33%
Strawberry French C'Cake-frozen				
(Sara Lee)	1 slice	11	200	50%
Stawberry Short Cake-frozen				
(Sara Lee)	1 slice	8	190	38%
frozen (Weight Watchers)	3 oz	4	160	23%
Torte				
chocolate (8½" dia)/homemade	1/16 cake	22	317	63%
Vanilla-frozen-(Pepperidge Farm)	15⅝ oz	8	190	38%
White cake-homemade-				
w/white frosting (9" dia)	1/16 cake	9	260	28%
w/coconut frosting (9" dia)	1/16 cake	10	289	31%
Yellow cake-homemade				
w/caramel frosting (9" dia)	1/16 cake	9.5	293	29%
w/choc frosting (9" dia)	1/16 cake	11	245	40%
Donettes (Hostess)				
Chocolate-coated	1 piece	3	60	45%
Powdered	1 piece	1	40	23%
Donut Sticks (Little Debbie)	1 pkg/2.5 oz	18	330	49%
	1 pkg/			
	1.67 oz	13	230	51%
SNACK MIX				
(Lawry's)-Flavor Tree-Party Mix	¼ cup	11	163	61%
no salt	¼ cup	10.8	163	60%
(Ralston)-Chex Mix Brand				
Golden Cheddar	1 oz	5	130	35%
Sour Cream & Onion	1 oz	5	130	35%
Traditional	1 oz	5	120	38%
Snackn' Bag				
Barbeque	1 oz	5	130	35%
Golden CHeddar Cheese	1 oz	5	130	35%
Sour Cream & Onion	1 oz	5	130	35%

Food and Description	Amount	Fat Grams	Total Calories	% Fat Calories
SNACKS (*See also* CHEESE SNACKS, CORN CHIPS, POPCORN, POTATO CHIPS, POTATO SNACKS, PRETZELS)				
(Bugles)-Nacho Cheese	1 oz	9	160	51%
Plain	1 oz	8	150	48%
Carrot Chips (Hain)				
barbecue	1 oz	8	140	51%
plain	1 oz	9	150	54%
no salt	1 oz	7	150	42%
(Combos)-Cracker Cheddar Cheese	1 oz	8	150	48%
Nacho Cheese	1 oz	6	130	42%
Peanut Butter	1 oz	9	150	54%
Pizza-Cheese	1 oz	5	130	35%
Extra Cheese	1 oz	7	140	45%
Pepperoni	1 oz	7	140	45%
Pretzel	1 oz	6	130	42%
(Cornnuts)				
barbecue	1 oz	4	110	33%
cheddar cheese	1 oz	4	110	33%
original	1 oz	4	120	30%
(Crunch'N Munch)				
Candied	1.25 oz	7	170	37%
Caramel	1.25 oz	5	160	28%
Maple Walnut	1.25 oz	6	160	34%
Toffee	1.25 oz	5	160	28%
(Eagle)-Mexican Snack Mix	1 oz	9	160	51%
(Guy's)-Tasty Mix	1 oz	7	130	49%
(Health Valley)-Carrot Lites	½ oz	1	70	13%
(Keebler)-Pizza Chips Pizzarias				
Cheese	1 oz	6	140	39%
Zesty Pepperoni	1 oz	6	140	39%
(Lawry's)-Flavor Tree				
Cajun Hot Sticks	¼ cup	9	133	61%
Cheddar Sticks	¼ cup	8	129	56%
Honey Roasted	¼ cup	9	138	59%
Jalapeno & Cheddar	¼ cup	8	129	56%
Oat Bran	¼ cup	7.5	124	54%
Sesame Sticks	¼ cup	9	133	61%
Sesame Sticks-no salt	¼ cup	8	131	55%
Sour Cream & Onion	¼ cup	8	127	57%
(Lawry's)-Sesame Chips	¼ cup	9	163	50%
(Lite Munchies)				
Bar B Que	.5 oz	2	60	30%
Nacho Cheese	.5 oz	2	60	30%
Toasted Onion	.5 oz	2	60	30%

Food and Description	Amount	Fat Grams	Total Calories	% Fat Calories
(Nabisco)				
Doo Dads				
original	1 oz	6	140	39%
zesty cheese	1 oz	6	140	39%
Twigs-Sesame & Cheese Sticks	.5 oz	4	70	51%
(Pepperidge Farm)-Cheese Sticks	8 pieces	6	130	42%
Original	8 pieces	5	130	35%
Pumpernikel	8 pieces	5	130	35%
Rye	8 pieces	4	130	28%
Sesame	8 pieces	5	130	35%
(Planter's)-Sour Cream & Onion Puffs	1 oz	10	160	56%
Pork skins	1 oz	10	160	56%
Skinny Munchies (Skinny Haven)				
Chocolate Fudge	.5 oz	2	66	27%
Nacho Cheese	.5 oz	2	59	31%
Smokey Bar B Q	.5 oz	2	59	31%
Toasted Onion	.5 oz	2	59	31%
Snack Mix (Snyder's)	1 oz	5	130	35%
Weight Watchers)-Snacks				
Bar-Be-Que	.5 oz	3	60	45%
Cheddar Cheese	.5 oz	3	60	45%
Toasted Onion	.5 oz	3	60	45%
SNAIL/(Escargot)				
cooked-moist heat	3 oz	1	230	4%
raw	3 oz	< 1	117	4%
SNAPPER				
cooked-dry heat	3 oz	1	109	8%
raw	3 oz	1	85	11%
SNOW PEA	1 cup	–	30	–
frozen (La Choy)	½ pkg	< 1	35	13%
SOCKEYE				
canned (Libby's)	7¾ oz	21	380	50%
cooked-dry heat	3 oz	9	183	44%
raw	3 oz	7	143	44%
SODA (See also PUNCH)				
Apple				
(Crush)	12 fl oz	–	180	–
Diet	12 fl oz	–	20	–
(Slice)	12 fl oz	–	196	–
Diet	12 fl oz	–	20	–
(Welch's)	12 fl oz	–	180	–
(Big Red)	12 fl oz	–	163	–
Birch Beer				
(Canada Dry)	12 fl oz	–	166	–

Food and Description	Amount	Fat Grams	Total Calories	% Fat Calories
(Shasta) diet	12 fl oz	–	4	–
Bitter Lemon				
(Canada Dry)	12 fl oz	–	150	–
(Schweppes)	12 fl oz	–	156	–
Black Cherry				
(Cragmont)	12 fl oz	–	180	–
(Diet-Rite)	12 fl oz	–	4	–
(Shasta)	12 fl oz	–	162	–
(Bubble Up)	12 fl oz	–	145	–
Diet	12 fl oz	–	2	–
Sugar free	12 fl oz	–	2	–
Cactus Cooler (Canada Dry)	12 fl oz	–	180	–
Cherry (Crush)	12 fl oz	–	150	–
Cherry Cola				
(Cragmont)	12 fl oz	–	158	–
(RC)	12 fl oz	–	171	–
Diet	12 fl oz	–	–	–
(Shasta)	12 fl oz	–	140	–
Chocolate-flavored	12 fl oz	–	155	–
Diet	12 fl oz	–	7	–
(Barons)	9.5 oz	–	142	–
(Canfield's)-fudge-diet	6 oz	–	2	–
Yoo Hoo	9 oz	< 1	95	5%
Citrus Mist				
(Shasta)	12 oz	–	70	–
Club Soda	12 oz	–	–	–
(Canada Dry)	12 oz	–	–	–
(Schweppes)	12 oz	–	–	–
(Shasta)	12 oz	–	–	–
(Coca Cola)	6 oz	–	77	–
Caffeine Free	6 oz	–	77	–
Cherry	12 oz	–	154	–
	6 oz	–	76	–
diet	12 oz	–	2	–
Classic	6 oz	–	72	–
Diet	6 oz	–	1	–
Cola				
(Canada Dry)	12 oz	–	–	–
(Diet Rite)	6 oz	–	–	–
(Like)	12 oz	–	162	–
sugar free	12 oz	–	1	–
(RC)	6 oz	–	86	–
100 caffeine-free	6 oz	–	87	–
diet	6 oz	–	–	–

Food and Description	Amount	Fat Grams	Total Calories	% Fat Calories
(Shasta)	12 oz	–	147	–
diet	12 oz	–	–	–
Collins (Shasta)	12 oz	–	118	–
Cream Soda	12 oz	–	191	–
(A&W)-diet	12 oz	–	–	–
(Barqs) Red Creme	12 oz	–	175	–
(Cragmont)	12 oz	–	168	–
diet	12 oz	–	–	–
(Crush)-vanilla cream	12 oz	–	180	–
(Dad's)-diet	12 oz	–	2	–
(Shasta)	12 oz	–	154	–
Dr Diablo (Shasta)	12 oz	–	140	–
(Dr Pepper)	12 oz	–	156	–
Diet	12 oz	–	1	–
Pepper-Free	12 oz	–	156	–
Sugar-free Pepper-Free	12 oz	–	1	–
(Fresca)	12 oz	–	4	–
Fruit Punch	12 oz	–	200	–
(Nehi)	12 oz	–	200	–
(Shasta)	12 oz	–	173	–
Ginger Beer (Schweppes)	6 oz	–	68	–
Gingsing Ginger	12 oz	–	137	–
Gingerale	12 oz	–	124	–
low-cal	12 oz	–	7	–
(Canada Dry)	12 oz	–	140	–
diet	6 oz	–	2	–
golden	12 oz	–	150	–
(Cragmont)	6 oz	–	63	–
(Fanta)	6 oz	–	63	–
(Health Valley)	13 oz	1	153	6%
(Nehi)	12 oz	–	152	–
(Schweppes)	6 oz	–	63	–
diet	6 oz	–	–	–
(Shasta)	8 oz	–	120	–
diet	8 oz	–	–	–
Grape	12 oz	–	161	–
low-cal	12 oz	–	3	–
(Canada Dry)	12 oz	–	195	–
(Cragmont)	12oz	–	192	–
(Crush)	12 oz	–	200	–
(Fanta)	6 oz	–	86	–
(Nehi)	12 oz	–	192	–
diet	12 oz	–	3	–
(Schweppes)	6 oz	–	92	–

Food and Description	Amount	Fat Grams	Total Calories	% Fat Calories
(Shasta)	12 oz	–	177	–
(Welch's)-Sparkling	12 oz	–	180	–
Grapefruit/				
(Cragmont)	12 oz	–	168	–
(Schweppes)	6 oz	–	77	–
(Wink)	12 oz	–	180	–
(Kool-Aid) Kool Busters				
Cherry	6.75 oz	–	130	–
Grape	6.75 oz	–	130	–
Orange	6.75 oz	–	130	–
Tropical Punch	6.75 oz	–	130	–
Rock-A-Dile Red	6.75 oz	–	130	–
Lemon-Lime	12 oz	–	149	–
(Cragmont)	12 oz	–	148	–
diet	12 oz	–	–	–
(Minute Maid)	6 oz	–	71	–
diet	6 oz	–	10	–
(Nehi)-diet	12 oz	–	5	–
(Schweppes)	12 oz	–	142	–
(7-Up)	12 oz	–	144	–
diet	12 oz	–	4	–
Gold	12 oz	–	155	–
diet	12 oz	–	4	–
(Shasta)	12 oz	–	146	–
diet	12 oz	–	–	–
(Slice)-diet	12 oz	–	16	–
(Sprite)	12 oz	–	142	–
diet	12 oz	–	4	–
Lemon-Lime-Cherry				
(Cragmont)	12 oz	–	164	–
diet	12 oz	–	–	–
(7-Up)	12 oz	–	155	–
diet	12 oz	–	4	–
Lemon Sour (Schweppes)	12 oz	–	149	–
Mandarin Orange (Slice)	12 oz	–	193	–
low-cal	12 oz	–	12	–
(Mello Yellow)	12 oz	–	174	–
Mineral Water (Perrier)				
With-A-Twist Lemon	12 oz	–	–	–
With-A-Twist Lime	12 oz	–	–	–
(Mountain Dew)	12 oz	–	171	–
diet	12 oz	–	4	–
(Mr. Pibb)	6 oz	–	71	–
Orange	12 oz	–	177	–

Food and Description	Amount	Fat Grams	Total Calories	% Fat Calories
low-cal	12 oz	–	2	–
(Canada Dry)-diet	12 oz	–	3	–
Sunripe	12 oz	–	195	–
(Cragmont)	12 oz	–	178	–
(Crush)	12 oz	–	200	–
sugar free	12 oz	–	24	–
(Minute Maid)	12 oz	–	174	–
diet	12 oz	–	8	–
(Nehi)	12 oz	–	209	–
diet	12 oz	–	2	–
(Schweppes)-Sparkling	12 oz	–	172	–
(Shasta)	12 oz	–	177	–
(Welch's)-Sparkling	12 oz	–	180	–
Peach	12 oz	–	203	–
(Pepsi) Cola	12 oz	–	160	–
diet	6 oz	–	–	–
diet caffeine free	6 oz	–	–	–
(Pepsi) Free	12 oz	–	160	–
diet	12 oz	–	2	–
(Pepsi) Light	12 oz	–	1	–
(Pepsi) Wild Cherry-diet	12 oz	–	1	–
Pineapple (Canada Dry)	12 oz	–	166	–
(Crush)	12 oz	–	200	–
Pink Grapefruit (Diet-Rite)	12 oz	–	4	–
Purple Passiion (Canada Dry)	12 oz	–	180	–
Punch (Cragmont)-sparkling	12 oz	–	198	–
Quinine Water	12 oz	–	142	–
Red Berry (Shasta)	12 oz	–	158	–
Red Raspberry (Diet-Rite)	12 oz	–	4	–
Red Pop (Shasta)	12 oz	–	158	–
Rootbeer	12 oz	–	152	–
(A&W)-low-cal	12 oz	–	–	–
(Barrelhead)-diet	6 oz	–	2	–
(Canada Dry)-Barrelhead	12 oz	–	166	–
diet	12 oz	–	3	–
(Cragmont)	12 oz	–	168	–
diet	12 oz	–	–	–
(Dad's)-diet	12 oz	–	2	–
(Fanta)	12 oz	–	156	–
(Health Valley)	13 oz	1	120	8%
(Hires)	12 oz	–	180	–
sugar free	12 oz	–	4	–
(IBC)-diet	12 oz	–	2	–
(New Century)-Mug Old Fashioned	12 oz	–	168	–

Food and Description	Amount	Fat Grams	Total Calories	% Fat Calories
(Ramblin')	12 oz	–	176	–
sugar free	12 oz	–	1	–
(Schweppes)	12 oz	–	150	–
(Shasta)	12 oz	–	154	–
Sarsaparilla (Health Valley)	13 oz	–	153	–
Seltzer Water	12 oz	–	–	–
Lemon Flavored	12 oz	–	–	–
Lime Flavored	12 oz	–	–	–
Orange Flavored	12 oz	–	–	–
Strawberry Flavored	12 oz	–	–	–
(Crystal Geyser)-Light -				
Black CherryCider	6 oz	–	60	–
Cranberry-Raspberry	6 oz	–	60	–
Kiwi Lemonade	6 oz	–	60	–
Natural Peach	6 oz	–	60	–
Vanilla Creme	6 oz	–	60	–
Strawberry	6 oz	–	192	–
low-cal	6 oz	–	3	–
(Canada Dry)	6 oz	–	180	–
(Cragmont)	6 oz	–	176	–
(Crush)	6 oz	–	180	–
(Nehi)	6 oz	–	192	–
diet	6 oz	–	3	–
(Shasta)	6 oz	–	147	–
(Welch's)-Sparkling	6 oz	–	180	–
(Tab)	6 oz	–	–	–
Tangerine (Diet-Rite)	6 oz	–	4	–
Tonic Water	6 oz	–	125	–
low cal	6 oz	–	2	–
(Canada Dry)	6 oz	–	135	–
diet	6 oz	–	4	–
(Schweppes)	6 oz	–	128	–
sugar free	6 oz	–	3	–
Vanilla Cream (Canada Dry)	12 oz	–	195	–
Wild Berry (Health Valley)	13 oz	1	142	6%
Wild Cherry (Canada Dry)	12 oz	–	195	–
SOLE (See also SEAFOOD ENTREE/DINNER)				
baked w/butter	3 oz	6	120	45%
cooked-dry heat	3 oz	1	80	11%
raw	3 oz	< 1	58	8%
SORGHUM	1 Tbs	–	53	–
	1 cup	–	848	–
Cane and Maple	1 Tbs	–	50	–
	1 cup	–	794	–

Food and Description	Amount	Fat Grams	Total Calories	% Fat Calories
Table blend	1 Tbs	–	59	–
	1 cup	–	951	–
SORGHUM GRAIN	4 oz	4	380	10%

SOUP

(NOTE: Condensed soups were prepared as directed on packaging w/water, unless otherwise stated. When prepared with milk, whole milk was used. If you use low-fat or skim milk, refer to the Quick Reference-Milk below to adjust your fat and calorie data. Ready-To-Serve (RTS) soups were heated as directed w/no added liquid.)

QUICK REFERENCE: MILK	Amount	Fat Grams	Total Calories	% Fat Calories
Whole	½ cup	4	75	48%
	¼ cup	2	38	47%
2% lowfat	½ cup	2.5	61	37%
	¼ cup	1	31	29%
1% lowfat	½ cup	1	55	16%
	¼ cup	.5	26	17%
Skim	½ cup	–	45	–
	¼ cup	–	23	–

Food and Description	Amount	Fat Grams	Total Calories	% Fat Calories
(Andersen's)				
Cream of Asparagus	7.5 oz	7	150	42%
Cream of Broccoli	7.5 oz	7	150	42%
Cream of Potato	7.5 oz	11	220	45%
Split Pea	7.5 oz	–	140	–
Split Pea w/ham	7.5 oz	1	150	6%
Tomato	7.5 oz	4	140	26%
Asparagus				
(Campbell's) Creamy Natural	1 cup	5	100	45%
prepared w/milk	1 cup	9	170	48%
Asparagus, Cream of	1 pkg/2.2 oz	7	234	27%
	1 cup	1.7	59	26%
	1 cup	4	87	41%
prepared w/milk	1 cup	8	161	45%
Bacon, Lettuce, & Tomato				
(Pepperidge Farm)	5.3 oz	12	170	64%
5-Bean Vegetable/chunky				
(Health Valley)	7.5 oz	2	100	18%
Bean, Black	1 cup	1.5	116	12%
(Campbell's)	1 cup	2	110	16%
(Health Valley)	7.5 oz	4	160	23%
Bean, Black Turtle	1 cup	–	218	–
Bean, Black w/Sherry				
(Pepperidge Farm)	5.3 oz	1.7	109	14%

Food and Description	Amount	Fat Grams	Total Calories	% Fat Calories
Bean, Navy				
(Pritikin)	7⅜ oz	–	130	–
Bean W/Bacon	1 pkg/1 oz	2	105	17%
	1 cup	2	105	17%
(Campbell's)				
Special Request	1 cup	4	120	30%
Bean W/Franks	1 cup	6.98	187	34%
condensed not prepared	11.25 oz	17	454	34%
Bean W/Ham				
(Campbell's)				
Old Fashioned Soup For One	11 oz	7	220	29%
Bean W/Ham Chunky Old Fashioned				
(Campbell's) RTS	11 oz	9	290	28%
	9⅝ oz	8	250	29%
Beans, Red & Rice w/sausage				
Chunky Creole Style				
ready-to-serve (Campbell's)	9.5 oz	13	300	39%
Beef				
(Campbell's)	1 cup	2	80	23%
(Right Time)	6 oz	–	8	–
ready-to-serve (Progresso)	9.5 oz	6	160	34%
Beef Barley				
ready-to-serve (Progresso)	9.5 oz	4	150	24%
Beef Broth				
(College Inn)	1 cup	–	18	–
(Health Valley)	7.5 oz	–	8	–
(Pritikin)	7.25 oz	–	20	–
ready-to-serve	14 oz	1	27	33%
(Swanson)	7¼ oz	1	18	50%
Beef Broth or Bouillon/ready-to-serve	1 cup	.5	16	28%
Beef Broth & Barley(Campbell's)	1 cup	1	59	15%
Beef Cabbage (Manischewitz)	1 cup	–	62	–
Beef Chunky				
(Campbell's) ready-to serve	10¾ oz	5	190	24%
	9.5 oz	4	170	21%
Beef, Hearty				
(Campbell's) Home Cookin' RTS	10¾ oz	3	140	19%
	9.5 oz	3	130	21%
Beef Minestrone				
ready-to-serve				
(Progresso)	9.5 oz	4	160	23%
Beef Mushroom	1 cup	3	73	37%
Beef Noodle				
(Campbell's)	1 cup	3	70	39%

Food and Description	Amount	Fat Grams	Total Calories	% Fat Calories
(Campbell's) Home Cookin' RTS	10.76 oz	3.8	144	24%
microwave (Lunch Bucket)	8.25 oz	2	120	15%
(Weight Watchers) RTS	10.5 oz	2	90	20%
Beef Noodle-homestyle				
(Campbell's)	1 cup	3	80	34%
Beef Ravioli Romano				
ready-to-serve				
(Campbell's)	9.49 oz	8	231	31%
Beef Stroganoff Style				
(Campbell')				
Home Cookin' RTS	10¾ oz	16	320	45%
Beef Vegetable				
ready-to-serve				
(Progresso)	9.5 oz	4	160	23%
Beefy Mushroom				
(Campbell's)	1 cup	3	60	45%
Borscht				
(Gold's)	1 cup	–	100	–
(Manischewitz) w/beets	1 cup	–	80	–
low cal	1 cup	–	20	–
Borscht				
(Mother's)				
Old Fashioned	1 cup	–	96	–
(Pepperidge Farm)	5.3 oz	–	89	–
Borscht Beverage (Mother's)-low cal	8 oz	–	25	–
Broccoli				
(Campbell's) Creamy Natural	1 cup	3	70	39%
prepared w/milk	1 cup	7	140	45%
(Pepperidge Farm) Cream of	5.3 oz	6	100	54%
Cauliflower				
(Campbell's) Creamy Natural	1 cup	9	130	62%
prepared w/milk	1 cup	13	200	59%
Cauliflower, Creamy	1 cup	5.9	97	55%
Celery, Cream of				
condensed not prepared	10.75 oz	14	219	58%
prepared w/milk	1 cup	9.68	165	53%
prepared w/water	1 cup	5.59	90	56%
prep w/water (Campbell's)	1 cup	7	100	63%
Cheddar Cheese				
(Campbell's)	1 cup	8	130	55%
Cheese				
condensed not prepared	11 oz	25	377	60%
prepared w/milk	1 cup	14.56	230	57%
prepared w/water	1 cup	10.5	155	61%

Food and Description	Amount	Fat Grams	Total Calories	% Fat Calories
Chickarina				
ready-to-serve (Progresso)	9.5 oz	5	110	41%
Chickarina W/Tiny Meatballs				
ready-to-serve (Progresso)	9.5 oz	6	90	60%
Chicken				
(Clear)/(Manischewitz)	1 cup	–	46	–
Chicken & Dumplings	1 cup	5.5	97	51%
(Campbell's)	1 cup	3	80	34%
Chicken & Stars (Campbell's)	1 cup	2	60	30%
Chicken Alphabet (Campbell's)	1 cup	2	70	26%
Chicken Barley (Campbell's)	1 cup	1.8	70	23%
Chicken Broth	1 cup	1	39	23%
condensed unprepared	10.75 oz	3	94	29%
(Campbell's)	1 cup	2	35	51%
(Campbell's) Low Sodium RTS	10.5 oz	2	40	45%
(College Inn)	1 cup	3	35	77%
(Health Valley)	7.5 oz	2	34	53%
(Manischewitz)	1 cup	–	83	–
(Pritikin)	6⅞ oz	–	14	–
(Swanson) RTS	7¼ oz	2	30	60%
Chicken Broth & Noodles (Campbell's)	1 cup	2	60	30%
Chicken Broth & Rice (Campbell's)	1 cup	1	50	18%
Chicken/Chunky Old Fashioned				
(Campbell's) RTS	10¾ oz	5	180	56%
	9.5 oz	4	150	24%
Chicken Corn Chowder/Chunky				
ready-to-serve (Campbell's)	10¾ oz	22	350	57%
Chicken Curry (Pepperidge Farm)	5.3 oz	8	170	42%
Chicken Gumbo				
(Campbell's)	1 cup	2	60	30%
(Pritikin)	7⅜ oz	1	60	15%
Chicken, Cream of				
(Campbell's)	1 cup	7	110	57%
(Campbell's)prepared w/milk	1 cup	14.97	191	71%
(Campbell's) Special Request	1 cup	7	110	57%
ready-to-serve (Campbell's)	7.27 oz	5.5	85	58%
Chicken, Cream of w/mushrooms				
ready-to-serve (Progresso)	9.5 oz	11	180	55%
Chicken, Creamy Mushroom (Campbell's)	1 cup	7	111	57%
Chicken, Golden & Noodles (Campbell's)				
Soup For One	11 oz	4	120	30%
Chicken, Hearty				
microwave				
(Lunch Bucket)	8.25 oz	3	110	25%

Food and Description	Amount	Fat Grams	Total Calories	% Fat Calories
ready-to-serve (Progresso)	9.5 oz	4	140	26%
Chicken Homestyle/ready-to-serve	9.5 oz	3	90	30%
Chicken Minestrone/ready-to-serve	9.5 oz	6	160	34%
Chicken Mushroom	1 cup	9	132	61%
Chicken Mushroom-creamy				
(Campbell's)	1 cup	8	120	60%
Chunky-RTS	9.38 oz	21.5	272	71%
Chicken-Curly Noodle (Campbell's)	1 cup	3	80	34%
Chicken Noodle				
(Campbell's) Special Request	1 cup	2	70	26%
microwave (Lunch Bucket)	8.25 oz	4	110	33%
ready-to-serve (Campbell's)	7.27 oz	2	60	30%
ready-to-serve (Progresso)	9.5 oz	4	130	28%
ready-to-serve (Weight Watchers)	10.5 oz	2	80	23%
Chunky/(Campbell's)ready-to-serve	10¾ oz	7	200	32%
	9.5 oz	6	180	30%
Chicken Noodle-Homestyle (Campbell's)	1 cup	3	70	39%
(Lipton) Hearty Ones Microwave	11 oz	4	230	16%
Chicken Noodle W/Meatballs				
ready-to-serve	1 cup	3.57	99	33%
	20 oz	8	227	32%
Chicken Noodle-O's (Campbell's)	1 cup	2	70	26%
Chicken Nuggets w/Veg. & Noodles/Chunky				
(Campbell's) ready-to-serve	10¾ oz	9	210	39%
	9.5 oz	8	190	38%
Chicken Rice				
(Manischewitz)	1 cup	–	47	–
Ready-to-serve				
(Campbell's)	7.27 oz	2	52	35%
(Progresso)	9.5 oz	3	120	23%
Ready-to-serve-chunky	1 cup	3	127	21%
(Campbell's)	9.5 oz	4	140	26%
Chicken Rice W/Veg				
ready-to-serve	9.5 oz	3	140	19%
Chicken W/Noodles				
(Campbell's)				
Home Cookin' RTS	10¾ oz	4	140	26%
	9.5 oz	3	120	23%
(Campbell's) Low Sodium RTS	10¾ oz	5	160	28%
Chicken W/Noodles & Mushrooms				
ready-to-serve				
(Campbell's)	10.76 oz	6.6	195	31%
Chicken w/Ribbon Pasta	7.25	.5	60	8%

Food and Description	Amount	Fat Grams	Total Calories	% Fat Calories
Chicken W/Rice				
(Campbell's)	1 cup	2	60	30%
(Campbell's) Special Request	1 cup	2	60	30%
Chicken W/Wild Rice				
(Pepperidge Farm)	5.3 oz	3	85	32%
Chicken Vegetable				
(Campbell's)	1 cup	3	70	39%
(Estee)	7.25 oz	7	130	49%
(Manischewitz)	1 cup	–	55	–
(Pritikin)	7.25 oz	.5	70	6%
ready-to-serve	9.5 oz	4.8	167	26%
ready-to-serve (Progresso)	9.5 oz	3	140	19%
Chicken Vegetable, Chunky				
(Campbell's) RTS	9.5 oz	6	170	32%
(Campbell's) Low Sodium RTS	10¾ oz	11	240	41%
Chicken Vegetable W/Wild Rice				
(Campbell's) Golden Classic	1 cup	3	80	34%
Chicken Vegetable-w/rice				
ready-to-serve (Campbell's)	10.76 oz	2.7	131	19%
Chili (*See* (Lipton) Kettle Ready in this listing, and also MEXICAN FOODS)				
Chili Beef	1 cup	6.6	169	35%
condensed unprepared	11.25 oz	16	411	35%
(Campbell's)	1 cup	5	140	32%
Chili Beef, Chunky				
ready-to-serve (Campbell's)	9.75 oz	6	260	21%
	11 oz	7	290	22%
Clam Chowder-Manhattan				
(Campbell's)	1 cup	2	70	26%
(Health Valley)	7.5 oz	3	110	25%
(Pepperidge Farm)	5.3 oz	2	80	23%
(Pritikin)	7⅜ oz	–	70	–
ready-to-serve				
(Campbell's)	7.27 oz	1.8	67	24%
(Progresso)	9.5 oz	2	120	15%
(Snow's)	7.5 oz	2	70	26%
Chunky/ready-to-serve	1 cup	3	133	21%
Chunky (Campbell's) RTS	10¾ oz	5	160	28%
	9.5 oz	4	150	24%
Clam Chowder-New England				
(Campbell's)	1 cup	3	80	34%
(Campbell's) Soup For One	11 oz	4	130	28%
prepared w/milk				
(Campbell's) Soup for One	11 oz	7	190	33%
(Snow's)	7.5 oz	6	140	39%

Food and Description	Amount	Fat Grams	Total Calories	% Fat Calories
(Pepperidge Farm)	5.3 oz	6	133	41%
(Pritikin)	7⅜ oz	–	118	–
ready-to-serve (Progresso)	9.5 oz	12	220	49%
(Stouffer's)-frozen	8 oz	9	180	45%
Clam Chowder-New England, Chunky/ready-to-serve				
(Campbell's)	10¾ oz	17	290	53%
	9.5 oz	15	250	54%
(Gorton's)	¼ can	5	140	32%
Consomme (Beef) W/Gelatin				
condensed-not prepared	10.5 oz	–	71	–
(Campbell's)	1 cup	–	25	–
Consomme, Madrilene				
(Pepperidge Farm)	5.3 oz	–	40	–
Corn Chowder				
(Pepperidge Farm)	5.3 oz	12	170	64%
Corn Chowder-New England				
(Snow's)				
prepared w/milk	7.5 oz	6	150	36%
Corn Potage				
(Campbell's)	1 cup	2	93	19%
Crab				
(Pepperidge Farm)	5.3 oz	1.7	80	19%
ready-to-serve	1 cup	1.5	76	18%
Creole-style - see Beans, Red				
Escarol				
ready-to-serve	1 cup	2	27	67%
ready-to-serve				
(Progresso)	9.25 oz	1	30	30%
	19.5 oz	4	61	59%
Fish Chowder-New England				
(Snow's) prepared w/milk	7.5 oz	6	130	42%
Fisherman's Chowder/Chunky				
(Pepperidge Farm)	5.3 oz	6	150	36%
ready-to-serve (Campbell's)	9.5 oz	13	230	51%
	10¾ oz	14	260	49%
French Onion				
(Campbell's)	1 cup	2	60	30%
(Pepperidge Farm)	5.3 oz	4.7	71	60%
ready-to-serve (Campbell's)	9.5 oz	8	120	60%
Gazpacho				
(Campbell's)	1 cup	–	41	–
(Pepperidge Farm)	5.3 oz	2	68	27%
ready-to-serve	1 cup	2	57	32%
	13 oz	3	87	31%

Food and Description	Amount	Fat Grams	Total Calories	% Fat Calories
Greek-homemade	1 cup	2.5	85	27%
(Hain)				
Chicken Broth	8¾ oz	6	70	77%
no salt	8¾ oz	5	60	75%
Chicken Noodle	9.5 oz	4	120	30%
no salt	9.5 oz	4	110	33%
Creamy Mushroom	9¼ oz	4	110	33%
Italian Vege-Pasta	9½ oz	5	160	28%
low sodium	9½ oz	6	140	39%
Minestrone	9½ oz	2	170	11%
no salt	9½ oz	4	160	23%
Mushroom Barley	9½ oz	2	100	18%
New England Clam Chowder	9¼ oz	4	180	20%
Turkey Rice	9½ oz	3	100	27%
no salt	9½ oz	3	100	27%
Vegetable Chicken	9½ oz	4	120	30%
no salt	9½ oz	3	120	23%
Vegetarian Lentil	9½ oz	3	160	17%
no salt	9½ oz	3	160	17%
Split Pea	9½ oz	1	170	5%
no salt	9½ oz	1	170	5%
Vegetarian Vegetable	9½ oz	4	140	26%
no salt	9½ oz	5	150	30%
Ham & Bean				
ready-to-serve (Progresso)	9.5 oz	2	180	10%
Ham & Butter Beans/Chunky				
ready-to-serve (Campbell's)	10¾ oz	10	280	32%
Hunter's				
(Pepperidge Farm)	5.3 oz	4	105	34%
Italian Pasta, Classice				
(Lipton) Hearty Ones Microwave	11 oz	3	190	14%
Lentil				
(Health Valley)	7.5 oz	2.5	160	14%
(Pritikin)	7⅜ oz	–	100	–
(Progresso)-ready-to-serve	9.5 oz	4	170	21%
Lentil, Hearty				
(Campbell's)				
Home Cookin' RTS	10¾ oz	1	170	5%
	9.5 oz	1	150	6%
Lentil W/Ham				
ready-to-serve	1 cup	2.78	140	18%
	13 oz	6	320	17%
Lentil W/Sausage				
ready-to-serve (Progresso)	9.5 oz	7	180	35%

Food and Description	Amount	Fat Grams	Total Calories	% Fat Calories
(Lipton) Kettle Ready-frozen				
Black Bean w/Ham	6 oz	6	154	35%
Boston Clam Chowder	6 oz	7	131	48%
Chicken Gumbo	6 oz	3.5	94	34%
Chicken Noodle	6 oz	2.9	94	28%
Chili-Jalapeno	6 oz	7.8	173	41%
Traditional	6 oz	6.5	161	36%
Corn & Broccoli Chowder	6 oz	5	102	44%
Cream of Asparagus	6 oz	4	62	58%
Cream of Cauliflower	6 oz	6.9	93	67%
Cream of Cheddar Broccoli	6 oz	11	137	72%
Cream of Cheddar Cheese	6 oz	12.5	158	71%
Cream of Chicken	6 oz	6	98	55%
Cream of Mushroom	6 oz	6	85	64%
French Onion	6 oz	2	42	43%
Garden Vegetable	6 oz	2.8	85	30%
Hearty Beef Vegetable	6 oz	2.8	85	30%
Hearty Minestrone	6 oz	4	104	35%
Manhattan Clam Chowder	6 oz	2.6	69	34%
New England Clam Chowder	6 oz	6.5	116	50%
Savory Bean w/Ham	6 oz	3.6	113	29%
Split Pea w/Ham	6 oz	4	155	23%
Tortellini in Tomato	6 oz	5	122	37%
Lobster Bisque (Pepperidge Farm)	5.3 oz	10.9	158	62%
Macaroni & Bean				
ready-to-serve (Progresso)	9.5 oz	4	170	21%
Meatball Alphabet (Campbell's)	1 cup	4	100	36%
Minestrone				
(Campbell's)	1 cup	2	80	23%
(Health Valley)	7.5 oz	2.5	120	19%
(Pepperidge Farm)	5.3 oz	4	110	33%
(Pritikin)	7⅜ oz	.5	110	4%
ready-to-serve (Campbell's)	7.27 oz	2	70	26%
ready-to-serve (Progresso)	9.5 oz	3	160	17%
Minestrone/Chunky-ready-to-serve	1 cup	2.8	127	20%
(Campbell's) RTS	9.5 oz	5	170	27%
(Estee)	7.5 oz	8	165	44%
Minestrone, Extra Zesty				
ready-to-serve (Progresso)	9.5 oz	8	180	40%
Minestrone, Old World				
(Campbell's) Home Cookin' RTS	10¾ oz	4	150	24%
	9.5 oz	3	130	21%
Minestrone W/Italian Sausage				
ready-to-serve	9.49 oz	8	169	43%

Food and Description	Amount	Fat Grams	Total Calories	% Fat Calories
Mushroom (Pritikin)	7⅜ oz	–	60	–
Mushroom Barley	1 cup	2	73	25%
(Health Valley)	7.5 oz	3	110	25%
(Manischewitz)	1 cup	–	72	–
Mushroom, Cream of				
condensed unprepared	10.75 oz	23	313	66%
prepared w/milk	1 cup	13.59	203	60%
preparedw/water	1 cup	8.97	129	63%
(Campbell's)	1 cup	7	100	63%
(Campbell's) Low Sodium RTS	10.5 oz	13	190	62%
(Campbell's) Special Request	1 cup	7	100	63%
ready-to-serve				
(Progresso)	9.25 oz	8	140	51%
(Weight Watchers)	10.5 oz	2	90	20%
Mushroom, Creamy/Chunky				
(Campbell's) RTS	10.5 oz	21	260	73%
	9⅜ oz	19	240	71%
Mushroom, Creamy Chicken/Chunky				
(Campbell's) RTS	10.5 oz	25	320	70%
	9⅜ oz	23	290	71%
Mushroom, Golden				
(Campbell's)	1 cup	3	80	34%
Mushroom W/Beef stock	1 cup	4	85	42%
Mushroom, Savory Cream of (Campbell's)				
Soup For One	11 oz	13	180	65%
Nacho Cheese				
(Campbell's)	1 cup	8	110	66%
(Campbell's) prepared w/milk	1 cup	12	180	60%
Noodles & Ground Beef				
(Campbell's)	1 cup	3.5	90	35%
Onion	1 cup	1.7	57	27%
condensed unprepared	10.5 oz	4	138	26%
Onion, Cream of				
(Campbell's)	1 cup	5	100	45%
(Campbell's)prepared w/milk	1 cup	7	140	45%
Oyster Stew				
prepared w/milk	10.5 oz	19	325	53%
(Campbell's)	1 cup	5	80	56%
(Campbell's) prepared w/milk	1 cup	9	150	54%
(Pepperidge Farm)	5.3 oz	6	110	49%
Pea, Green				
prepared w/milk	1 cup	7	239	26%
prepared w/water	1 cup	2.9	164	16%

Food and Description	Amount	Fat Grams	Total Calories	% Fat Calories
(Campbell's)	1 cup	3	160	17%
(Pepperidge Farm)	5.3 oz	7	210	30%
ready-to-serve (Campbell's)	7.5 oz	2.6	136	17%
Pea, Green Split				
(Health Valley)	7.5 oz	1.7	160	10%
ready-to-serve(Progresso)	9.5 oz	3	180	15%
Pea, Split				
(Campbell's) Low Sodium RTS	10¾ oz	5	240	19%
(Manischewitz)	1 cup	–	133	–
(Pritikin)	7.5 oz	–	130	–
Pea, Split W/Ham				
(Campbell's) Home Cookin' RTS	10¾ oz	4	210	17%
	9.5 oz	4	190	19%
microwave (Lunch Bucket)	8.25 oz	3	130	21%
ready-to-serve(Progresso)	9.5 oz	4	170	21%
Chunky/ready-to-serve(Campbell's)	1 cup	3.98	184	20%
	10¾ oz	6	240	23%
	9.5 oz	5	210	21%
Pea, Split w/Ham & Bacon (Campbell's)	1 cup	4	150	24%
Pepper Pot				
(Campbell's)	1 cup	4	90	40%
condensed not prepared	10.5 oz	11	251	39%
Pepper Steak/Chunky-(Campbell's) RTS	10¾ oz	3	180	15%
	9.5 oz	3	160	17%
Potato				
(Campbell's) Creamy Natural	1 cup	7	120	53%
prepared w/milk	1 cup	11	190	52%
(Health Valley) RTS	4 oz	1	70	13%
homemade	1 cup	12	201	54%
Potato, Cream of (Campbell's)	1 cup	3	70	39%
prepared w/2 oz milk & 2 oz water	1 cup	4	110	33%
Potato Leek (Health Valley)	7.5 oz	2.5	110	21%
Schav (Manischewitz)	1 cup	–	11	–
Scotch Broth (Campbell's)	1 cup	3	80	34%
condensed not prepared	10.5 oz	6	195	28%
Seafood Chowder-New England/(Snow's)				
prepared w/milk	7.5 oz	6	130	42%
Shiitake Mushroom (Pepperidge Farm)	5.3 oz	2.7	73	33%
Shrimp, Cream of				
(Campbell's)	1 cup	6	90	60%
(Campbell's) prep w/milk	1 cup	10	160	56%
condensed-not prepared	10.75 oz	13	219	53%
Sirloin Beef				
(Campbell's) Golden Classic	1 cup	3	70	39%

Food and Description	Amount	Fat Grams	Total Calories	% Fat Calories
Sirloin Burger/Chunky-ready-to-serve				
(Campbell's)	9.5 oz	8	200	36%
	10¾ oz	9	230	35%
Spinach				
(Campbell's) Creamy Natural	1 cup	6	90	60%
(Campbell's) Creamy Natural				
prepared w/milk	1 cup	10	160	56%
Spinach, Cream of (Stouffer's)-frozen	8 oz	15	210	64%
Steak & Potato-Chunky				
ready-to-serve (Campbell's)	1 cup	3.8	169	20%
	10¾ oz	5	200	23%
	9.5 oz	4	170	21%
Stockpot	1 cup	3.9	100	35%
condensed-not prepared	11 oz	9	242	34%
(Tabatchnick) frozen				
Barley/Bean	8 oz	2	63	29%
Cabbage	8 oz	2	53	34%
Chicken Noodle	8 oz	2	58	31%
Cream of Broccoli	8 oz	1-3	90	10%-30%
Cream of Spinach	8 oz	1-3	90	10%-30%
Lentil	8 oz	1.5	90	15%
Manhattan Chowder	8 oz	1.5	94	14%
Minestrone	8 oz	1.5	90	15%
Mushroom Barley	8 oz	2	90	20%
New England Chowder	8 oz	1	97	9%
Northern Bean	8 oz	2	80	23%
Pea	8 oz	2	180	10%
Potato	8 oz	1	95	10%
Vegetable	8 oz	1	90	10%
Tomato				
(Campbell's)	1 cup	2	90	20%
prepared w/milk	1 cup	6	160	34%
Special Request	1 cup	2	90	20%
(Health Valley)	7.5 oz	2.8	100	25%
(Manischewitz)	1 cup	–	60	–
ready-to-serve	7.27 oz	1.7	106	14%
Tomato W/Tomato Pieces				
(Campbell's) Low Sodium RTS	10.5 oz	5	180	25%
(Pritikin)	7.5 oz	–	70	–
Tomato W/Vegetables				
ready-to-serve				
(Progresso)	9.5 oz	2	110	16%
(Progresso)	9.25 oz	5	140	32%

Food and Description	Amount	Fat Grams	Total Calories	% Fat Calories
Tomato Beef				
W/Noodles				
prepared w/water	1 cup	4	140	26%
w/Rotini				
ready-to-serve (Progresso)	9.5 oz	6	170	32%
Tomato Bisque				
prepared w/milk	1 cup	6.6	198	30%
(Campbell's)	1 cup	3	120	23%
Tomato, Cream of				
Homestyle/(Campbell's)	1 cup	3	110	25%
(Campbell's) prepared w/milk	1 cup	7	180	35%
Tomato Garden				
(Campbell's) Home Cookin' RTS	10¾ oz	3	150	18%
	9.5 oz	3	130	21%
Tomato Garden-Crispy (Campbell's)	1 cup	–	78	–
Tomato Rice				
Old Fashioned (Campbell's)	1 cup	2	110	16%
Tomato Royale				
(Campbell's) Soup For One	11 oz	3	180	15%
Tomato, Zesty (Campbell's)	1 cup	1	90	10%
Tortellini				
ready-to-serve (Progresso)	9.5 oz	3	80	34%
Tortellini & Vegtable				
(Campbell's) Golden Classic	1 cup	2	79	23%
Tortilla/Chunky				
ready-to-serve (Campbell's)	10.76 oz	9.6	293	30%
Turkey				
(Weight Watchers) RTS	10.5 oz	2	70	26%
Turkey/Chunky				
ready-to-serve	1 cup	4	136	27%
Turkey Noodle (Campbell's)	1 cup	3	70	39%
Turkey Rice				
(Hain) RTS	9.5 oz	3	100	27%
Turkey Vegtable				
(Campbell')	1 cup	3	70	39%
Chunky (Campbell's) RTS	9⅜ oz	6	150	36%
(Weight Watchers) RTS	10.5 oz	2	70	26%
Turkey Vegetable w/Ribbon Pasta				
(Pritikin)	7⅜ oz	.5	50	9%
Vegetable				
(Campbell's)	1 cup	2	80	23%
(Campbell's) Special Request	1 cup	2	80	23%
(Health Valley)	7.5 oz	1	100	9%
homemade	1 cup	–	70	–

Food and Description	Amount	Fat Grams	Total Calories	% Fat Calories
(Manischewitz)	1 cup	–	63	–
(Pritikin)	7⅜ oz	–	70	–
ready-to-serve (Progresso)	9.5 oz	3	100	27%
Chunky-(Health Valley)	7.5 oz	7	120	52%
ready-to-serve (Campbell's)	1 cup	3.7	122	27%
	10¾ oz	5	160	28%
	9.5 oz	4	140	26%
(Weight Watchers)	10.5 oz	2	100	18%
Vegtable Beef				
(Campbell's)	1 cup	2	70	26%
(Campbell's) Special Request	1 cup	2	70	26%
Chunky (Estee)	7.5 oz	7	140	45%
homemade	1 cup	25	320	70%
microwave (Lunch Bucket)	8.25 oz	5	140	32%
Vegetable Beef, Old Fashioned (Campbell's)				
Home Cookin' RTS	10¾ oz	3	140	19%
	9.5 oz	3	140	19%
Chunky (Campbell's) RTS	9.5 oz	5	160	28%
	10¾ oz	5	180	25%
Vegetable Chicken/chunky (Health Valley)	4 oz	7	120	53%
Vegetable, Country (Campbell's)				
Home Cookin'RTS	10¾ oz	2	120	15%
	9.5 oz	2	110	16%
microwave (Lunch Bucket)	8.25 oz	1	90	10%
Vegetable, Garden (Campbell's)	1 cup	1.8	63	26%
Vegetable, Homestyle (Campbell's)	1 cup	2	60	30%
Vegetable, Mediterranean/Chunky (Campbell's) RTS	9.5 oz	5	160	28%
Vegetable, Old Fashioned (Campbell's)	1 cup	1.6	60	24%
Vegetable, Old World (Campbell's) Soup for One	11 oz	4	130	28%
Vegetable, Vegetarian (Campbell's)	1 cup	2	80	23%
Vichyssoise	1 cup	6	148	37%
(Pepperidge Farm)	5.3 oz	6.9	114	55%
Watercress (Pepperidge Farm)	5.3 oz	3	90	30%
Won Ton				
(Campbell's)	1 cup	1	45	20%
homemade	1 cup	3	205	13%
Won Ton Imperial/Chunky ready-to-serve (Campbell's)	9.49 oz	3	121	22%

Food and Description	Amount	Fat Grams	Total Calories	% Fat Calories
SOUP/DEHYDRATED:				
(NOTE: Prepared as directed with water, unless otherwise stated. Pkg, pkt, or cube servings are unprepared.)				
Beef Broth or Bouilon	1 cup	.7	19	33%
Beef Broth (Cubed)	1 cube	–	8	–
with water	1 cup	–	8	–
Beef Noodle	1 cup	.79	41	17%
Broth				
(G. Washington's)				
Brown Seasoning	1 pkg	–	48	–
	1 serving	–	6	–
Brown Seasoning				
Kosher for Passover	1 pkg	–	48	–
	1 serving	–	6	–
Golden Seasoning	1 pkg	–	48	–
Golden Seasoning				
Kosher for Passover	1 serving	–	6	–
Onion Seasoning	1 pkg	–	96	–
	1 serving	–	12	–
Vegetable Seasoning	1 pkg	–	96	–
	1 serving	–	12	–
Romanoff (M B T)				
beef	1 pkt	.5	12	38%
chicken	1 pkt	.5	14	32%
onion	1 pkt	.5	16	28%
vegetable	1 pkt	.5	12	38%
Caldo Pronto				
(Sanwa)				
Albondigas Meatball w/noodles	1 cup	17	333	46%
Sabor A Camaron Shrimp	1 cup	14	310	41%
Sabor A Pollo Chicken	1 cup	13	310	38%
Sabor A Res Beef	1 cup	12	310	35%
(Campbell's)				
Chicken Noodle	8 oz	2	100	18%
Hearty Noodle	8 oz	2	100	18%
Vegetable	8 oz	1	60	15%
(Campbell's) Cup 2 Minute Soup Mix				
Broccoli	6 oz	3	70	39%
Chicken Noodle w/white meat	6 oz	2	90	20%
Chicken Vegetable	6 oz	2	90	20%
Creamy Chicken w/white meat	6 oz	5	120	38%
Noodle w/chicken broth	6 oz	2	100	18%
Tomato	6 oz	.5	90	5%
Vegetable Beef w/Sirloin Beef	6 oz	2	110	16%

Food and Description	Amount	Fat Grams	Total Calories	% Fat Calories
Cauliflower	1 pkg/.7 oz	1.7	68	23%
	1 cup	1.7	68	23%
Celery, Cream of	1 cup	1.6	63	23%
Chicken/(Right Time)	6 oz	–	14	–
Chicken Broth, Bouilon, Consomme	1 Pkt.	.8	16	45%
with water	1 cup	1	21	43%
Chicken Broth (Cubed)	1 cube	–	8	–
with water	1 cup	–	8	–
Chicken, Cream of	1 pkg/.6 oz	4	80	45%
	1 cup	5	107	42%
Chicken Noodle	1 cup	1	53	17%
(Campbell's)	1 cup	2	100	18%
Chicken Rice	1 cup	1	60	15%
Chicken Rice w/white meat				
(Campbell's)	1 cup	2	90	20%
Chicken Vegtable	1 cup	.79	49	15%
Clam Chowder-Manhattan	1 cup	1.55	65	22%
Clam Chowder-New England	1 cup	3.67	95	35%
Consomme W/Gelatin	1 pkg/2 oz	–	77	–
	1 cup	–	17	–
(Estee)				
Beef Noodle	6 oz	.5	20	23%
Chicken Noodle	6 oz	.5	25	18%
Mushroom	6 oz	2	40	45%
Onion	6 oz	.5	25	18%
Tomato	6 oz	.5	40	11%
Golden Mushroom	6 oz	1	60	15%
(Hain)				
Natural Classics Soup & Sauce				
Cheese	1/3 pkt	2	90	20%
	3/4 cup	16	250	58%
Minestrone	1/3 pkt	–	90	–
Onion	1/3 pkt	–	45	–
Potato Leek	1/3 pkt	–	50	–
Savory Soup				
Lentil	3/4 cup	2	130	8%
Minestrone	3/4 cup	1	110	8%
Potato Leek	3/4 cup	18	260	62%
Split Pea	3/4 cup	10	310	29%
Vegetable	3/4 cup	1	80	11%
no salt	3/4 cup	1	80	11%
Savory Soup & Recipe				
Cheese & Broccoli	3/4 cup	22	310	64%
Mushroom	3/4 cup	15	210	64%

Food and Description	Amount	Fat Grams	Total Calories	% Fat Calories
no salt	¾ cup	20	250	72%
Tomato	¾ cup	14	220	57%
Savory Soup, Dip & Recipe				
Onion	¾ cup	2	50	36%
no salt	¾ cup	1	50	18%
(Herb-Ox)				
Bouillon Cubes				
beef	1 cube	–	6	–
chicken	1 cube	–	6	–
Instant Broth				
beef	1 pkt	–	8	–
chicken	1 pkt	–	12	–
onion	1 pkt	–	14	–
Instant Broth, Low Sodium				
beef	1 pkt	–	12	–
chicken	1 pkt	–	12	–
onion	1 pkt	–	12	–
(Knorr) Soup mix				
Asparagus	8 oz	2	60	30%
Cauliflower	8 oz	2	80	23%
Chick'N Pasta	8 oz	2	90	20%
Chicken Noodle	8 oz	2	100	18%
Country Barley	8 oz	2	110	16%
Fine Herbs	8 oz	5	110	41%
French Onion	8 oz	1	45	20%
Leek	8 oz	2	70	26%
Minestrone	8 oz	2	110	16%
Mushroom	8 oz	3	80	34%
Oxtail Hearty Beef	8 oz	3	70	39%
Spinach	8 oz	2	70	26%
Tomato Basil	8 oz	3	90	30%
Vegetable	8 oz	1	35	26%
Leek	6 oz	2	71	25%
(Lipton)				
Cup-A-Soup				
Chicken & Noodles	6 oz	1	120	8%
Chicken-Flavored Broth	6 oz	.6	20	27%
Chicken'N Rice	6 oz	.8	47	15%
Chicken Noodle				
w/white meat	6 oz	1	50	18%
Chicken Vegetable	6 oz	.7	47	13%
Country Style Chicken				
flavor Supreme	6 oz	5.9	107	50%

Food and Description	Amount	Fat Grams	Total Calories	% Fat Calories
Country Style Chicken w/sweet corn	6 oz	5.5	133	37%
Country Style Harvest Vegetable	6 oz	1	90	10%
Country Style Hearty Chicken	6 oz	1	70	13%
Cream of Chicken	6 oz	4	80	45%
Cream of Mushroom	6 oz	3	70	39%
Creamy Broccoli	6 oz	2	60	30%
Creamy Broccoli & Cheese	6 oz	4	90	40%
Creamy Chicken w/vegetables	6 oz	6	110	49%
Creamy Onion	6 oz	3	70	39%
Green Pea	6 oz	4	113	32%
Lite Chicken Dijon	6 oz	1	50	18%
Lite Chicken Florentine	6 oz	.5	42	11%
Lite Creamy Broccoli	6 oz	1	50	18%
Lite Creamy Tomato & Herb	6 oz	< 1	65	7%
Lite Golden Broccoli	6 oz	1	42	21%
Lite Lemon Chicken	6 oz	1	45	20%
Lite Oriental	6 oz	1.7	45	34%
Lite Tomato & Herb	6 oz	1	60	15%
Onion	6 oz	.5	27	17%
Ring Noodle	6 oz	.7	47	13%
Spring Vegetable	6 oz	.8	33	22%
Tomato	6 oz	.9	103	8%
Vegetable Noodle Meatball	6 oz	2	100	18%
Lots-A-Noodles				
Beef	7 oz	1	110	8%
Hearty Garden Vegetable	7 oz	1.5	130	10%
Hearty Chicken	7 oz	1.5	118	11%
Hearty Chicken Noodle	7 oz	1	120	8%
Hearty Creamy Chicken	7 oz	8	180	40%
Lots-A-Noodles Single Serving				
Beef	9 oz	< 1	170	3%
Chicken	9 oz	2	180	10%
Oriental	9 oz	1	200	5%
Recipe & Soup Mix				
Beef Flavor Mushroom	8 oz	.5	38	12%
Beefy Onion	8 oz	1	30	30%
Golden Onion w/real chicken broth	8 oz	1.5	62	22%
Onion	8 oz	< 1	18	25%
Onion Mushroom	8 oz	.9	40	20%
Vegetable	8 oz	.5	39	12%
Soup Mix				
Country Vegetable	8 oz	.7	80	8%

Food and Description	Amount	Fat Grams	Total Calories	% Fat Calories
Giggle Noodle w/ real chicken broth	8 oz	2	77	23%
Hearty Beef Noodle	8 oz	.9	85	10%
Hearty Chicken Noodle	8 oz	1	83	11%
Hearty Noodle w/vegetables	8 oz	1.6	75	19%
Noodle w/real chicken broth	8 oz	2	70	26%
Ring-O-Noodle w/real chicken broth	8 oz	2	71	25%
(Lite-Line) Bouillon				
Low Sodium				
Beef	1 tsp	–	12	–
Chicken	1 tsp	–	12	–
(Mayacamas) Soup Mix				
Avgholemono	6 oz	1	59	15%
Cheddar Cheese	6 oz	5	83	54%
Chicken Style	6 oz	1	52	17%
Cockie Leekie	6 oz	1	59	15%
Cream of Mushroom	6 oz	1	52	17%
Cream of Tomato	6 oz	1	53	17%
Cream Soup Base	6 oz	1	55	16%
Creamy Clam	6 oz	1	65	14%
French Onion	6 oz	1	48	19%
Garden Pea	6 oz	1	65	14%
Lentil	6 oz	1	64	14%
Minestrone	6 oz	1	72	13%
Mock Turtle	6 oz	1	48	19%
Mulligatawny	6 oz	1	53	17%
Potato Leek	6 oz	1	60	15%
Senegalese	6 oz	1	54	17%
Minestrone	8 oz	1.7	79	19%
(Manischewitz)	6 oz	–	45	–
Mushroom	8 oz	4.86	96	46%
(Nile Spice)				
Lentil Curry	10.5 oz	–	200	–
Tomato Minestrone	10.5 oz	–	190	–
Vegetable Chicken	10.5 oz	–	190	–
Vegetable Parmesan	10.5 oz	1	200	5%
Noodle-Hearty				
(Campbell's)	8 oz	2	110	16%
Onion	1 Pkt	.5	35	13%
(Campbell's)	1 cup	–	50	–
(Lipton)	1 cup	1	35	26%
Onion Mushroom	8 oz	.5	80	6%
(Campbell's)	8 oz	1	50	18%
Oxtail	1 cup	2.55	71	32%
Pea, Green or Split	1 cup	1.58	133	11%

Food and Description	Amount	Fat Grams	Total Calories	% Fat Calories
(Manischewitz)	6 oz	.5	45	10%
(Soup Break) Instant				
Black Bean	6 oz	1	95	10%
Broccoli	6 oz	1	80	11%
Chicken Leek	6 oz	2	85	21%
Garden Pea	6 oz	1	85	11%
New England Clam	6 oz	2	105	17%
Potato Leek	6 oz	1	85	11%
Tomato	1 pkg/.7 oz	2	77	23%
	1 cup	2	102	18%
Tomato Vegetable	1 pkg/1.4 oz	2	125	14%
	1 cup	.87	55	14%
Vegetable				
(Campbell's)	1 cup	1	60	15%
(Manischewitz)	6 oz	–	50	–
Vegtable Beef	1 cup	1	53	17%
Vegtable, Cream of	1 cup	5.69	105	49%
(Wyler's) Bouillon				
Beef	1 tsp	–	6	–
	1 cube	–	6	–
Chicken	1 tsp	–	8	–
	1 cube	–	8	–
Onion	1 tsp	–	10	–
Vegetable	1 tsp	–	6	–
SOUP/MICROWAVE				
(Campbell's)				
Bean with Bacon'n Ham	8 oz	5	230	20%
Chicken Noodle	7.75 oz	4	100	36%
Chicken w/rice	7.75 oz	4	100	36%
Chili Beef	7 oz	4	190	19%
Vegetable Beef	7.75 oz	2	100	18%
SOUP GREENS (Durkee) - Jar	2.5 oz	3	216	13%
SOUR CREAM				
(Kemps)	1 cup	42	450	84%
Potato Topping	1 cup	41	450	82%
(Kemps)				
Light	1 cup	16	250	58%
Tator Topper	1 cup	16	250	58%
(Knudsen)				
Hamshire	4 Tbs	13	130	90%
Nice N'Light	4 Tbs	6	90	60%
(Land O'Lakes)				
regular	1 Tbs	2	32	56%
low-fat	1 Tbs	1	20	45%

Food and Description	Amount	Fat Grams	Total Calories	% Fat Calories
low-fat-Light Sour Cream				
Dairy Blend	1 Tbs	1	20	45%
low-fat-Light Sour Cream (Nice N Light)	4 Tbs	6	90	60%
regular (cultured)	1 Tbs	2.5	26	87%
	1 cup	48	493	87%
Sour Cream-half & half	1 Tbs	1.8	20	81%
(Weight Watchers)-Light	2 Tbs	2	35	51%
SOUR CREAM SUBSTITUTES				
Sour Cream-flavored sprinkle products:				
Best of Butter	½ tsp	< 1	4	100%
Molly McButter	½ tsp	< 1	4	100%
Sour Cream/substitute				
non-butterfat	1 oz	4	42	86%
	1 cup	39	417	84%
non-dairy	1 oz	6	59	92%
(Chivo)	1 Tbs	3	30	90%
(Dean's)-Sour Delite	1 oz	5	50	90%
(IMO)	1 Tbs	3	30	90%
(Land O'Lakes)				
Light Dairy Blend	1 Tbs	1	20	45%
(Slender Choice)	1 Tbs	2	26	69%
SOURSOP/pureed	1 cup	.7	146	4%
SOY MEAL/defatted	½ cup	1	206	4%
SOY MILK				
Dry (Soyamel)	1 oz	7	130	49%
Fluid	1 cup	4.58	79	52%
(Edensoy)				
Carob	1 cup	4.5	160	25%
Original	1 cup	5	140	32%
Vanilla	1 cup	2	150	12%
(Health Valley)-Soy Moo	8.5 oz	6	120	45%
(Isomil)-infant formula w/iron	5 oz	5	100	45%
(ISoyalac)-infant formula	5 oz	5.5	100	50%
(Soyalac)-infant formula	5 oz	5.5	100	50%
(Vitasoy)				
Creamy Original	6 oz	1	105	9%
Vanilla Delite	6 oz	4	150	24%
(Westsoy)-nondairy	1 cup	7	170	37%
SOY PROTEIN CONCENTRATE	1 oz	–	92	–
SOY SAUCE (*See also* SAUCE)				
(Shoyu)	1 Tbs	–	9	–
	¼ cup	–	30	–
(Tamari)	1 Tbs	–	11	–
	¼ cup	–	35	–

Food and Description	Amount	Fat Grams	Total Calories	% Fat Calories
SOYA GRANULES (Feam)	¼ cup	–	140	–
SOYBEAN (See also individual products of, such as MISO PASTE, TOFU, etc.)				
Green				
boiled	½ cup	5.8	127	41%
canned (La Loma)				
w/liquid	~ 4 oz	7	120	53%
raw	½ cup	19	387	44%
roasted	½ cup	21.8	405	48%
SOYBEAN NUTS				
roasted-dry	½ cup	18.6	387	43%
roasted-salted or unsalted	1 oz	6.8	129	47%
	½ cup	21.8	405	48%
roasted & toasted	1 oz	6.8	129	47%
SOYBEAN SPROUTS				
cooked	½ cup	2	38	47%
raw	10 sprouts	.6	12	45%
stir-fried	4 oz	8	143	50%
SPAGHETTI (See PASTA)				
SPAGHETTI DINNERS (See also PASTA DINNERS)				
Spaghetti w/meat sauce				
Box (Kraft)	1 cup	14	360	35%
Canned (Franco-American)	7.5 oz	8	211	34%
Spaghetti w/meatballs & meat sauce				
Canned	1 cup	10	260	35%
(Chef Boyardee)	7 oz	8	210	34%
(Estee)	7.5 oz	14	240	53%
(Franco-American)	7⅜ oz	8	220	33%
Standard Home Recipe (USDA)	1 cup	12	330	33%
Spaghetti w/meatballs & tomato sauce				
canned	1 cup	10.8	258	38%
homemade	1 cup	11.7	332	32%
Spaghetti w/tomato sauce & cheese				
canned	1 cup	1.5	190	7%
homemade	1 cup	8.8	280	28%
SPAGHETTI SAUCE (See SAUCE)				
SPAGHETTIO'S				
Canned (Franco-American)				
w/Meat balls	7⅜ oz	8	210	34%
w/Sliced beef franks	7⅜ oz	9	220	33%
SPICE BLENDS				
(Lawry's)				
Bacon Onion	1 tsp	–	10	–
Garlic Pepper	¼ tsp	–	2	–
Garlic Powder w/parsley	1 tsp	–	12	–

Food and Description	Amount	Fat Grams	Total Calories	% Fat Calories
Garlic Salt	1 tsp	–	4	–
Hot'N Spicy Seasoned Salt	1 tsp	–	3	–
Lemon Pepper	1 tsp	–	6	–
Minced Onion	1 tsp	–	7	–
Pinch of Herbs	1 tsp	.5	9	50%
Salt Free 17	1 tsp	–	10	–
Seasoned Pepper	1 tsp	–	9	–
Seasoned Salt	1 tsp	–	4	–
Seasoned Salt Free	1 tsp	–	3	–
Seasoned Lite Salt	1 tsp	–	8	–
(Mrs. Dash)				
Extra Spicy	1 tsp	–	12	–
Lemon & Herb	1 tsp	–	12	–
Low Pepper	1 tsp	–	12	–
No Garlic	1 tsp	–	12	–
Original	1 tsp	–	12	–
Table Blend	1 tsp	–	9	–
SPICES (See individual listings)				
SPINACH				
Spinach				
canned	½ cup	< 1	25	18%
canned-chopped or whole leaf- (Del Monte)	½ cup	–	25	–
canned-Premium Northwest (S&W)	½ cup	–	25	–
fresh-boiled	½ cup	–	21	–
frozen-(Green Giant)	½ cup	–	25	–
(Harvest Fresh)	½ cup	–	25	–
(Pictsweet)-Leaf	3.3 oz	–	20	–
Express-Microwave	2.4 oz	–	18	–
frozen-boiled	½ cup	–	27	–
raw/chopped	½ cup	–	6	–
Spinach-New Zealand				
boiled	½ cup	–	12	–
raw	1 lb	1	86	11%
SPINACH DISHES				
Creamed Spinach/frozen (Green Giant)	½ cup	3	80	34%
Cut Leaf Spinach in butter sauce /frozen (Green Giant)	½ cup	2	45	40%
Spinach, creamed/frozen (Birds Eye)	½ cup	4	60	60%
Spinach Quiche/hommade	~ 5 oz	25.7	337	69%
Spinach Souffle w/whole milk, butter, and cheese/homemade	1 cup	18	218	74%
SPOT FISH				
cooked-dry heat	3 oz	18.6	252	66%

Food and Description	Amount	Fat Grams	Total Calories	% Fat Calories
raw	3 oz	13.5	188	65%
SQUAB (Pigeon)				
breast meat only-raw	~ 4 oz	4.57	135	30%
giblets-raw	3 oz	6	132	41%
meat & skin-raw	~ 7 oz	47	584	72%
meat only-raw	~ 6 oz	12.6	239	47%
SQUASH				
Summer/fresh-boiled	½ cup	–	18	–
Crookneck/fresh-boiled	½ cup	–	18	–
/frozen	½ cup	–	24	–
Scallop/fresh-boiled	½ cup	–	14	–
mashed	½ cup	–	19	–
Zucchini & Cocozelle/raw	½ cup	–	9	–
canned (S&W) Italian Style	½ cup	–	45	–
fresh				
boiled	½ cup	–	14	–
mashed	½ cup	–	15	–
frozen	½ cup	–	19	–
Winter/fresh-baked	½ cup	.6	39	14%
fresh-boiled-mashed	½ cup	–	47	–
frozen-cooked (Birds Eye)	½ cup	–	45	–
Acorn/fresh-baked	½ cup	–	57	–
fresh-boiled-mashed	½ cup	–	41	–
Butternut/fresh-baked	½ cup	–	41	–
fresh-boiled-mashed	½ cup	–	50	–
frozen	½ cup	–	47	–
Hubbard/fresh-baked	½ cup	.6	51	11%
fresh-boiled-mashed	½ cup	–	37	–
Spaghetti/boiled or baked	½ cup	–	23	–
SQUASH DISHES				
Zucchini, Breaded/frozen (Stilwell)	3.3 oz	10	200	45%
(Ore Ida)	3 oz	9	150	54%
Zucchini, Italian style/canned	½ cup	–	33	–
Zucchini Sticks-Light Batter/frozen -				
(Pepperidge Farm)	3 oz	12	200	54%
SQUID				
breaded & fried	3 oz	6	149	36%
dried	3 oz	4.6	260	16%
pickled	1 oz	–	23	–
raw	3 oz	1	78	12%
SQUIRREL/raw-boneless	3 oz	8.5	182	42%
STEAK SAUCE				
(French's)	1 Tbs	–	16	–

Food and Description	Amount	Fat Grams	Total Calories	% Fat Calories
STRAWBERRY				
fresh	1 cup	.56	45	11%
	1 pint	1	97	9%
frozen lite syrup (Birds Eye)	5 oz	< 1	90	5%
frozen syrup-halved (Birds Eye)	5 oz	< 1	120	4%
frozen				
sweetened				
sliced	1 cup	< 1	245	2%
whole	1 cup	< 1	200	2%
unsweetened	3.5 oz	< 1	50	9%
unsweetened-unthawed	1 cup	< 1	52	9%
STRAWBERRY-BANANA JUICE				
Nectar/bottled	6 oz	–	100	–
STRAWBERRY DRINK	8 oz	–	125	–
with Vitamin C	8 oz	–	89	–
(Juice Works)	6 oz	–	94	–
STRAWBERRY JUICE				
Strawberry (Smucker's)	8 oz	–	130	–
Strawberry Delight/bottled	6 oz	–	80	–
Stawberry Nectar/bottled (Kern's)	6 oz	–	110	–
Strawberry, Ripe Nectar (Libby's)	8 oz	–	150	–
STUFFING				
(Betty Crocker)-mix				
Chicken/dry	¼ pkg	1	110	8%
Chicken/prepared	¼ pkg	9	180	45%
Corn Bread/dry	¼ pkg	1	110	8%
Corn/prepared	¼ pkg	9	180	45%
Pork/dry	¼ pkg	.5	110	4%
Pork/prepared	¼ pkg	9	190	43%
Traditional Herb/dry	¼ pkg	.5	110	4%
Traditional Herb/prepared	¼ pkg	9	190	43%
Corn Bread				
(Pepperidge Farm)-dry	1 oz	1	110	8%
(Golden Grains) mix				
prepared as directed				
All Flavors	½ cup	9	180	45%
(Oven Stuffin')-mix				
Chicken/dry	1 oz	1	120	8%
Chicken/prepared	½ cup	9	190	43%
Cornbread Flavor/dry	~ 1 oz	1	120	8%
Cornbread/prepared	½ cup	9	190	43%
(Pepperidge Farms)-dry-pkg				
Corn Bread,Cubed, Country Style, &				
Herb Seasoned	1 oz	1	110	8%

Food and Description	Amount	Fat Grams	Total Calories	% Fat Calories
Distinctive Stuffing-				
Apples & Raisin	1 oz	2	100	18%
Country Garden Herb	1 oz	3	110	25%
Harvest Veg & Almond	1 oz	4	110	33%
Wild Rice & Mushroom	1 oz	2	100	18%
(Pillsbury) Stuffing Originals				
Chicken	½ cup	7	170	37%
Cornbread	½ cup	6	170	32%
Mushroom	½ cup	7	150	42%
Wild Rice	½ cup	7	160	39%
(Stove Top Stuffing) Microwave				
Broccoli & Cheese/mix	1 serving	5	140	32%
/prepared	1 serving	8	170	42%
Homestyle Cornbread/mix	1 serving	3	120	23%
/prepared	1 serving	7	160	39%
Mushroom & Onion/mix	1 serving	3	130	21%
/prepared	1 serving	7	170	37%
Regular				
prepared w/butter	½ cup	7	160	39%
prepared w/o butter	½ cup	4	130	28%
(Stove Top Stuffing) Mix				
prepared w/butter				
Americana New England	½ cup	9	180	45%
Americana San Francisco	½ cup	9	170	48%
Beef	½ cup	9	180	45%
Chicken Flavor	½ cup	9	180	45%
Chicken Flavor -(Flexible Serving)	½ cup	9	170	48%
Cornbread	½ cup	9	170	48%
Cornbread -(Flexible Serving)	½ cup	8	170	48%
Homestyle Herb -(Flexible Serving)	½ cup	9	170	48%
Long Grain & Wild Rice	½ cup	9	180	45%
Pork	½ cup	9	170	48%
Savory Herbs	½ cup	9	180	45%
Turkey	½ cup	9	170	48%
With Rice	½ cup	9	180	45%
prepared w/o butter				
Chicken Flavor	½ cup	1	110	8%
regular	½ cup	1	110	8%
stuffing w/beef broth	½ cup	9	180	45%
(Stove Top Stuffing)15 minute Mix				
Long Grain & Wild Rice mix	1 serving	1	110	8%
prepared	1 serving	9	180	45%
Mushroom & Onion mix	1 serving	1	110	8%
prepared	1 serving	9	180	45%

Food and Description	Amount	Fat Grams	Total Calories	% Fat Calories
STURGEON				
cooked-dry heat	3 oz	4	115	31%
raw	3 oz	3	90	30%
smoked	3 oz	3.7	147	23%
steamed	3 oz	4.8	135	32%
SUCCOTASH (*See also* VEGETABLES, MIXED)				
Country Style-canned				
(Libby)	½ cup	1	80	11%
(S & W)	½ cup	1	80	11%
Homemade	½ cup	–	110	–
SUCKER/raw				
White	3 oz	1.97	79	22%
SUET/raw	1 Tbs	13	121	100%
SUGAR				
Brown	1 cup	–	541	–
Firmly packed	1 cup	–	821	–
	1 Tbs	–	52	–
	1 tsp	–	18	–
Maple	1 piece/			
	1 oz	–	99	–
	1 Tbs	–	52	–
Powdered	1 cup	–	462	–
	1 Tbs	–	31	–
	1 tsp	–	10	–
White-granulated	1 cube	–	25	–
	1 tsp	–	15	–
	1 Tbs	–	46	–
	1 cup	–	770	–
SUGAR APPLE/raw				
(Sweetsop)	1 cup	.8	235	3%
SUGAR SUBSTITUTE				
(Equal)	1 pkt	–	4	–
	1 tablet	–	.5	–
Fructose	1 tsp	–	12	–
(Superose)	1 pkt	–	12	–
(Nutradiet) Sweetener	any amount	–	–	–
(Nutrasweet)	1 pkt	–	4	–
Sprinkle Sweet	1 tsp	–	–	–
Sucaryl	1 tsp	–	–	–
Sugar Twin	1 tsp	–	–	–
	1 pkt	–	< 4	–
brown sugar	1 tsp	–	1.5	–
Sweet * 10	⅛ tsp	–	–	–
Sweet'n It (Estee)	6 drops	–	–	–

Food and Description	Amount	Fat Grams	Total Calories	% Fat Calories
Sweet'N Low	1 tsp	–	12	–
	1 packet	–	4	–
	1 tablet	–	–	–
brown sugar	1/10 tsp	–	2	–
Sweet'N Low-liquid	10 drops	–	–	–
Sweet'ner (Weight Watchers)	1 pkt	–	3.5	–
	1 measuring spoon	–	4	–
SUNFISH/raw	3 oz	.6	76	7%
SUNFLOWER BUTTER	1 Tbs	8	92	78%
(Hain)	2 Tbs	15	180	75%
SUNFLOWER NUTS (PLANTERS)				
dry roasted	1 oz	14	160	79%
unsalted	1 oz	15	170	79%
oil roasted	1 oz	15	170	79%
SUNFLOWER SEED				
(Frito Lay's)	1oz	16	170	85%
Kernels	1 oz	17	180	85%
kernels-dried	1 oz	14	162	78%
	1 cup	71	821	78%
(Planters)	1 oz	14	160	79%
kernels-dry roasted	1 oz	14	165	76%
	1 cup	63.7	745	77%
kernels-oil roasted	1 oz	16	175	82%
	1 cup	77.56	830	84%
kernels-toasted	1 oz	16	176	82%
	1 cup	76	829	83%
(Laura Scudder's)				
dry roasted	1 oz	8.5	144	53%
oil roasted	1 oz	17	190	81%
roasted in shell	1 oz	7	86	73%
SUNFLOWER SEED BUTTER	1 oz	13.6	165	74%
	1 Tbs	7.6	93	74%
SUNFLOWER SEED FLOWER				
(partially defatted)	1 cup	1	261	3%
SURIMI	3 oz	.8	84	9%
SWAMP CABBAGE/fresh-boiled	½ cup	–	10	–
SWEET 'N SOUR SAUCE (*See* SAUCE)				
SWEET POTATO				
boiled-no skin-mashed	½ cup	.5	172	3%
canned-mashed	1 cup	.5	258	2%
pieces	1 cup	< 1	183	3%
w/syrup	1 cup	< 1	212	2%
dehydrated flakes/dry	½ cup	< 1	228	2%

Food and Description	Amount	Fat Grams	Total Calories	% Fat Calories
prepared w/water	1 cup	< 1	242	2%
fresh-baked-mashed	½ cup	< 1	103	4%
frozen-baked	½ cup	< 1	88	5%
raw whole potato	½ cup	1	118	5%
SWEET POTATO DISHES				
Candied w/butter and brown sugar				
homemade	~ 3.5 oz	3	144	19%
Candied Sweets'N Apples-frozen				
(Pepperidge Farm)	4 oz	–	160	–
Candied Sweet Potatoes-frozen				
(Pepperidge Farm)	4 oz	–	190	–
(Birds Eye) Specialty Classics	5 oz	9	220	37%
(Mrs. Paul's) microwavable	4 oz	–	190	–
SWEET POTATO LEAVES				
cooked	1 cup	< 1	22	21%
raw-chopped	1 cup	< 1	12	38%
SWEETENER, ARTIFICIAL (*See* SUGAR SUBSTITUTE)				
SWORDFISH				
breaded & fried	3 oz	11.9	207	52%
cooked-dry heat	3 oz	4	132	27%
raw	3 oz	3	103	26%
SYRUP (*See also* PANCAKE/WAFFLE SYRUP)				
Cane	1 Tbs	–	53	–
Corn	1 Tbs	–	59	–
(Karo)				
Dark	1 Tbs	–	60	–
	½ cup	–	480	–
Light	1 Tbs	–	60	–
	½ cup	–	480	–
Maple	1 Tbs	–	50	–

T

Food and Description	Amount	Fat Grams	Total Calories	% Fat Calories
TABASCO SAUCE (*See* SAUCE)				
TABOULI (TABOULE, TABOULY)				
(Casbah) mix-prepared	1 Serving	1	148	6%
(Near East) wheat salad mix	⅞ oz	–	80	–
TACO SAUCE (*See* SAUCE)				

Food and Description	Amount	Fat Grams	Total Calories	% Fat Calories
TAMARIND/fresh	1	–	5	–
TANGELO/fresh	1	–	39	–
TANGELO JUICE/fresh	8 oz	–	101	–
TANGERINE				
fresh	1	–	37	–
canned				
in juice	½ cup	–	46	–
in syrup	½ cup	–	76	–
TANGERINE JUICE				
Mandarin Tangerine Juice				
(Dole) Pure & Light	6 oz	–	100	–
Tangerine Juice				
canned	8 oz	–	107	–
canned (sweetened)	1 cup	.5	125	4%
fresh	8 oz	–	108	–
from frozen concentrate	8 oz	–	114	–
undiluted	6 oz	< 1	345	1%
TAPIOCA (*See also* PUDDING)				
(Minute)	1 Tbs	–	30	–
	3.5 oz	–	352	–
TARO				
chips	10	5.86	110	48%
fresh-cooked-slices	½ cup	–	94	–
leaves-raw	½ cup	–	12	–
steamed	½ cup	< 1	17	27%
raw	½ cup	–	56	–
shoots	~ 3 oz	< 1	9	50%
Tahitian				
cooked-sliced	½ cup	< 1	30	15%
raw-sliced	½ cup	1	25	36%
TARRAGON/ground	1 tsp	–	5	–
TARTAR SAUCE (*See also* SAUCE)				
Generic	1 Tbs	8	75	96%
TAVERN NUTS				
(Planters)	1 oz	15	170	79%
TEA				
Brewed	6 oz	–	2	–
(Bigelow) Regular/all flavors	6oz	–	1	–
(Celestial Seasonings)				
all flavors	1cup	–	1-7	–
Kafree (Worthington)				
caffeine free	1bag	–	1	–
(Lipton) Herbal tea bags				
all flavors	1 bag	–	4	–

Food and Description	Amount	Fat Grams	Total Calories	% Fat Calories
(Nestea) tea bags	1 bag	–	2	–
Canned w/sugar	12 oz	–	146	–
Instant-mixes				
(Crystal Light)-diet	8 oz	–	4	–
(Lipton)	6 oz	–	–	–
decaffeinated	6 oz	–	–	–
sugar-free	8 oz	–	1	–
decaffeinated	8 oz	–	1	–
with Nutrasweet	8 oz	–	5	–
decaffeinated	8 oz	–	5	–
lemon flavored-sweetened	6 oz	–	55	–
lemon flavored-unsweetened	8 oz	–	3	–
(Maxwell House) concentrate-				
sweetened	8 oz	–	80	–
unsweetened	8 oz	–	2	–
(Maxwell House) instant	6 oz	–	2	–
(Nestea)-decaffeinated	6 oz	–	–	–
decaffeinated ice tea mix				
sugar-free	8 oz	–	6	–
Iced tea mix-sugar-free	8 oz	–	6	–
Iced tea mix w/sugar &				
lemon	8 oz	–	70	–
Purepak iced tea w/sugar &				
lemon	8 oz	–	70	–
Purepak iced tea-sugar-free				
w/lemon	8 oz	–	2	–
(Nestea) Ice Teasers-Citrus	8 oz	–	6	–
Lemon	8 oz	–	6	–
Orange	8 oz	–	6	–
Tropical	8 oz	–	6	–
WildCherry	8 oz	–	6	–
sugar-free/all flavors	8 oz	–	4	–
sugar sweetened w/lemon	12 oz	–	120	–
(Wyler's)-fruit tea punch				
bottle	6 oz	–	118	–
canned	6 oz	–	118	–
Russian tea	8 oz	–	111	–
TEACLE/black	1 Tbs	–	53	–
TEMPEH	½ cup	6	165	33%
TEMPURA BATTER MIX				
Krusteaz	1 oz	–	102	–
S&B Sunbird	1 pkg	.5	112	4%
TEQUILA (*See* DISTILLED LIQUOR)				
TERIYAKI SAUCE (*See* SAUCE)				

Food and Description	Amount	Fat Grams	Total Calories	% Fat Calories
TERRAPIN/baked	3/4 cup	4	161	22%
THYME/ground	1 tsp	–	4	–
TILEFISH				
cooked-dry heat	3 oz	3	117	23%
raw	3 oz	2	80	23%
TOASTER PASTRY (*See* PASTRY, TOASTER)				
TOFU				
dried-frozen	~ ½ oz	5	82	55%
fried	~ ½ oz	2.6	35	67%
Okara	½ cup	1	47	19%
raw-firm	¼ block	7	118	53%
	½ cup	10.98	183	54%
(Hinoichi)-Chinese	4 oz	3	70	39%
raw-regular	¼ block	5.55	88	57%
	½ cup	5.9	94	57%
(Hinoichi) Japanese	4 oz	2	60	30%
salted & fermented-fuyu	1 block	1	13	69%
soft-(Hinoichi)-Kinugoshi	4 oz	2	50	36%
TOFU FROZEN DESSERT PRODUCTS				
Dreamy Tofu	½ cup	4.8	135	32%
Le Tofu				
chocolate	3.5 oz	7.7	155	45%
strawberry	3.5 oz	8.5	163	47%
vanilla	3.5 oz	7.8	155	45%
Tofulite	4 oz	7	150	42%
Tofutti				
(hard)	4 oz	13	220	53%
(soft)	4 oz	8	158	46%
(soft)-Lite				
Hi-Lite chocolate	4 oz	1	100	9%
Hi-Lite vanilla	4 oz	1	90	10%
Cappuccino Love Drops	4 oz	12	230	47%
Chocolate Cuties	4 oz	5	140	32%
Chocolate Love Drops	4 oz	13	220	53%
chocolate supreme	4 oz	13	210	56%
vanilla	4 oz	11	200	50%
vanilla almond bark	4 oz	14	230	55%
Vanilla Cuties	4 oz	5	130	35%
Vanilla Love Drops	4 oz	12	220	49%
Wildberry	4 oz	12	210	51%
Tofutti Cutie				
chocolate sandwich	1	5	140	32%
vanilla sandwich	1	5	130	35%

Food and Description	Amount	Fat Grams	Total Calories	% Fat Calories
Tofutti Lite lite				
chocolate-vanilla twirl	4 oz	< 1	90	5%
vanilla,chocolate,strawberry	4 oz	< 1	90	5%
Tofruzen (non-dairy)				
strawberry	4 oz	8	160	5%
praline pecan	4 oz	8	180	40%
vanilla almond	4 oz	8	180	40%
TOMATO				
Green	1	–	30	–
Red	1	–	24	–
canned-California Sliced-				
(Contadina)	½ cup	–	40	–
canned-crushed (Hunt's)	½ cup	< 1	25	18%
canned-Italian Style (pear)-				
(Contadina)	½ cup	–	25	–
(S&W)	½ cup	–	25	–
canned-Italian Style Stewed-				
(Contadina)	½ cup	–	35	–
(S&W)	½ cup	–	35	–
canned-ready cut-peeled (S&W)	½ cup	–	25	–
canned-stewed (Contadina)	½ cup	–	35	–
(Del Monte)	½ cup	–	35	–
(Hunt's)	½ cup	–	35	–
(S&W)	½ cup	–	35	–
canned-stewed-50% less salt				
(S&W)	½ cup	–	35	–
canned-stewed-Mexican Style				
(S&W)	½ cup	–	40	–
canned-wedges (Del Monte)	½ cup	–	30	–
canned-whole (Hunt's)	½ cup	–	20	–
(Nutradiet)	½ cup	–	25	–
canned-whole-peeled (Contadina)	½ cup	–	25	–
(Del Monte)	½ cup	–	25	–
(S&W)	½ cup	–	25	–
TOMATO ASPIC/canned				
Supreme (S&W)	½ cup	–	60	–
TOMATO DISHES				
Stewed Tomatoes				
homemade	1 cup	2	60	30%
TOMATO JUICE				
canned	6 oz	–	32	–
(Campbell's)	6 oz	–	35	–
(Hunt's)-no salt added	6 oz	–	30	–
(Nutradiet)	6 oz	–	35	–

Food and Description	Amount	Fat Grams	Total Calories	% Fat Calories
(S&W)-California	6 oz	–	35	–
Tomato w/beef broth/canned	5.5 oz	–	61	–
Tomato & Chile Cocktail (Del Monte)-				
Snap-E-Tom	6 oz	–	40	–
Tomato & Clam/canned	5.5 oz	–	77	–
TOMATO MARINARA SAUCE/canned	1 cup	8	171	42%
TOMATO PASTE/canned	½ cup	1	110	8%
(Contadina)	2 oz	–	50	–
canned Italian style	2 oz	1	65	14%
(Del Monte)	¾ cup	1	150	6%
(Hunt's)	2 oz	–	45	–
Italian Style	2 oz	–	50	–
(S&W)	6 oz	–	150	–
TOMATO POWDER	4 oz	< 1	342	1%
TOMATO PUREE/canned	1 cup	–	102	–
canned (Contadina)	½ cup	–	40	–
w/crushed tomatoes	½ cup	–	30	–
(Hunt's)	4 oz	–	45	–
(S&W)	4 oz	–	60	–
w/diced tomatoes	4 oz	–	35	–
TOMATO SAUCE (See also SAUCE)				
canned (Contadina)	½ cup	–	30	–
Italian	½ cup	–	30	–
Thick & Zesty	½ cup	–	40	–
canned (Del Monte)	1 cup	1	70	13%
w/onions	1 cup	1	100	9%
canned (Hunt's)	4 oz	–	30	–
Italian	4 oz	2	60	30%
(S&W)	½ cup	–	40	–
TOMATO SOUP (See SOUP)				
TONIC WATER (See SODA)				
TORTELLINI SOUP (See SOUP)				
TORTILLA				
corn				
(Azteca)	1	–	45	–
(El Charrito)	2	1	95	10%
(Old El Paso)	1	1	60	15%
taco shell	1	2	50	36%
tostada shell	1	2	50	36%
flour				
(7") (Azteca)	1	2	85	21%
(9") (Azteca)	1	3	130	21%
taco salad shell (Azteca)	1	12	200	54%

ood and Description	Amount	Fat Grams	Total Calories	% Fat Calories
whole wheat tortilla	1-1.5 oz	1.8	93	17%
ix				
Corn Masa Harina-De Maiz				
(Quaker) 6" dia	2	1	140	6%
Wheat Masa Trigo				
(Quaker) 6" dia	2	4	150	24%
Quaker				
Corn-Masa Harina De Maiz	1 cup	5	411	11%
Wheat-Masa Trigo	1 cup	12	445	24%
ROUT				
ixed				
raw	3 oz	5.6	126	40%
ainbow				
broiled with butter	3 oz	9	175	46%
cooked-dry heat	3 oz	3.66	129	26%
raw	3 oz	2.85	100	26%
smoked	3 oz	3	153	18%
UMERIC/ground	1 tsp	–	8	–
UNA (See also SEAFOOD ENTREE/DINNER)				
luefin				
fresh-raw	3 oz	4	122	30%
cooked-dry heat	3 oz	5	157	29%
ght				
canned in oil	3 oz	6.98	169	37%
canned in water	3 oz	< 1	111	4%
ght Chunk				
canned in oil				
(Bumble Bee)	2 oz	12	160	68%
(Carnation)	2 oz	8	125	58%
(Chicken of the Sea)	2 oz	13	170	69%
(S&W)-Fancy	2 oz	10	140	64%
(Star Kist)	2 oz	13	150	78%
ght Chunk				
canned in water				
(Carnation)	2 oz	2	70	26%
(Chicken of the Sea)	2 oz	1	60	5%
(Chicken of the Sea)	3.5 oz	1	105	9%
(Featherweight)	2 oz	1	60	15%
(S&W)-Fancy	2 oz	1	60	15%
(Star Kist)	2 oz	.5	60	8%
canned in distilled water				
(Star Kist)	2 oz	.5	65	7%
kipjack				
fresh-raw	3 oz	1	88	10%

Food and Description	Amount	Fat Grams	Total Calories	% Fat Calories
White				
canned in oil	2 oz	6.87	158	39%
canned in water	2 oz	2	116	16%
White-chunk				
canned in water				
(Bumble Bee)	2 oz	2	70	26%
White-solid				
canned in oil				
(Star Kist)	2 oz	13	150	78%
canned in water				
(Bumble Bee)	2 oz	2	70	26%
White-solid Albacore				
canned Fancy				
in oil (S&W)	2 oz	12	160	68%
canned in water				
(Chicken of the Sea)	3.5 oz	2	120	15%
(Star Kist)	2 oz	.5	70	6%
Yellowfin				
fresh-raw	3 oz	1	90	10%
TUNA HELPER (*See also* SEAFOOD ENTREE/DINNER)				
(Betty Crocker) prepared				
Cheesy Noodles	⅕ pkg	9	250	32%
Cold Salad	⅕ pkg	27	420	58%
Creamy Noodles	⅕ pkg	14	300	42%
Fettuccine Alfredo	⅕ pkg	14	300	42%
Pot Pie	⅙ pkg	27	420	58%
Romanoff	⅕ pkg	9	290	28%
Tetrazzini	⅕ pkg	8	240	30%
Tuna Au Gratin	⅕ pkg	11	280	35%
TUNA SALAD				
commercial				
(Carnation)				
The Spreadables	1.875 oz	6	90	60%
homemade-includes salad dressing,				
tuna canned in oil, & NO EGG	1 cup	19	375	46%
TURBINADO SUGAR				
(Hain)	1 Tbs	–	50	–
TURBOT/raw	3 oz	2.5	81	28%
TURKEY				
(NOTE: All turkey meat is roasted, unless otherwise stated.)				
all classes/meat, skin, giblets,				
and neck-roasted-1 whole turkey	~ 9 lb	379.97	8245	42%
dark meat w/skin	~ 2 lb	93	1789	47%
dark meat w/o skin	~ 5 oz	10	262	34%

Food and Description	Amount	Fat Grams	Total Calories	% Fat Calories
giblets /simmered	~ 5 oz	7	243	26%
gizzard/simmered	~ 5 oz	5.6	236	21%
heart/simmered	~ 5 oz	8	257	28%
light meat w/skin	2¼ lb	87	206	38%
light meat w/o skin	~ 5 oz	4.5	219	19%
liver/simmered	~ 5 oz	8	237	30%
meat & skin-dark & light-no giblets				
or neck	~ 4 lb	180.6	3857	42%
(Butterball)-Deep basted	3.5 oz	9-10	190-200	42%-45%
meat only (dark & light)	~ 5 oz	6.95	238	26%
(Louis Rich)-fresh whole	1 oz	3	55	49%
(Armour Star)				
Broth basted w/sugar	4 oz	10	180	50%
w/o sugar	4 oz	10	180	50%
Butter basted	4 oz	10	190	47%
(Butterball)				
boneless-light & dark-meat				
only-cooked	3.5 oz	7	140	45%
Deep Basted-dark meat w/o skin	3.5 oz	10	195	46%
light meat w/o skin	3.5 oz	4	160	23%
Li'L Butterball/frozen				
light & dark-meat only-				
cooked	3.5 oz	7	175	36%
Stuffed/frozen-light-meat only-				
cooked	3.5 oz	3.5	140	23%
dark meat only-cooked	3.5 oz	7	175	36%
(Butterball)-cooked parts w/o skin				
breast fillet	3.5 oz	3.5	140	23%
breast half	3.5 oz	7	175	36%
breast slices	3.5 oz	3.5	140	23%
drumsticks	3.5 oz	7	175	36%
thighs	3.5 oz	14	245	51%
wing drumettes	3.5 oz	10	280	32%
wings	3.5 oz	10.5	210	45%
(Land O'Lakes)-Fresh				
Breast	3 oz	1	100	9%
Drumsticks	3 oz	5	120	38%
Thighs	3 oz	10	150	60%
Wings	3 oz	5	120	38%
Butter-basted young turkey	3 oz	8	140	51%
Plain young turkey	3 oz	7	130	49%
Self-(broth) basting young	3 oz	5	120	38%
Turkey Hindquarters Roast	3 oz	8	140	51%

Food and Description	Amount	Fat Grams	Total Calories	% Fat Calories
(Louis Rich)-Fresh Turkey Cuts				
Turkey Breast-cooked	1 oz	2	45	40%
Turkey Breast Roast-cooked	1 oz	1	40	23%
Turkey Breast Slices-cooked	1 oz	1	40	23%
Turkey Breast Steaks-cooked	1 oz	1	40	23%
Turkey Breast Tenderloins-cooked	1 oz	.5	40	11%
Turkey Drumsticks	1 oz	3	55	49%
Turkey Thighs	1 oz	4	65	55%
Turkey Wings	1 oz	3	55	49%
Turkey Wing Drumettes	1 oz	2	50	36%
Turkey Wing Portions	1 oz	3	55	49%
Turkey Back/meat only-simmered	~ 5 oz	11	274	36%
Turkey Breast/meat & skin (½ breast)	~ 2 lb	64	1637	35%
Turkey Breast/(Armour)				
Turkey Selects-boneless -				
Breast Roast	3 oz	5	120	38%
Breast slices	3 oz	1	90	10%
Breast Tenderloins	3 oz	1	90	10%
Turkey Strips	3 oz	4	100	36%
Turkey Breast/meat only (Butterball) frozen-cooked	3.5 oz	7	175	36%
Turkey Breast of/boneless meat only (Butterball)-cooked	3.5 oz	3.5	140	23%
Turkey Drumsticks (Butterball)-Fresh'N Easy Drumettes cooked	1 oz	3	80	34%
Turkey Drumsticks/(Butterball)-Fresh'N Easy-cooked	1 oz	2	50	36%
Turkey/flesh only				
dark meat	1 cup	9	223	36%
light meat	1 cup	4	194	19%
Turkey/ground-packaged	2 oz	7	122	52%
(Armour)-Golden Star-raw	1 oz	4	50	72%
(Armour)-Turkey Selects	3 oz	6	120	45%
Turkey Leg/meat & skin	~ 1 lb	55	1133	41%
Turkey Wing/meat & skin	~ 6.5 oz	23	426	49%
(Butterball)-Fresh'N Easy-cooked	1 oz	2	60	30%
(Louis Rich)-85% lean	1 oz	4	60	60%
90% lean	1 oz	3	50	54%
(Swift Premium)-dark meat w/skin-cooked	3.5 oz	14	245	51%
(Swift Premium)-cooked	1 oz	5	70	64%
TURKEY ENTREE/DINNER (See also FROZEN ENTREE/DINNER)				
Turkey and Gravy/frozen	5 oz	3.7	95	35%

Food and Description	Amount	Fat Grams	Total Calories	% Fat Calories
(Banquet)	8 oz	8	150	48%
(Banquet-Cook'n Bags)	5 oz	6	100	54%
Turkey Dijon/frozen (Lean Cuisine)	9.5 oz	10	270	33%
Turkey Loaf/homemade	5 oz	15	280	48%
Turkey/(Louis Rich)-breaded-frozen -				
Turkey Nuggets-prepared	~ 1 oz	4	65	55%
Turkey Patties-prepared	~ 3 oz	13	220	53%
Turkey Sticks	1 oz	5	80	56%
Turkey Pie/frozen (Stouffer's)	10 oz	36	540	60%
Turkey Pot Pies & meat pies -				
frozen (Banquet)	7 oz	31	500	56%
(Banquet)-supreme microwave	7 oz	26	423	55%
(Morton)	7 oz	27	420	58%
(Swanson)	7 oz	22	390	51%
(Swanson) Hungry Man	16 oz	42	750	50%
homemade 9"dia	⅓ serving/			
	~ 8 oz	31	550	51%
Turkey Roast/frozen-light & dark	~ 7 oz	11	304	33%
	3 oz	5	130	35%
Turkey, Scalloped/homemade	~ 7 oz	5.6	253	20%
Turkey/(Schwan's)-home delivery-frozen-partially or fully cooked unless otherwise stated.				
Roll	3.5 oz	8	140	51%
Breast w/Gravy	3.5 oz	5	110	41%
Turkey Breast	3.5 oz	2	100	18%
Turkey, Sticks/homemade-breaded/battered and fried	5 oz	24	397	54%
Turkey, Stuffed Breast/frozen				
(Weight Watchers)	8.5 oz	10	260	35%
Turkey/(Tyson)-frozen Gourmet				
Selection Entree	11.5 oz	11	380	26%
Turkey Tetrazzini/frozen	~ 7 oz	16.6	282	53%
TURKEY PRODUCTS (*See also* LUNCHEON MEATS)				
Turkey Bacon				
(Armour) Turkey Selects	1 strip	2	40	45%
Turkey Bologna	2 slices/2 oz	8.6	113	69%
Turkey Breakfast Strips/(Armour)-Golden				
Star-raw	1 strip	4	50	72%
(Armour)-Turkey Selects	1 strip	4	50	72%
(Armour)				
barbequed-packaged	1 oz	1	39	23%
(Butterball)-Deli-no salt added	1 oz	–	45	–
Fresh Half-cooked	1 oz	2	50	36%
Fresh'N Easy slices-cooked	1 oz	1	40	23%

Food and Description	Amount	Fat Grams	Total Calories	% Fat Calories
Oven Prepared Deli				
w/caramel-skinless	1 oz	–	25	–
Slice'N Serve Hickory Smoked-				
Breast of turkey	1 oz	1	35	26%
Slice'N Serve BBQ Seasoned-				
Breast of Turkey	1 oz	2	40	45%
Slice'N Serve oven-prepared w/broth	1 oz	1	30	30%
Slice'N Serve oven-prepared smoked	1 oz	1	30	30%
Slice'N Serve oven-prepared				
skinless young w/broth	1 oz	1	30	30%
Slice'N Serve oven-roasted				
Breast of turkey	1 oz	1	35	26%
turkey breast	1 oz	2	40	45%
(Louis Rich)-fully cooked				
Barbecued	1 oz	1	35	26%
Hickory Smoked	1 oz	1	35	26%
Hickory Smoked Dark				
Roast of Turkey	1 oz	.5	35	13%
Honey Roasted	1 oz	1	35	26%
Oven Roasted	1 oz	1	30	30%
Roast of Turkey-Breast & Dark	1 oz	.5	30	15%
(Oscar Meyer)-Oven roasted				
97% fat-free	1 slice	.5	20	23%
Smoked-98% fat-free	1 slice	.5	20	23%
Turkey, canned/boned w/broth	2.5 oz	4.87	116	38%
(Hormel)-Chunk	6¾ oz	10	230	39%
(Swanson)-Premium Chunk White	2.5 oz	2	90	20%
(Swanson)-Premium Chunk				
White & Dark	2.5 oz	3	90	30%
Turkey Frankfurter	2.5 oz	8	102	71%
Turkey Ham	2 slices/2 oz	2.88	73	36%
(Butterball)-Slice'N Serve	1 oz	2	35	51%
Slice'N Serve-Honey cured	1 oz	2	40	45%
(Louis Rich)	1 oz	1	35	26%
w/water added	1 oz	1	35	26%
Turkey Loaf	2 slices/2 oz	.67	47	13%
Turkey Pastrami	2 oz	3.5	80	39%
(Butterball)-Slice'N Serve	1 oz	1	35	26%
Turkey Patties/breaded-battered-fried	1(2¼ oz)	11.5	181	57%
Turkey Roll/light	1 oz	2	42	43%
light & dark	2 slices/2 oz	1.98	42	42%
Turkey Salami	2 slices/2 oz	7.8	111	63%
(Butterball)-Slice'N Serve	1 oz	4	50	72%
Turkey Sausage-smoked-packaged	1 oz	3.8	55	62%

Food and Description	Amount	Fat Grams	Total Calories	% Fat Calories
(Armour)-Golden Star-raw				
links or patties	1 oz	4	60	60%
(Armour)-Turkey Selects-Heat'N Serve	1 oz	6	80	68%
(Louis Rich) Turkey-Ground Breakfast	1 oz	4	55	66%
TURKEY SOUP (*See* SOUP)				
TURNIP				
fresh-boiled	½ cup	–	14	–
frozen	½ cup	–	26	–
raw	½ cup	–	18	–
TURNIP GREENS				
fresh-boiled	½ cup	–	15	–
canned	½ cup	–	17	–
canned-w/diced turnips-seasoned				
w/pork-(Luck's)	7.5 oz	6	90	60%
frozen	½ cup	–	24	–
frozen (Pictsweet) w/diced turnips	3.3 oz	–	20	–
raw	½ cup	–	7	–
TURTLE/Green				
canned	3 oz	.6	91	6%
raw	3 oz	< 1	76	6%

V

Food and Description	Amount	Fat Grams	Total Calories	% Fat Calories
VEAL CUTS:				
Breast/lean and fat-braised	3 oz	18	258	63%
Chop				
Lean and fat-fried				
w/ bone-raw	6.5 oz	18.6	282	59%
Lean only w/bone-raw	6.5 oz	6.6	177	34%
Chuck/lean and fat-cooked	3 oz	10.9	200	49%
Cutlet, Steak/Lean				
Lean and fat				
Boneless-broiled/braised	3 oz	9.4	182	47%
Lean only				
Boneless-broiled/braised	3 oz	3.5	140	23%
Loin/lean and fat				
Braised or broiled	3 oz	13	199	59%

Food and Description	Amount	Fat Grams	Total Calories	% Fat Calories
Rib Roast/lean and fat				
Roasted	3 oz	14	230	55%
Round with Rump				
Roasts & leg cutlets				
Braised or broiled	3 oz	9.6	184	47%
VEAL CUTS, OTHER				
Calf				
Heart/braised-chopped	1 cup	13	302	39%
Liver/fried	3 oz	11	222	45%
Sweetbreads/braised	3 oz	2.7	143	17%
Tongue/braised-sliced	~ 1 oz	1.7	45	34%
VEAL DISHES-FROZEN & HOMEMADE				
(NOTE: The data listed in this table may vary slightly, pending the fat content of the veal cuts used in preparation.)				
Veal Parmigiana/Breaded				
Frozen				
(Banquet)	5 oz	11	230	43%
w/sauce & cheese	~ 6.5 oz	18	282	57%
(Swanson's)	~ 12 oz	22	450	44%
Standard Home Recipe (USDA)	~ 6.5 oz	20	351	51%
Veal Patty Parmigiana				
Frozen (Weight Watchers)	8.44 oz	10	220	41%
Veal Scallopini w/Sauce				
Standard Home Recipe (USDA)	~ 3.5 oz	19	255	67%
VEAL STEAKS/Frozen				
Breaded (Hormel)	4 oz	13	240	49%
Unbreaded (Hormel)	4 oz	4	130	28%
VEGETABLE DISHES (*See also* individual listings of vegetable dishes)				
Broccoli, carrots, & pasta w/lightly seasoned sauce				
frozen (Birds Eye)	⅔ cup	4	87	41%
Broccoli, cauliflower, carrots w/butter sauce				
frozen (Green Giant)	½ cup	1	30	30%
Broccoli, Cauliflower, Carrots w/cheese sauce				
frozen				
(Birds Eye)	5 oz	5	100	45%
(Green Giant)	½ cup	2	60	30%
(Stokely)				
Singles	4 oz	3	70	39%
Broccoli, Cauliflower, Carrots in Cheese Sauce				
One serving-frozen (Green Giant)	5 oz	3	70	39%
Broccoli, Cauliflower in Creamy Itailian Cheese Sauce				
frozen (Birds Eye)	½ cup	6	90	60%

Food and Description	Amount	Fat Grams	Total Calories	% Fat Calories
Corn, green beans, & pasta curls w/light cream sauce				
frozen (Birds Eye)	½ cup	4.9	108	41%
Garden Salad				
canned (Joan of Arc)	½ cup	–	70	–
Micro Quick				
frozen (Freshlike)				
Broccoli, Pasta, Carrots in Cheese Sauce	4.5 oz	3	100	27%
Corn, Italian Green Beans, Red Peppers in Butter Sauce	5 oz	2	90	20%
Peas, Carrots, Onions-Cheese Sauce	5 oz	3	90	30%
Peas, Cauliflower, Red Peppers in Butter Sauce	5 oz	2	90	20%
Mixed vegetables in butter sauce				
frozen (Green Giant)	½ cup	2	80	23%
Mixed vegetables in onion sauce				
frozen (Birds Eye)	2.6 oz	5	100	45%
Pizza-cheese & veg				
homemade/thin crust	1 sl/~ 2 oz	6	163	33%
Stew Vegetables				
frozen (Ore Ida)	3 oz	–	60	–
Sweet Corn, Pinto Beans, Red Bell Pepper in savory sauce microwave Vegetable Classics				
(Del Monte)	3⅓ oz	4	110	33%
Vegetables in Authentic Oriental Sauce				
frozen (Birds Eye) Custom Cuisine	3.5 oz	3	70	39%
Vegetables in Creamy Cheese Sauce				
frozen (Birds Eye) Custom Cuisine	3.5 oz	5	210	21%
Vegetables in Delicate Herb Sauce				
frozen (Birds Eye) Custom Cuisine	3.5 oz	4	60	60%
Vegetables & Pasta in Creamy Stroganoff Sauce				
frozen (Birds Eye) Custom Cuisine	4.6 oz	5	130	35%
Vegetable Medley				
breaded/frozen (Ore Ida)	3 oz	9	160	51%
Vegetable Lasagna				
(Impromtu Lite) box mix-microwave	10.6 oz	11	290	34%
Vegetables & rice w/butter				
frozen (Banquet)	½ cup	9	183	44%
Vegetarian Medley				
frozen (Kibun)	10 oz	2	240	8%

Food and Description	Amount	Fat Grams	Total Calories	% Fat Calories
VEGETABLE JUICE COCKTAIL				
V-8 (Campbell's)	6 oz	–	35	–
–no salt added	6 oz	–	40	–
–Spicy Hot	6 oz	–	35	–
Vegetable Juice Cocktail/canned	6 oz	–	34	–
Very Veggi/low-cal	8 oz	–	40	–
VEGETABLE SOUP (*See* SOUP)				
VEGETABLES, MIXED				
Canned				
Beets w/onions	½ cup	–	80	–
Chop Suey Vegetables (La Choy)	½ cup	–	10	–
Fancy Chinese Vegetables				
(La Choy)	½ cup	–	12	–
Hot & Spicy Garden Mix (Vlasic)	1 oz	–	4	–
Mixed vegetables (Del Monte)	½ cup	–	40	–
Mixed vegetables-Old Fashioned Harvest				
Time (S&W)	½ cup	–	35	–
Peas & carrots	½ cup	–	48	–
(Libby)	½ cup	–	50	–
Peas & onions	½ cup	–	30	–
Succotash (lima beans & corn) -				
(Libby)	½ cup	1	80	11%
country style (S & W)	½ cup	1	80	11%
w/cream-style corn	½ cup	.7	102	6%
w/whole kernel corn	½ cup	.6	81	7%
Veg-All-Homestyle (Larsen's)	½ cup	–	35	–
Lite (Larsen's)	½ cup	–	35	–
Regular (Larsen's)	½ cup	–	35	–
Dehydrated Flakes (French's)	1 Tbs	–	12	–
Frozen (Birds Eye)-				
Baby carrots, peas, pearl onions	~ ½ cup	–	50	–
Broccoli, baby carrots,				
water chestnuts	~ ½ cup	–	35	–
Broccoli, carrots, & pasta twists	~ ½ cup	4	9	40%
Broccoli, carrots, water chestnuts	¾ cup	–	45	–
Broccoli, cauliflowr, carrots	~ ½ cup	–	25	–
Broccoli, corn, & red peppers	~ ½ cup	–	50	–
Broccoli, green beans, pearl onions,				
red peppers	~ ½ cup	–	25	–
Broccoli, red peppers, bamboo shoots,				
straw mushrooms	~ ½ cup	–	25	–
Brussels sprouts, cauliflower, carrots	~ ½ cup	–	30	–
Carrots & pasta	~ ½ cup	4	90	40%
Carrots, peas, & pearl onions	~ ½ cup	–	48	–

Food and Description	Amount	Fat Grams	Total Calories	% Fat Calories
Cauliflower & carrots	~ ½ cup	2.9	60	44%
Cauliflower, baby carrots, snow peas	~ ½ cup	–	30	–
Chinese style - International Recipe	~ ½ cup	3.9	68	52%
Chinese style - Stir Fry	~ ½ cup	–	36	–
Chow Mein Style - International Recipe	~ ½ cup	4	90	40%
Corn, green beans, & pasta curls	~ ½ cup	5	110	41%
Custom Cuisine-Creamy Mushroom	~ ½ cup	6	107	51%
Vegetables w/herb sauce	~ ½ cup	6	107	51%
Green beans, French, toasted almond	~ ½ cup	2	50	36%
Green peas, pearl onions	~ ½ cup	–	70	–
Italian Style - International Recipe	~ ½ cup	5.5	102	49%
Japanese Style - International Recipe	~ ½ cup	6	100	54%
Japanese Style - Stir Fry	~ ½ cup	–	30	–
Mandarin style - International Recipe	~ ½ cup	4	90	40%
Mixed vegetables-regular	~ ½ cup	–	60	–
New England style - International Recipe	~ ½ cup	6	125	43%
Pasta primavera style -International Recipe	~ ½ cup	5	120	38%
Peas & carrots	~ ½ cup	–	38	–
Peas & onions	~ ½ cup	–	40	–
Rice, green peas, mushrooms	~ ½ cup	–	110	–
San Francisco style - International Recipe	~ ½ cup	5	100	45%
(Freshlike)				
California Blend	3.3 oz	–	30	–
Chuckwagon Blend	3.3 oz	–	70	–
Italian Blend	3.3 oz	–	30	–
Midwestern Blend	3.3 oz	–	40	–
Mixed Vegetables	3.3 oz	–	70	–
Oriental Blend	3.3 oz	–	25	–
Winter Blend	3.3 oz	–	95	–
Wisconsin Blend	3.3 oz	–	50	–
Scandinavian Blend	3.3 oz	–	45	–
Vegetables For Soup	3.3 oz	–	50	–
Vegetables for Stew	3.3 oz	–	50	–
(Green Giant)				
Broccoli, Cauliflower, Carrots One Serving Veg.	4 oz	–	25	–
Broccoli, Peas, Carrots One Serving Veg.	4 oz	–	50	–
Microwaveable/Pantry Express				
Corn, Green Beans, Carrots, Pasta	½ cup	2	80	23%
Green Beans, Potatoes, Mushrooms	½ cup	2	50	36%

Food and Description	Amount	Fat Grams	Total Calories	% Fat Calories
Mixed Vegetables	½ cup	1	35	26%
Mixed Vegetables	4 oz	–	50	–
(Harvest Fresh)-Mixed Vegetables	4 oz	–	45	–
(Ore Ida)- Stew Vegetables	4 oz	–	60	–
(Pictsweet)				
Express-microwave				
Broccoli, carrots, cauliflower	2.5 oz	–	20	–
Broccoli, carrots, water chestnuts	2.5 oz	–	25	–
Broccoli, cauliflower	2.5 oz	–	20	–
Broccoli, corn, red peppers	2.5 oz	–	25	–
Broccoli, French Beans, Onions, & Red Peppers	2.5 oz	–	20	–
Peas, Pearl Onions, & Mushrooms	2.5 oz	–	45	–
Squash, onion, peppers	2.5 oz	–	18	–
Mixed Vegetables	3.2 oz	–	60	–
Succotash	3.3 oz	1	100	9%
Vegetables California	3.2 oz	–	25	–
Vegetables Belgian	3.2 oz	–	30	–
Vegetables Cantonese	3.2 oz	–	35	–
Vegetables Del Sol	3.2 oz	–	30	–
Vegetables for Stir Fry	3.5 oz	–	35	–
prepared as directed	3.5 oz	4	75	48%
Vegetables Grande	3.2 oz	–	45	–
Vegetables Italian	3.2 oz	–	20	–
Vegetables Japanese	3.2 oz	–	25	–
Vegetables Milano	3.2 oz	–	40	–
Vegetables New England	3.2 oz	–	40	–
Vegetables Oriental	3.2 oz	–	25	–
Vegetables Prisian	3.2 oz	–	30	–
Vegetables Romano	3.2 oz	–	50	–
Vegetables Swiss	3.2 oz	–	25	–
Vegetables Western	3.2 oz	–	50	–
(Stokely)				
Singles Broccoli, carrots, Water Chestnuts	3 oz	1	30	30%
Singles Broccoli, cauliflower	3 oz	1	20	45%
Singles Broccoli, Cauliflower, Carrots	3 oz	1	25	36%
(Valley Combinations) - Pillsbury				
Broccoli Cauliflower Supreme	½ cup	–	20	–
Broccoli Carrot Fanfare	½ cup	–	20	–
Corn Broccoli Bounty	½ cup	1	45	20%
Sweet Pea Cauliflower Medley	½ cup	–	30	–
Cauliflower Green Bean Festival	½ cup	–	16	–

Food and Description	Amount	Fat Grams	Total Calories	% Fat Calories
(Valley Combinations) - Pillsbury-Dual Pouch				
American Style w/o sauce	½ cup	–	50	–
w/sauce	½ cup	2	70	26%
Broccoli Cauliflower Medley				
w/o sauce	½ cup	–	30	–
w/sauce	½ cup	1	50	18%
Broccoli Fanfare w/o sauce	½ cup	–	50	–
w/sauce	½ cup	2	70	26%
Italian Style w/o sauce	½ cup	–	18	–
w/sauce	½ cup	2	40	45%
Japanese Style w/o sauce	½ cup	–	30	–
w/sauce	½ cup	1	45	20%
Le Sueur Style w/o sauce	½ cup	–	50	–
w/sauce	½ cup	2	60	30%
Mexican Style w/o sauce	½ cup	–	90	–
w/sauce	½ cup	5	140	32%

VEGETARIAN FOOD

(La Loma)

Food and Description	Amount	Fat Grams	Total Calories	% Fat Calories
Canned & Dry Packed - Meatless				
Bacon-Like Bits	3.2 grams	1	10	90%
Big Franks	1.8 oz	6	110	49%
Chicken Supreme	~ 1 oz	.76	100	7%
Dinner Cuts	3.5 oz	1	110	49%
no salt	3.5 oz	1	110	49%
Fried Chicken w/Gravy	2.7 oz	17	230	67%
Linketts	2.5 oz	8	140	51%
Little Links	1.6 oz	5	90	50%
Nuteena-luncheon loaf	2.3 oz	12	160	68%
Ocean Platter	~ 1 oz	.8	100	7%
Patty Mix	~ 1 oz	2	120	15%
Proteena-nut loaf	2.5 oz	7	150	42%
Rediburger	2.4 oz	6	130	42%
Sandwich Spread	1.7 oz	4	70	51%
Savory Dinner Loaf				
mix unprepared	~ 1 oz	.68	100	6%
Sizzle Franks	2.4 oz	13	170	69%
Stew Pack	2 oz	3	90	30%
Swiss Steak w/Gravy	3.3 oz	10	170	53%
Tastee Cuts	2.2 oz	1	60	15%
Tender Bits	2 oz	3	80	34%
Tender Rounds	2.6 oz	4	120	30%
Vege Scallops	2.7 oz	2	90	20%
Vege-burger mix	3.8 oz	2	110	16%
no salt	3.8 oz	2	110	16%

Food and Description	Amount	Fat Grams	Total Calories	% Fat Calories
Vegelona	2.4 oz	1	100	9%
Vegetein Beef	3.1 oz	15	360	38%
Vegetein Chicken	3.1 oz	15	370	37%
Vegetein Chorizo	3.1 oz	15	370	37%
Vegetein Taco Mix	3.1 oz	14	360	35%
Vegetein Unflavored	2 oz	11	250	40%
Vitaburger Chunks	¾ oz	< 1	70	6%
Vitaburger Granules	¾ oz	< 1	70	6%
Frozen Products - Meatless				
Bologna Slices	2 oz	8	150	48%
Bologna Roll	2.5 oz	10	180	50%
Chicken Slices	2 oz	4	100	36%
Chicken Roll	2.5 oz	5	120	38%
Chicken Nuggets	~ 3 oz	20	270	67%
Chicken Patties	2.5 oz	13	200	59%
Corn Dogs	2.5 oz	8	190	38%
Fried Chicken	2 oz	14	180	70%
Griddle Steaks	2 oz	6	140	39%
Ocean Fillets	2 oz	9	140	58%
Olive Loaf Slices	2 oz	6	120	45%
Olive Loaf	2.5 oz	7	150	42%
Roast Beef Slices	2 oz	4	100	36%
Roast Beef Roll	2.5 oz	6	140	39%
Salami Slices	2 oz	4	110	33%
Salami Roll	2.5 oz	5	130	35%
Savoy Meatball	2.5 oz	8	190	38%
Sizzle Burger	2.5 oz	12	220	49%
Spicy Chicken	~ 3 oz	13	230	51%
Turkey Slices	2 oz	4	100	36%
Turkey Roll	2.5 oz	5	120	38%
Miscellaneous				
Vege-Beans	~ 4 oz	.5	90	5%
Vegeburger	3.8 oz	2	110	16%
Wheat Fries	2.5 oz	1	60	15%
(Worthington)				
Canned & Dry Packed - Meatless				
Chik				
Diced-drained	¼ cup	8	90	80%
Sliced-drained	2 slices	8	90	80%
Chili	⅔ cup	10	190	47%
Choplets	2 slices	2	100	18%
Country Stew	9.5 oz	10	220	41%
Fri Chik	2 pieces	13	180	65%
Granburger	6 Tbs	1	110	8%

Food and Description	Amount	Fat Grams	Total Calories	% Fat Calories
Natural Touch Mix				
dry-Loaf	4 oz	7	180	35%
Spicy Chili	⅔ cup	12	190	57%
Stroganoff	4 oz	3	90	30%
Taco	2 Tbs	2	90	20%
Non Meat Balls	3	6	100	54%
Numete	½" slice	11	160	62%
Prime Stakes	1 piece	10	160	56%
Protose	½" slice	8	180	40%
Saucettes	2 links	9	140	58%
Savory Slices	2 slices	6	100	54%
Super Links	1 link	7	100	63%
Turkee Slices	2 slices	9	130	62%
Vegetable Skallops	½ cup	2	90	20%
no salt	½ cup	1	80	11%
Vegetable Steaks	2½ pieces	2	110	16%
Vegetarian Burger	½ cup	4	150	24%
no salt added	½ cup	6	160	34%
Veja-Links	2 links	10	140	64%
Frozen Products - Meatless				
Beef Pie-Vegetarian	8 oz	16	360	40%
Beef Style Roll	4 slices	6	130	42%
Bolono	2 slices	2	60	30%
Chic-ketts roll	½ cup	7	160	39%
Chicken				
diced	½ cup	13	190	62%
roll	~ 2.5 oz	10	150	60%
slices	2 slices	9	130	62%
Chicken Pie-Vegetarian	8 oz	20	380	47%
Chik Stiks	1 piece/ 1.6 oz	7	110	57%
Corned Beef				
roll	2.5 oz	7	150	42%
slices	4 slices	6	120	45%
Crispy Chik	3 oz	19	280	61%
patties	1 pattie	15	220	61%
Dinner Roast	2 oz	8	120	60%
Dixie Dogs	1	10	200	45%
Egg Rolls-Vegetarian	1	6	160	34%
Fillets-Vegetarian	2 fillets	9	180	45%
Fripats	1 piece	12	180	60%
Harvest Bake Lentil Rice Loaf	2½ slices	9	190	43%
Leanies	1 link	6	100	54%
Natural Touch Dinner Entree	1 pattie	14	230	55%

Food and Description	Amount	Fat Grams	Total Calories	% Fat Calories
Okara Patties	1 pattie	10	160	56%
Prosage				
links	3 links	14	190	66%
patties	2 patties	14	210	60%
roll	~ 2.5 oz	12	180	60%
Salami				
roll	2 slices	5	90	50%
slices	2 slices	4	80	45%
Smoked Beef	3 slices	6	120	45%
Smoked Turkey				
roll	4 slices	12	180	60%
slices	4 slices	12	180	60%
Stakelets	1 piece	8	150	48%
Stripples	4 strips	9	120	68%
Tofu Garden Patties	1 pattie	4	90	40%
Tuno-roll	2 oz	7	100	63%
Wham				
roll	3 slices	7	120	53%
slices	3 slices	7	120	53%
Morningstar Farms Frozen Products - Meatless				
Breakfast Links	3 links	14	190	66%
Breakfast Patties	2 patties	12	190	57%
Breakfast Strips	3 strips	6	80	68%
Country Breakfast				
Cinnamon Swirl French Toast & Patties	6.5 oz	15	380	36%
Scramblers, Links, & Hash Browns	7 oz	23	360	58%
Scramblers, Links, & Pancakes	6.8 oz	19	380	45%
Country Crisp Patties	1 pattie	15	220	61%
Grillers	1 pattie	12	180	60%
Homestyle Country Crisps	3 oz	16	250	58%
Scramblers	¼ cup	3	60	45%
Zesty Country Crisps	3 oz	19	280	61%
VENISON				
cured-boneless	3 oz	5	151	30%
raw-boneless steaks	3 oz	5	153	29%
raw-lean meat	3 oz	3	107	25%
stewed-boneless	3 oz	5	153	29%
VICHYSSOISE (*See* SOUP)				
VINEGAR				
Cider	1 oz	–	–	–
	½ cup	–	15	–
Distilled	1 Tbs	–	2	–
	1 cup	–	29	–

Food and Description	Amount	Fat Grams	Total Calories	% Fat Calories
(Regina) Wine Vinegars				
red	1 oz	–	4	–
red/garlic	1 oz	–	4	–
white	1 oz	–	4	–
VITA JUICE-including Beta Carotene	8 oz	–	90	–
VODKA (*See* DISTILLED LIQUOR)				

W

ood and Description	Amount	Fat Grams	Total Calories	% Fat Calories
WAFFLE				
Belgian Waffle Mix				
Classique Fare/dry	1.66 oz	1	172	5%
Box-Mix (*See also* PANCAKE MIX)				
(Aunt Jemima)				
Buckwheat	¼ cup	1	107	8%
Buttermilk	⅓ cup	1	75	12%
Original	¼ cup	1	108	8%
Whole wheat	⅓ cup	1	142	6%
Frozen				
(Aunt Jemima)				
Apple & Cinnamon	2	6	180	30%
Blueberry	2	5	180	25%
Buttermilk	2	6	180	30%
Original	2	7	230	27%
Raisin	2	4	200	18%
Whole Grain	2	3	150	18%
(Belgian Chef)				
Original	1	2	90	10%
w/oat bran	1	6	140	39%
(Downyflake)				
Blueberry	2	4	180	20%
Buttermilk				
Jumbo regular	2	4	170	21%
Oat bran	2	13	260	45%
Plain/jumbo	2	4	170	21%
Plain/regular	2	3	120	23%

Food and Description	Amount	Fat Grams	Total Calories	% Fat Calories
(Eggo)				
Apple Cinnamon	1	5	130	35%
Blueberry	1	5	130	35%
Buttermilk	1	5	120	38%
Homestyle	1	5	120	38%
Mini's	4	3	90	30%
Nut & honey	1	6	130	42%
Oat Bran	1	4	110	33%
Special K-fat free	1	–	80	–
(Nutri-Grain)	1	5	130	35%
Strawberry	1	5	130	35%
(Roman Meal)-plain	2	14	280	45%
(Swanson) Great Starts				
Belgian w/sausage	2⅞ oz	19	280	61%
Shake 'N Pour Mix (Bisquick)				
Original	2	6	280	19%
Standard Home Recipe (USDA)				
7" round	~ 2½ oz	7	209	30%
9" square	11 oz	19.6	558	32%
WAFFLE SYRUP (*See* PANCAKE/WAFFLE SYRUP)				
WALNUT				
Black				
dried	1 oz	16	172	84%
dried-chopped	1 cup	70.7	759	84%
(Planters)	1 oz	17	180	85%
English or Persian				
(Azar)-pieces	1 oz	19	190	90%
(Diamond)-pieces	1 oz	19	190	90%
dried	1 oz	17.57	182	87%
dried-pieces	1 cup	74	770	87%
(Planters)	1 oz	20	190	95%
WATER				
Flavored				
Coor's Rocky Mountain Sparkling Water				
Cherry	8 fl oz	–	–	–
Lemon Lime	8 fl oz	–	–	–
Original	8 fl oz	–	–	–
Perrier/all flavors	8 fl oz	–	–	–
Plain/all types		–	–	–
WATER CHESTNUT, CHINESE				
canned-sliced	½ cup	–	35	–
(Chun King)				
sliced	8 oz	.5	179	3%
whole	8.5 oz	.5	190	2%

Food and Description	Amount	Fat Grams	Total Calories	% Fat Calories
raw-sliced	½ cup	–	66	–
WATERCRESS				
chopped	½ cup	–	2	–
raw	1 sprig	–	–	–
WATERCRESS SOUP (*See* SOUP)				
WATERMELON				
fresh-10" diameter	1/16 wedge	2	152	12%
	1 cup	.68	50	12%
Kernels-dried	1 oz	13	158	74%
	1 cup	51	602	76%
WAX BEAN				
canned	½ cup	–	25	–
(Del Monte)				
cut	½ cup	–	20	–
French style	½ cup	–	20	–
(Festal)	½ cup	–	20	–
(Joan of Arc)	½ cup	–	25	18%
(S&W) Premium Golden cut	½cup	–	20	–
WAX GOURD				
fresh-boiled	1 cup	–	23	–
raw	1 cup	–	17	–
WEAKFISH				
broiled w/butter or margarine	3 oz	9.6	177	49%
WHALE/raw	3 oz	6	130	42%
WHEAT				
Buglar Hard Red Winter Wheat				
Canned				
Seasoned	1 cup	4.5	246	17%
Unseasoned	1 cup	.9	227	4%
Dry	1 cup	3	600	5%
Cracked Wheat	1 slice	1	75	12%
(Pepperidge Farm)	1 slice	1	65	14%
(Roman Meal)	1 slice	–	66	–
WHEAT GERM				
Kretschmer				
Honey crunch	¼ cup	3	110	25%
Plain	¼ cup	3	100	27%
Krusteaz	1 oz	2	103	18%
WHELK (*See* SNAILS)				
WHEY				
dried				
acid	1 Tbs	–	10	–
sweet	1 cup	2.5	792	3%
	1 Tbs	–	26	–

Food and Description	Amount	Fat Grams	Total Calories	% Fat Calories
fluid				
acid	1 cup	< 1	60	8%
sweet	1 cup	.7	65	10%
WHIPPED TOPPING (See also CREAM, DESSERT TOPPING)				
frozen	1 Tbs	1	15	60%
frozen-non dairy	1 Tbs	.8	11	66%
powdered-with whole milk	1 Tbs	–	10	–
	1 cup	10	150	60%
powdered-low-calorie	1 Tbs	1	8	100%
pressurized-cream	1 Tbs	1	8	100%
	½ cup	7	75	84%
non dairy	1 Tbs	1	10	81%
	1 cup	16	185	78%
WHISKEY (See DISTILLED LIQUOR)				
WHITE BEANS				
boiled	½ cup	–	125	–
canned	½ cup	–	153	–
Small				
boiled	½ cup	.58	127	4%
WHITE PERCH/raw	3 oz	3	100	27%
WHITE SAUCE (See SAUCE)				
WHITEFISH				
Mixed				
jellied (Mother's)	1 fishball	1	46	20%
jellied in broth (Mother's)	1 fishball	1	70	13%
raw	3 oz	4.98	114	39%
smoked	3 oz	.79	92	8%
WHITEFISH & PIKE				
jar (Manischewitz)	3.5 oz	3.57	99	33%
sweet	3.5 oz	4	129	28%
jellied (Rokeach)	1 fishball	1	60	15%
jellied in broth (Mother's)	1 fishball	1	60	15%
WHITING (See also SEAFOOD ENTREE/DINNER)				
breaded & fried	3 oz	9.7	171	51%
cooked-dry heat	3 oz	1	98	9%
raw	3 oz	1	77	12%
WINE				
(NOTE: Percent refers to alcohol content.)				
Barbera, white	4 fl oz	–	91	–
Beaujolais-12%	4 fl oz	–	96	–
Bordaux-red-12%	4 fl oz	–	96	–
Burgundy				
Cooking	¼ cup	–	2	–
Red-12%	4 fl oz	–	96	–

Food and Description	Amount	Fat Grams	Total Calories	% Fat Calories
Sparkling-12%	4 fl oz	–	116	–
White-12%	4 fl oz	–	90	–
Cabernet Sauvignon	4 fl oz	–	88	–
Chablis	4 fl oz	–	84	–
Emerald	4 fl oz	–	102	–
Gold	4 fl oz	–	97	–
Pink	4 fl oz	–	98	–
Ruby	4 fl oz	–	104	–
Champagne				
Brut	4 fl oz	–	100	–
Extra Dry	4 fl oz	–	105	–
Pink	4 fl oz	–	98	–
Domestic	4 fl oz	–	84	–
Chardonnay	4 fl oz	–	88	–
Chenin Blanc	4 fl oz	–	86	–
Chianti	4 fl oz	–	100	–
Cold Duck	4 fl oz	–	108	–
Desert	4 fl oz	–	180	–
Dubonnet	4 fl oz	–	160	–
French Colombard	4 fl oz	–	88	–
Liebfraumilch-10%	4 fl oz	–	84	–
Madeira-19%	4 fl oz	–	160	–
Muscatelle (Muscatel)	3.5 fl oz	–	158	–
Port				
Ruby-20%	4 fl oz	–	184	–
Tawny-20%	4 fl oz	–	184	–
White	4 fl oz	–	172	–
Reising-12%	4 fl oz	–	90	–
Rhine-11%	4 fl oz	–	96	–
Rhone-125	4 fl oz	–	96	–
Rose'	4 fl oz	–	90	–
Sauterne				
Cooking	¼ cup	–	2	–
12%	4 fl oz	–	116	–
12% dry	4 fl oz	–	108	–
Sauvignon Blanc	4 fl oz	–	80	–
Sherry				
Cooking	¼ cup	–	20	–
Cream-19.5%	4 fl oz	–	200	–
Dry-19%	4 fl oz	–	162	–
Sweet Wines	4 fl oz	–	165	–
Sylvaner-12%	4 fl oz	–	90	–
Table				
Red	3.5 fl oz	–	74	–

Food and Description	Amount	Fat Grams	Total Calories	% Fat Calories
Rose	3.5 fl oz	–	73	–
White	3.5 fl oz	–	70	–
Tokay	4 fl oz	–	164	–
Vermouth				
Dry-17%	4 fl oz	–	136	–
Sweet-17%	4 fl oz	–	180	–
Wine Cooler	7 fl oz	–	101	–
	12 fl oz	–	192	–
(Bartles & Jaymes)				
Light	6 oz	–	67	–
Light Berry	6 oz	–	75	–
Wine Spritzer	5 fl oz	–	61	–
Zinfandel	4 fl oz	–	92	–
White	4 fl oz	–	82	–
WINGED BEAN/boiled	½ cup	5	126	36%
WOLF FISH/raw	3 oz	2	80	23%
WON TON SOUP (See SOUP)				
WORCESTERSHIRE SAUCE (See also SAUCE)				
regular	1 Tbs	–	10	–
smokey	1 Tbs	–	10	–

Y

Food and Description	Amount	Fat Grams	Total Calories	% Fat Calories
YAM				
canned-candied (S&W)	½ cup	–	180	–
heavy syrup	½ cup	–	120	–
light syrup	½ cup	–	110	–
mashed	½ cup	–	90	–
w/pineapple orange sauce	½ cup	–	190	–
canned-whole Southern in extra heavy				
syrup (S&W)	½ cup	1	139	7%
fresh-boiled or baked	1 cup	–	158	–
Mountain Yam-Hawaii				
cooked-cubed	½ cup	–	59	–
raw-cubed	½ cup	–	46	–
raw	1 cup	–	177	–

Food and Description	Amount	Fat Grams	Total Calories	% Fat Calories
YAM BEAN-TUBER				
boiled	4 oz	–	52	–
raw w/skin	½ lb	< 1	85	5%
w/o skin	4 oz	< 1	47	10%
YARDLONG BEAN				
boiled	½ cup	–	102	–
YEAST				
Active dry-baker's	1 pkg	–	20	–
	1 oz	.5	80	6%
Brewer's	1 Tbs	–	25	–
	1 oz	–	80	–
(Louis Labatories)	2 Tbs	1	114	8%
Compressed-baker's	1 oz	1	24	38%
(Fleischmann's)	1 cube	–	15	–
Torula	1 oz	–	79	–
YELLOW BEAN				
baked-canned	½ cup	3	180	15%
boiled	½ cup	.95	126	7%
Snap				
cooked	½ cup	–	22	–
canned	½ cup	–	13	–
frozen	½ cup	–	18	–
YELLOWEYE BEAN				
canned-Seasoned w/Pork (Luck's)	7.5 oz	6	220	25%
YELLOWTAIL/raw	3 oz	4.5	124	33%
YOGURT				
(NOTE: The yogurt listed below is found in either your grocer's dairy department or frozen food section.)				
Bon Lait (Fromage Frais)				
peach	6 oz	5	200	23%
raspberry	6 oz	5	200	23%
strawberry	6 oz	5	200	23%
(Breyers)				
black cherry	8 oz	5	270	17%
blueberry	8 oz	6	260	21%
mixed berry	8 oz	5	270	17%
mixed berry-low fat	8 oz	2	250	7%
peach	8 oz	5	270	17%
peach-low fat	8 oz	2	250	7%
pineapple	8 oz	5	270	17%
plain	8 oz	8	190	38%
red raspberry	8 oz	6	260	21%
strawberry	8 oz	5	270	17%
strawberry banana	8 oz	6	280	19%

Food and Description	Amount	Fat Grams	Total Calories	% Fat Calories
strawberry banana-low fat	8 oz	2	250	7%
vanilla bean	8 oz	7	230	27%
(Carnation)-Smooth N'Creamy-all flavors	3 oz	3	230	12%
(Dannon)				
banana	8 oz	3	240	11%
blueberry	8 oz	3	240	11%
blueberry-Fresh Flavors	8 oz	4	200	18%
boysenberry	8 oz	3	240	11%
cherry	8 oz	3	240	11%
coffee-Fresh Flavors	8 oz	3	200	14%
dutch apple	8 oz	3	240	11%
exotic fruit-Fresh Flavors	8 oz	3	240	11%
lemon-Fresh Flavors	8 oz	4	210	17%
mixed berry	8 oz	3	240	11%
nonfat	8 oz	–	110	–
peach	8 oz	3	240	11%
pina colada	8 oz	3	240	11%
plain	8 oz	4	140	26%
raspberry-Fresh Flavors	8 oz	4	200	18%
strawberry	8 oz	3	240	11%
strawberry-Fresh Flavors	8 oz	4	200	18%
strawberry-banana	8 oz	3	240	11%
vanilla-Fresh Flavors	8 oz	3	200	14%
(Dannon)-Light				
blueberry	8 oz	–	100	–
peach	8 oz	–	100	–
raspberry	8 oz	–	100	–
strawberry	8 oz	–	100	–
strawberry-banana	8 oz	–	100	–
(Del Monte) Yogurt Cup 1½% milkfat				
awesome peach	4¾ oz	2	140	13%
cool blueberry	4¾ oz	2	140	13%
rad raspberry	4¾ oz	2	140	13%
totally strawberry	4¾ oz	2	140	13%
(Johnston's) Premium				
black cherry	6 oz	5	260	17%
boysenberry	6 oz	5	260	17%
lemon Chiffon	6 oz	5	225	20%
peach	6 oz	5	260	17%
raspberry trifle	6 oz	5	225	20%
strawberry	6 oz	5	260	17%
vanilla	6 oz	7	200	32%
(Kissle)-Creamy Blend (No yogurt culture)				
blackberry	6 oz	3	180	15%

Food and Description	Amount	Fat Grams	Total Calories	% Fat Calories
blueberry	6 oz	3	180	15%
cherry	6 oz	3	180	15%
chocolate	6 oz	4	200	18%
French vanilla	6 oz	3	180	15%
lemon	6 oz	3	180	15%
milk chocolate	6 oz	4	200	18%
mixed berry	6 oz	3	180	15%
peach	6 oz	3	180	15%
raspberry	6 oz	3	180	15%
strawberry	6 oz	3	180	15%
strawberry/banana	6 oz	3	180	15%
(La Carona)-Low Fat				
all fruit flavors	8 oz	4	230	16%
plain	8 oz	5	160	28%
non fat/plain	8 oz		120	4%
(La Yogurt)/all fruit flavors	6 oz	4	190	19%
plain	6 oz	6	140	39%
(La Yogurt-25)/all flavors	8 oz	–	200	–
(Light N'Lively)				
black cherry	6 oz	2	180	10%
blueberry	6 oz	2	180	10%
peach	6 oz	2	180	10%
pineapple	6 oz	2	180	10%
red raspberry	6 oz	2	170	11%
stawberry	6 oz	2	180	10%
strawberry banana	6 oz	2	200	9%
(Lite-Line)-lowfat Swiss Style-plain				
1½% milkfat	8 oz	2	140	13%
natural cherry vanilla-1% milkfat	8 oz	2	240	8%
natural peach -1% milkfat	8 oz	2	230	8%
natural strawberry-1% milkfat	8 oz	2	240	8%
(Lite N' Lively)- 99% fat free				
blueberry	5 oz	1	150	6%
peach	5 oz	2	150	12%
pineapple	5 oz	1	150	6%
red raspberry	5 oz	2	140	13%
strawberry	5 oz	2	150	12%
strawberry banana	5 oz	1	160	6%
strawberry fruit cup	5 oz	2	150	12%
(Lite N'Lively)-100-no sugar added				
all flavors	8 oz	–	100	–
(Lite N'Lively)-Fat & Cholesterol Free				
blueberry	4.4 oz	–	50	–
red raspberry	4.4 oz	–	50	–

Food and Description	Amount	Fat Grams	Total Calories	% Fat Calories
strawberry	4.4 oz	–	50	–
Lowfat				
coffee, vanilla-lowfat	4 oz	1	97	9%
fruit-lowfat	4 oz	1	115	8%
plain-lowfat	4 oz	1.8	72	23%
part skim (non-fat)	4 oz	–	63	–
whole milk	4 oz	3.7	70	48%
(Lucerne) Nonfat				
blueberry	8 oz	–	180	–
cherry	8 oz	–	180	–
peach	8 oz	–	180	–
plain	8 oz	–	130	–
strawberry	8 oz	–	180	–
(Meadow Gold)-lowfat-plain				
2% milkfat	8 oz	5	160	28%
sundae style-raspberry				
1.5% milkfat	8 oz	4	250	14%
(Mountain High)				
black cherry	8 oz	6	220	25%
blueberry	8 oz	6	220	25%
honey vanilla	8 oz	6	220	25%
honey vanilla blend	8 oz	8	210	34%
plain	8 oz	9	200	41%
plain/Acidophilus	8 oz	9	200	41%
raspberry	8 oz	6	220	25%
strawberry	8 oz	8	210	34%
(Mountain High)-Honey Light				
all flavors	8 oz	< 1	190	2%
(New Country)				
blue berry supreme	6 oz	2	150	12%
cherry supreme	6 oz	2	150	12%
fresh vanilla	6 oz	2	150	12%
mixed berries	6 oz	2	150	12%
orange supreme	6 oz	2	150	12%
peaches'n cream	6 oz	2	150	12%
raspberry supreme	6 oz	2	150	12%
strawberry banana supreme	6 oz	2	150	12%
strawberry supreme	6 oz	2	150	12%
(Quality Chekd-Kemps)				
all fruit flavors	8 oz	3	300	9%
plain	8 oz	3	160	17%
(Scandia)-all flavors	6 oz	2	160	11%
(Weight Watchers)/fruit				
all flavors	8 oz	1	150	6%

Food and Description	Amount	Fat Grams	Total Calories	% Fat Calories
plain	8 oz	1	150	6%
(Weight Watchers) Ultimate 90				
all fruit flavors	8 oz	–	90	–
(Whitney's)				
apples & raisins	6 oz	5	200	23%
blueberry	6 oz	5	200	23%
boysenberry	6 oz	5	200	23%
cherry	6 oz	5	200	23%
coffee	6 oz	6	200	27%
lemon	6 oz	6	200	27%
peach	6 oz	5	200	23%
pina colada	6 oz	7	210	30%
plain	6 oz	7	150	42%
raspberry	6 oz	5	200	23%
strawberry	6 oz	5	200	23%
strawberry banana	6 oz	5	200	23%
tropical fruits	6 oz	6	200	27%
vanilla	6 oz	6	200	27%
wild berries	6 oz	5	200	23%
(Yoplait)-custard style				
banana	6 oz	4	190	19%
cherry	6 oz	4	180	20%
strawberry	6 oz	4	190	19%
vanilla	6 oz	4	180	20%
(Yoplait)-Light/all flavors	6 oz	.5	90	5%
New Light				
blueberry	4 oz	–	60	–
raspberry	4 oz	–	60	–
strawberry	4 oz	–	60	–
strawberry-banana	4 oz	–	60	–
(Yoplait)-Low Fat				
blueberry	6 oz	4	230	16%
cherry	6 oz	3	210	13%
strawberry	6 oz	3	210	13%
strawberry-banana	6 oz	4	240	15%
(Yoplait)-Lowfat Breakfast				
apple cinnamon	6 oz	4	220	16%
berries	6 oz	3	220	12%
cherry w/almonds	6 oz	3	210	13%
sunrise peach	6 oz	3	230	12%
strawberry banana	6 oz	3	230	12%
strawberry w/almonds	6 oz	3	210	13%
tropical fruits	6 oz	4	230	16%

Food and Description	Amount	Fat Grams	Total Calories	% Fat Calories
(Yoplait)-Nonfat				
plain	8 oz	–	120	–
vanilla	8 oz	–	180	–
(Yoplait)-Original				
apple	6 oz	4	190	19%
blueberry	6 oz	4	190	19%
boysenberry	6 oz	4	190	19%
cherry	6 oz	4	190	19%
lemon	6 oz	4	190	19%
mixed berry	6 oz	4	190	19%
orange	6 oz	4	190	19%
peach	6 oz	4	190	19%
pina colada	6 oz	4	190	19%
plain	6 oz	5	130	35%
raspberry	6 oz	4	190	19%
strawberry	6 oz	4	190	19%
strawberry-banana	6 oz	4	190	19%
vanilla	6 oz	3	180	15%
(Yoplait 150)/all flavors	6 oz	–	150	–
YOGURT BARS				
(The Country's Best Yogurt)				
Yog-a-bar				
low-fat vanilla	1 3 oz bar	11	170	58%
sugar-free vanilla	1 3 oz bar	9	120	68%
vanilla w/heath	1 3 oz bar	14	220	57%
toasted almonds	1 3 oz bar	17	240	64%
YOGURT DESSERT (Sara Lee)				
frozen strawberry	1 slice	< 1	120	4%
YOGURT DRINKS				
(Dannon)/all flavors	8 oz	4	190	19%
(Glen Oaks)				
banana	8 oz	4	212	17%
raspberry	8 oz	4	212	17%
strawberry	8 oz	4	212	17%
tropical fruit	8 oz	4	212	17%
YOGURT, FROZEN				

(NOTE: Since the data for frozen yogurt varies from yogurt shop to yogurt shop, beginning at 0 for non-fat yogurt. I suggest you check with your favorite yogurt shop for the fat content in fat grams per ounce or serving, not in %, in the yogurts they serve. REMINDER—try to stick with the fruit toppings, as most other toppings are high in fat.)

Food and Description	Amount	Fat Grams	Total Calories	% Fat Calories
(Brice)				
cappuccino	3 oz	3	90	30%
chocolate	3 oz	3	100	27%

Food and Description	Amount	Fat Grams	Total Calories	% Fat Calories
strawberry	3 oz	3	100	27%
vanilla	3 oz	3	90	30%
(Dannon)-On A Stick				
all flavors	1.75 oz	1	50	18%
(Danny)-Yogurt Bars				
boysenberry-carob coated	1 bar	8	140	51%
chocolate	1 bar	1	60	15%
chocolate-chocolate coated	1 bar	8	130	55%
pina colada	1 bar	1	70	13%
raspberry-chocolate coated	1 bar	7	130	49%
strawberry-chocolate coated	1 bar	7	130	49%
vanilla	1 bar	1	60	15%
vanilla-chocolate coated	1 bar	8	130	55%
(Dreyer's) Inspirations				
low-fat				
blueberry	3 oz	1	80	11%
cherry	3 oz	1	80	11%
chocolate	3 oz	1	80	11%
chocolate sundae	3 oz	3	90	30%
citris height	3 oz	1	80	11%
marble fudge	3 oz	3	100	27%
mocha fudge	3 oz	3	100	27%
perfectly peach	3 oz	1	80	11%
raspberry	3 oz	1	80	11%
raspberry vanilla	3 oz	1	80	11%
strawberry	3 oz	1	80	11%
strawberry-banana	3 oz	1	80	11%
vanilla	3 oz	1	80	11%
non-fat				
cherry	3 oz	–	70	–
chocolate	3 oz	–	80	–
mocha	3 oz	–	80	–
strawberry	3 oz	–	70	–
vanilla	3 oz	–	80	–
(Haagen-Dazs)				
chocolate	3 oz	3	130	21%
peach	3 oz	3	120	23%
strawberry	3 oz	3	120	23%
vanilla	3 oz	3	130	21%
vanilla almond crunch	3 oz	5	150	30%
(Honey Hill)				
chocolate thunder	3 oz	3	110	25%
cookie jar	3 oz	5	130	35%
peach	3 oz	3	110	25%

Food and Description	Amount	Fat Grams	Total Calories	% Fat Calories
vanilla velvet	3 oz	4	110	33%
white almond chocolate	3 oz	5	120	38%
(Kemps)-all flavors	3 oz	1	80	11%
(Knudsen) Push Ups/all flavors	3 oz	1	90	10%
(La Corona)				
blueberry	3 oz	1	80	11%
chocolate	3 oz	2	90	20%
strawberry	3 oz	1	80	11%
strawberry-banana	3 oz	1	90	10%
(La Carona)/Frozen Yogurt On A Stick				
all flavors	1	1	50	18%
(Lite Time)				
french vanilla	3 oz	3	90	30%
strawberry	3 oz	3	90	30%
(Natural Nectar's) Fi-bar Yogurt-Lite				
all flavors	1 sandwich	7	190	33%
(Rhapsody Farms)				
mocha almond	4 oz	2	89	20%
red raspberry	4 oz	2	89	20%
vanilla	4 oz	2	89	20%
Non Fat				
chocolate peanut butter	3 oz	–	85	–
dutch chocolate	3 oz	–	85	–
mocha madness	3 oz	–	85	–
peach	3 oz	–	85	–
strawberry extravaganza	3 oz	–	85	–
(Sealtest)				
black cherry	1/4 pint	2	120	15%
red raspberry	1/4 pint	1	100	9%
strawberry	1/4 pint	2	110	16%
Tres Bein (Shamrock)				
french vanilla	3 oz	3	90	30%
honey nut	3 oz	3	100	27%
peach	3 oz	2	90	20%
raspberry	3 oz	2	90	20%
strawberry	3 oz	2	90	20%
(Yoplait)				
banana	3 oz	3	90	30%
chocolate	3 oz	2	90	20%
mixed berry	3 oz	3	90	30%
peach	3 oz	2	90	20%
raspberry	3 oz	3	90	30%
strawberry	3 oz	2	90	20%
vanilla	3 oz	2	90	20%

Z

Food and Description	Amount	Fat Grams	Total Calories	% Fat Calories

ZABAGLIONE (*See* CUSTARD)
ZUCCHINI (*See* SQUASH, SUMMER)

Fast food

Food and Description	Amount	Fat Grams	Total Calories	% Fat Calories
GENERIC LISTING (USDA Averages Derived From Several Restaurant Chains)				
BREAKFAST				
Biscuit-plain	1	13	276	42%
Croissant w/egg & cheese	1	24.7	369	60%
Croissant w/egg, cheese, & bacon	1	28	413	61%
Croissant w/egg, cheese, & ham	1	33.58	475	64%
Croissant w/egg, cheese, & sausage	1	38	524	65%
Danish-cheese	1	24.6	353	63%
Danish-cinnamon	1	16.7	349	43%
Danish-fruit	1	15.9	335	43%
Egg-scrambled	2 eggs	15	200	68%
English Muffin				
w/butter	1	5.76	189	27%
w/cheese & sausage	1	24	394	55%
w/egg, cheese, & Canadian bacon	1	19.76	383	46%
w/egg, cheese, & sausage	1	30.85	487	57%
French Toast w/butter	2 slices	18.76	356	47%
French Toast Sticks	5 sticks	29	479	55%
Omelet-ham & cheese	2 egg	17.7	255	62%
Pancakes w/syrup & butter	3 cakes	13.99	519	24%
Potatoes, hash brown	½ cup	9	151	54%
Sausage	1 patty	8	100	72%
CHICKEN, CHILI, SEAFOOD, PIZZA				
Chicken/breaded/fried/dark meat	2 pieces	26.7	430	56%
Chicken/breaded/fried/wing & breast	2 pieces	29.5	494	54%
Chicken nuggets				
plain	1 piece	2.95	48	55%
	6 pieces	17.7	290	55%
w/bar-b-q sauce	6 pieces	17.96	330	49%
w/honey	6 pieces	17.5	329	48%
w/mustard sauce	6 pieces	18.9	323	53%
w/sweet & sour sauce	6 pieces	17.95	346	47%
Chili Con Carne	1 cup	8	254	28%
Clams/breaded/fried	¾ cup	26	451	52%
Crab/baked	1 cake	1	88	10%

Food and Description	Amount	Fat Grams	Total Calories	% Fat Calories
Crab-soft shell/fried	1	17.86	334	48%
Crab/fried	1 cake	18.8	290	58%
Fish Fillet battered or breaded fried	1	11	211	47%
Oysters/battered or breaded/fried	6	17.9	368	44%
Pizza-cheese	⅛ of			
	12" pizza	2.5	109	21%
	12" pizza	20	873	21%
Pizza-meat & vegetable	⅛ of			
	12" pizza	4	152	24%
	12" pizza	35	1213	26%
Pizza-pepperoni	⅛ of			
	12" pizza	5	135	33%
	12" pizza	41.55	1081	35%
Pizza-supreme (thin & crispy)	½ of			
	10" pizza	21	510	37%
(thick & chewy)	½ of			
	10" pizza	22	640	31%
Scallops/breaded/fried	6 pieces	19	386	44%
Shrimp/breaded/fried	6-8 pieces	24.9	454	49%
CONDIMENTS				
Butter	1 pkt-½ oz	11	100	100%
Catsup	1 pkt-¼ oz	–	3	–
Half & Half	1 pkt-½ oz	1.6	18	80%
Honey	1 pkt-½ oz	–	43	–
Jelly	1 pkt-¾ oz	–	58	–
Lemon	1 pkt-½ oz	–	3	–
Lettuce	2 leaves	–	2	–
Mayonnaise	1 pkt-⅖ oz	9	81	100%
Mustard	1 pkt-⅕ oz	–	4	–
Nondairy Creamer	1 pkt-⅖ oz	3.5	55	57%
Onion	2 slices	–	7	–
Pickle	2 slices	–	2	–
Salad Dressings				
Bleu Cheese	1 pkt-2½ oz	34	342	90%
French	1 pkt-2 oz	20.6	228	81%
Italian	1 pkt-2 oz	34	326	94%
Low Calorie	1 pkt-2 oz	2	50	36%
Oriental	1 pkt-2 oz	1	102	9%
Thousand Island	1 pkt-2½ oz	39	396	89%
Wine Vinegar	1 Tbs	–	2	–
Sugar	1 pkt	–	25	–
Sugar Substitute	1 pkt	–	4	–

Food and Description	Amount	Fat Grams	Total Calories	% Fat Calories
Syrup	1 pkt-1½ oz	–	122	–
Tartar Sauce	1 pkt-½ oz	8	74	97%
Tomato	1 slice	–	5	–
DESSERTS				
Brownie	1	10	243	37%
Fried Pies	1	14	266	47%
Ice Cream Cone	Small	3	110	25%
	Medium	7	230	27%
	Large	10	340	27%
Ice Cream Cone dipped in chocolate	Small	7	150	42%
	Medium	13	300	39%
	Large	20	450	40%
Ice Cream Sandwich	1	4	140	26%
Ice Milk (soft serve w/cone)	1 oz	6	164	33%
Sundae				
carmel	1	9	303	27%
hot fudge	1	8.6	284	27%
strawberry	1	7.85	269	26%
MEXICAN FOODS				
Burritos				
bean	2	13.5	448	27%
bean & cheese	2	11.7	377	28%
bean & chili peppers	2	14.67	413	32%
bean & meat	2	17.8	508	32%
bean, cheese, & beef	2	13	331	35%
beef	2	20.8	523	36%
beef & chili peppers	2	16.5	426	35%
beef, cheese, & chili peppers	2	24.79	634	35%
Chimichanga				
beef	1	19.67	425	42%
beef & cheese	1	23.45	443	48%
beef & red chili peppers	1	19	424	40%
beef, cheese, & red chili peppers	1	17.55	364	43%
Enchilada				
cheese & beef	1	17.64	324	49%
cheese, beef, & beans	1	16	344	42%
cheese & sour cream	1	18.85	320	53%
Frijoles-cheese	1 cup	7.78	226	31%
Nachos				
cheese	6-8 pieces	18.95	345	49%
chese & jalapeno pepper	6-8 pieces	34	607	50%
cheese, ground beef, beans & jalapeno pepper	6-8 pieces	30.69	568	49%
cinnamon & sugar	6-8 pieces	35.98	592	55%

Food and Description	Amount	Fat Grams	Total Calories	% Fat Calories
Taco	1 small	20.55	370	50%
	1 large	31.6	569	50%
Taco Salad-lettuce, tomato, chili sauce, ground beef, cheese, & taco shell	1½ cup	14.77	279	47%
Taco Salad w/chili con carne	1½ cup	13	288	41%
Tostada				
bean & cheese	1	9.86	223	40%
bean, beef, & cheese	1	16.9	334	46%
beef & cheese	1	16	315	46%
beef, cheese, & guacomole	2	23	360	58%
SALADS & SALAD BAR MISC.				
Alfalfa Sprouts	1 oz	–	10	–
Bacon Bits	2 Tbs	3	54	50%
Broccoli	~ 2 oz	–	6	–
Carrots	~ 2 oz	–	12	–
Cauliflower	~ 2 oz	–	14	–
Cheese				
cheddar/shredded	3 Tbs	7	84	75%
cottage	½ cup	5	117	39%
parmesan	3 Tbs	4.5	70	58%
Cole Slaw	½ cup	8	90	80%
Croutons	18 pieces	1	35	26%
Cucumber-sliced	3 slices	–	2	–
Eggs-hard-cooked/chopped	2 Tbs	2	30	60%
Garbanzo Beans	1 Tbs	–	11	–
Green Peas	½ cup	–	60	–
Lettuce	½ cup	–	5	–
Mozzarella Cheese	1 oz	7	90	70%
Mushrooms-pieces	¼ cup	–	6	–
Onions	2 Tbs	–	4	–
Peppers, Green	2 Tbs	–	4	–
Salad Dressings (*See also* Condiments) REMEMBER: 2 oz = 4 LEVEL TBS!				
Salad-Chef-w/cheese, turkey, ham & egg	1½ cup	16	267	54%
Salad-tossed/no dressing w/lettuce, tomato, radishes, carrots, cabbage, cucumber & green pepper	1½ cup	–	32	–
Salad-tossed				
w/cheese & egg	1½ cup	5.79	102	51%
w/chicken	1½ cup	2	105	17%
w/pasta & seafood	1½ cup	20.85	380	49%
w/shrimp	1½ cup	2	107	17%

Food and Description	Amount	Fat Grams	Total Calories	% Fat Calories
Tomatoes	1 oz	6	–	–
SANDWICHES				

(NOTE: Meat patty sizes:Regular, single meat patty = 2 oz patty;
Regular, double meat patty = two 2 oz patties; Large, single meat
patty = 4 oz (¼ pound) patty. All sizes of meat patties are served)
on appropriate size buns.)

*Does not include condiments or garnishes such as pickle, catsup,
lettuce, onions, tomato, mustard, or mayonnaise/mayonnaise-type
dressing.

Food and Description	Amount	Fat Grams	Total Calories	% Fat Calories
Cheeseburger*	Regular/ Single	15	320	42%
Cheeseburger	Regular/ Double	28	457	55%
Cheeseburger*-double bun	Regular/ Double	21.6	461	42%
Cheeseburger*	Large/ Single	32.99	608	49%
Cheeseburger w/bacon	Large/ Single	36.76	609	60%
	Large/ Double	43.65	706	56%
Cheeseburger*	Large/ Triple	50.97	796	57%
Chicken Fillet*	1	29	515	51%
Chicken Fillet w/cheese*	1	38.76	632	55%
Egg & Cheese on bun*	1	19	340	50%
Fish Fillet*	1	22.77	431	48%
Fish Fillet w/tartar sauce/cheese*	1	28.6	524	49%
Hamburger*	Regular/ Single	11.8	275	39%
	Regular/ Double	27.9	544	46%
Hamburger	Regular/ Single	13	279	42%
	Regular/ Double	32	576	50%
Hamburger*	Large/ Single	22.9	400	52%
Hamburger	Large/ Single	27	511	48%
	Large/ Triple	41	693	53%
Ham & Cheese on Bun*	1	15	353	38%
Ham, Egg, & Cheese on Bun*	1	16	348	41%
Hot Dog*	1	14.5	242	54%

Food and Description	Amount	Fat Grams	Total Calories	% Fat Calories
Hot Dog w/chili*	1	17.5	324	49%
Hot Dog (i.e., corn dog)*	1	18.9	460	37%
Roast Beef on Bun*	1	13.77	346	36%
Roast Beef w/cheese*	1	18	402	40%
Roast Beef*	1 Super	28	620	41%
Sandwiches on sliced whole wheat bread w/average portions				
Bacon, Lettuce, Tomato	1	16	290	50%
Bologna/plain	1	16	305	47%
Chicken Salad	1	20	255	71%
Chicken-sliced w/lettuce	1	15	310	44%
Club-Chicken, bacon, & tomato	1	26	570	41%
Corned Beef/plain	1	10	296	30%
Cream Cheese & Jelly	1	16	370	39%
Egg Salad	1	13	285	41%
Ham/plain	1	16	285	51%
Ham & Cheese (Swiss)	1	24	390	55%
Ham Salad	1	17	321	48%
Liverwurst/plain	1	12	260	42%
Peanut Butter	1	20	350	51%
Peanut Butter & Jelly	1	15	385	35%
Roast Beef (hot w/gravy)	1	25	421	53%
Roast Pork (hot w/gravy)	1	31	503	56%
Steak/sirloin (lean & fat-3 oz)	1	12	325	33%
Tunafish Salad	1	14	275	46%
Turkey/plain	1	19	400	43%
SIDE ORDERS				
Chili	1 cup	9	268	30%
Coleslaw	¾ cup	10.97	147	67%
Corn on cob w/butter	1 ear	3	155	17%
Corn on cob w/o butter	1 ear	1	125	7%
Hush Puppies	5	11.59	256	41%
Macaroni Salad w/mayonnaise	½ cup	6	168	32%
Onion Rings	8-9	15.5	175	80%
Potato-baked				
w/cheese	1	28.7	475	54%
w/cheese & bacon	1	25.89	451	52%
w/cheese sauce & broccoli	1	21	402	47%
w/cheese sauce & chili	1	21.86	481	41%
w/sour cream & chives	1	22	394	50%
Potatoes-French Fried				
w/beef tallow	Regular	12	237	46%
	Large	18.5	358	47%
w/beef tallow & vegetable oil	Regular	12	237	46%
	Large	18.5	358	47%

Food and Description	Amount	Fat Grams	Total Calories	% Fat Calories
w/vegetable oil	Regular	12	235	46%
	Large	18.5	355	47%
Potatoes-mashed w/whole milk & margarine	⅓ cup	.97	66	13%
Potato Chips	10 chips	7	105	60%
	1 oz	10	148	61%
Potato Salad	⅓ cup	5.7	108	48%
Waldorf Salad	½ cup	5	90	50%

SUBS

[NOTE: Following subs are from 6 to 8 inches long (8 to 12 ounces).]

Food and Description	Amount	Fat Grams	Total Calories	% Fat Calories
Sub w/salami, ham, cheese, lettuce, tomato, onion, & roll	1	18.6	456	37%
Sub w/roast beef, lettuce, tomato and mayonnaise	1	12.96	411	28%
Sub-tuna salad	1	27.99	584	43%

FAST FOOD CHAINS BY NAME

ARBY'S

Food and Description	Amount	Fat Grams	Total Calories	% Fat Calories
Beef'N Cheddar	1	26.8	455	53%
Chicken Breast Sandwich	1	25	493	50%
Chicken (Roasted) Club Sandwich	1	33	610	49%
Chicken Salad	1	36	515	63%
Hot Ham'N Cheese Sandwich	1	13.7	292	42%
French Fries	Regular	13	246	48%
Potato Cakes	2 cakes	12.9	201	58%
Roast Beef, Giant Sandwich	1	23	531	39%
Roast Beef, Junior Sandwich	1	8.5	218	35%
Roast Beef, Regular Sandwich	1	14.8	353	38%
Roast Beef, Super	1	22	501	40%
Shake				
chocolate	12 oz	11.6	451	23%
jamocha	11.5 oz	10.5	368	26%
vanilla	11 oz	11.5	330	31%
Turkey Deluxe Sandwich	1	16.6	375	40%
Turnovers				
apple	1	18	303	54%
cherry	1	17.8	280	57%

BURGER KING

BEVERAGES

Food and Description	Amount	Fat Grams	Total Calories	% Fat Calories
Coffee	1	–	2	–
Milk				
2%	1	5	121	37%
whole	1	9	157	52%
Orange Juice	1	–	82	–
Shakes				
chocolate	Regular	12	320	34%

Food and Description	Amount	Fat Grams	Total Calories	% Fat Calories
chocolate syrup added	Regular	11	374	27%
vanilla	Regular	10	321	28%
vanilla syrup added	Regular	10	334	27%
Soft Drinks				
Diet Pepsi	Regular	–	1	–
Pepsi	Regular	–	159	–
7 UP	Regular	–	144	–
BREAKFAST				
Breakfast Bagel Sandwich				
bacon	1	19	438	39%
ham	1	15	418	32%
plain	1	14	387	33%
sausage	1	36	621	52%
Breakfast Croissan'wich				
bacon	1	24	355	61%
ham	1	20	335	54%
plain	1	19	304	56%
sausage	1	41	538	69%
French Toast Sticks	1 order	29	499	52%
Great Danish	1	40	500	72%
Scrambled Egg Platter	1	30	468	58%
w/bacon	1	36	536	60%
w/sausage	1	52	702	67%
CHICKEN				
Chicken Tenders	6 pieces	10	204	44%
DESSERTS				
Apple Pie	1	12	305	35%
SALADS				
Chef	1	9	180	45%
Chicken	1	4	140	26%
Garden	1	5	90	50%
Side	1	–	20	–
Salad Bacon Bits	1 pkt	1	16	56%
Salad Croutons	1 pkt	1	29	31%
Salad Dressing				
Bleu Cheese	1 pkt	31	300	93%
French	1 pkt	23	280	74%
House	1 pkt	26	260	35%
Reduced Calorie Italian	1 pkt	2	30	60%
Thousand Island	1 pkt	23	240	86%
SANDWICHES				
Bacon Double Cheeseburger	1	31	510	55%
Cheeseburger	1	15	317	43%
Chicken Specialty Sandwich	1	40	688	52%
Ham & Cheese Specialty Sandwich	1	23	471	44%

Food and Description	Amount	Fat Grams	Total Calories	% Fat Calories
Hamburger	1	12	275	39%
Whaler Fish Sandwich/tartar sauce	1	27	488	50%
Whopper Sandwich	1	36	628	52%
w/cheese	1	43	711	54%
Whopper Jr. Sandwich	1	17	322	48%
w/cheese	1	20	364	50%
SIDE ORDERS				
French fries	Regular	13	227	52%
Onion Rings	1 Order	16	274	53%
CARL'S JR.				
BAKERY PRODUCTS				
Blueberry Muffin	1	7	256	25%
Bran Muffin	1	6	220	25%
Chocolate Cake	1	20	380	47%
Chocolate Chip Cookies	1 Order	13	330	36%
Danish-variety	1	9	300	27%
BEVERAGES				
Carbonated	Regular	–	243	–
Diet Carbonated	Regular	–	2	–
Iced Tea	Regular	–	2	–
Milk-2% low-fat	10 oz	6	175	31%
Orange Juice	Small	1	94	10%
Shakes	Regular	7	353	18%
BREAKFAST				
Bacon	2 strips	4	50	72%
English Muffin w/margarine	1	6	180	30%
French Toast Dips	1 Order	25	480	47%
Hashed Brown Nuggets	1 Order	9	170	48%
Hot Cakes w/margarine	1 Order	12	360	30%
Sausage	1 Patty	17	190	81%
Scrambled Eggs	1 Order	9	120	68%
Sunrise Sandwich				
w/bacon	1	19	370	46%
w/sausage	1	32	500	58%
POTATOES				
Bacon & Cheese	1	34	650	47%
Broccoli & Cheese	1	17	470	33%
Cheese	1	22	550	36%
Fiesta	1	23	550	38%
Lite	1	3	250	11%
Sour Cream & Chive	1	13	350	33%
SALAD DRESSINGS				
Bleu Cheese	2 oz	14	150	84%
House	2 oz	17	186	82%
Italian Reduced-Calorie	2 oz	10	90	100%

Food and Description	Amount	Fat Grams	Total Calories	% Fat Calories
Thousand Island	2 oz	23	231	90%
SANDWICHES				
American Cheese	1	5	63	71%
California Roast Beef'n Swiss	1	8	360	20%
Charbroiler BBQ Chicken	1	5	320	14%
Charbroiler Chicken Club	1	22	510	39%
Country Fried Steak	1	33	610	49%
Double Western Bacon Cheeseburger	1	53	890	54%
Famous Star Hamburger	1	36	590	55%
Filet of Fish	1	26	550	43%
Happy Star Hamburger	1	8	220	33%
Old Time Star Hamburger	1	17	400	38%
Swiss Cheese	1	4	57	63%
Super Star Hamburger	1	50	770	58%
Western Bacon Cheeseburger	1	33	630	47%
SIDE ORDERS				
French Fries	Regular	17	360	43%
Onion Rings	1 Order	15	310	44%
Zucchini	1 Order	16	300	48%
SOUPS				
Boston Clam Chowder	1 Order	8	140	51%
Cream of Broccoli	1 Order	6	140	39%
Lumber Jack Mix Vegetable	1 Order	3	70	39%
Old Fashioned Chicken Noodle	1 Order	1	80	11%
CHICK-FIL-A				
DESSERTS/BEVERAGES				
Fudge Brownie w/nuts	1	19	369	46%
Icecream	1	4.9	134	33%
Lemon Pie	1 slice	5	329	14%
Lemonade	Regular	–	124	–
Iced Tea	Regular	–	3	–
SANDWICHES/NUGGETS				
Chick-fil-A Chicken Sandwich w/bun	1	8.8	426	19%
Chick-fil-A Chicken Deluxe Sandwich	1	8.9	435	18%
Chick-fil-A Nuggets	8 pack	15	287	47%
	12 pack	22.6	430	47%
Chicken Salad Sandwich w/wheat bread	1	26.5	449	53%
Chick-fil-A Chicken/no bun	1	6.8	219	28%
Chick-fil-A Chargrilled Chicken Sandwich	1	4.8	258	17%
Chick-fil-A Chargrilled Chicken Deluxe Sandwich w/lettuce & tomato	1	4.9	266	17%
SALADS/SIDE ORDERS				
Chargrilled Chicken Garden Salad	1	2	126	14%
Chicken Salad-Cup	1	28	309	82%

Food and Description	Amount	Fat Grams	Total Calories	% Fat Calories
Chicken Salad-Plate	1	43.5	475	82%
Cole Slaw-cup	1	14	175	72%
Carrot & Raisin Salad-Cup	1	4.8	116	37%
Hearty Breast of Chicken Soup-small	1	2.7	152	16%
Potato Salad-Cup	1	15	198	68%
Tossed Salad				
plain	1	–	21	–
w/Honey French	1	24	246	88%
w/Lite Italian	1	2	66	27%
w/Ranch dressing	1	16	177	81%
w/Thousand Island	1	21.9	231	85%
Waffle Potato Fries	Regular	13.5	270	45%
CHURCH'S FRIED CHICKEN				
Breast	1	17	287	64%
Breast w/wing	1	20	303	59%
Leg	1	9	147	55%
Thigh	1	22	306	65%
SIDE DISHES				
Corn w/butter spread	1	9	237	34%
French Fries	Regular	6	138	39%
DAIRY QUEEN				
BEVERAGES				
Malt-chocolate	Small	13	520	23%
	Regular	18	760	21%
	Large	25	1060	21%
Shake-chocolate	Small	13	490	24%
	Regular	19	710	24%
	Large	26	990	24%
MISCELLANEOUS SPECIALTIES				
Banana Split	1	11	540	18%
Blizzard-Heath	16 oz	24	800	27%
Buster Bar	1	29	460	57%
Chocolate Sundae	Small	4	190	19%
	Regular	8	310	23%
	Large	10	440	21%
Cone	Small	4	140	26%
	Regular	7	240	26%
	Large	10	340	27%
DQ Sandwich	1	4	140	26%
Dilly Bar	1	13	210	56%
Dipped Cone	Small	9	190	43%
	Regular	16	340	42%
	Large	24	570	38%
Double Delight	1	20	490	37%
Float	1	7	410	15%

Food and Description	Amount	Fat Grams	Total Calories	% Fat Calories
Freeze	1	12	500	22%
Frozen Dessert	4 oz	6	180	30%
Fudge Nut Bar	1	25	406	55%
Hot Fudge Brownie Delight Sundae	1	25	600	38%
Mr. Misty	Small	–	190	–
	Regular	–	250	–
	Large	–	340	–
Mr. Misty Float	1	7	390	16%
Mr. Misty Freeze	1	12	500	22%
Parfait	1	8	430	17%
Peanut Buster Parfait	1	34	740	41%
Queen's Choice				
chocolate	1	16	326	44%
vanilla	1	16	322	45%
Strawberry Shortcake	1	11	540	18%
SANDWICHES				
Chicken Fillet	1	41	670	55%
w/cheese	1	45	710	57%
Fish Fillet	1	17	400	38%
w/cheese	1	21	440	43%
Hamburger	Single	16	360	40%
	Double	28	530	48%
	Triple	45	710	57%
Hamburger-w/cheese	Single	20	410	44%
	Double	37	650	51%
	Triple	50	820	55%
Hot Dog	1	16	280	51%
w/cheese	1	21	330	57%
w/chili	1	20	320	56%
Super Hot Dog	1	27	520	47%
w/cheese	1	34	580	53%
w/chili	1	32	570	51%
SIDE ORDERS				
French Fries	Regular	10	200	45%
	Large	16	320	45%
Onion Rings	1 Order	16	280	51%
DOMINO'S				
CHEESE PIZZA				
12" - serves 4	2 slices	6	340	16%
16" - serves 6	2 slices	8	400	18%
Deluxe	2 slices	20	498	36%
PEPPERONI				
12" - serves 4	2 slices	12	380	28%
16" - serves 6	2 slices	14	440	29%
Double Cheese	2 slices	25	545	41%

Food and Description	Amount	Fat Grams	Total Calories	% Fat Calories
GODFATHER'S PIZZA				
ORIGINAL PIZZA				
Cheese				
Mini	¼ pizza	4	190	19%
Small	⅙ pizza	7	240	26%
Medium	⅛ pizza	8	270	27%
Large (Hot Slice)	⅛ pizza	11	370	27%
Large	⅒ pizza	9	297	27%
Combo				
Mini	¼ pizza	7	240	26%
Small	⅙ pizza	15	360	38%
Medium	⅛ pizza	17	400	38%
Large (Hot Slice)	⅛ pizza	24	550	39%
Large	⅒ pizza	19	437	39%
THIN CRUST				
Cheese				
Small	⅙ pizza	6	180	30%
Medium	⅛ pizza	7	210	30%
Large	⅒ pizza	7	228	28%
Combo				
Small	⅙ pizza	13	270	43%
Medium	⅛ pizza	14	310	41%
Large	⅒ pizza	16	336	43%
STUFFED PIE				
Cheese				
Small	⅙ pizza	11	310	32%
Medium	⅛ pizza	13	350	33%
Large	⅒ pizza	16	381	38%
Combo				
Small	⅙ pizza	20	430	42%
Medium	⅛ pizza	23	480	43%
Large	⅒ pizza	26	521	45%
HARDEE'S				
BREAKFAST				
Bacon Biscuit	1	21	360	53%
Bacon & Egg Biscuit	1	24	410	53%
Bacon, Egg, & Cheese Biscuit	1	28	460	55%
Big Country Breakfast				
w/bacon	1	40	660	55%
w/country ham	1	38	670	51%
w/ham	1	33	620	48%
w/sausage	1	57	850	60%
Biscuit'N'Gravy	1 Order	24	440	49%
Canadian Rise'N'Shine Biscuit	1	27	470	52%
Chicken Biscuit	1	22	430	46%

Food and Description	Amount	Fat Grams	Total Calories	% Fat Calories
Cinnamon'N'Raisin	1	17	320	48%
Country Ham Biscuit	1	18	350	46%
Country Ham & Egg Biscuit	1	22	400	50%
Ham Biscuit	1	16	320	45%
Ham & Egg Biscuit	1	19	370	46%
Ham, Egg, & Cheese Biscuit	1	23	420	49%
Hash Rounds	1 Order	14	230	55%
Margarine/Butter Blend	1	4	35	100%
Rise'N'Shine Biscuit	1	18	320	51%
Sausage Biscuit	1	28	440	57%
Sausage & Egg Biscuit	1	31	490	57%
Steak Biscuit	1	29	500	52%
Steak & Egg Biscuit	1	32	550	52%
Syrup	1	–	120	–
Three Pancakes	1 Order	2	280	6%
w/2 bacon strips	1 Order	9	350	23%
w/1 sausage pattie	1 Order	16	430	34%
HAMBURGERS & SANDWICHES				
All Beef Hotdog	1	17	300	51%
Bacon Cheeseburger	1	39	610	58%
Big Deluxe Burger	1	30	500	54%
Big Roast Beef	1	11	300	33%
Big Twin	1	25	450	50%
Cheeseburger	1	14	320	39%
Chicken Fillet	1	13	370	32%
Fisherman's Fillet	1	24	500	43%
Grilled Chicken Breast Sandwich	1	9	310	26%
Hamburger	1	10	270	33%
Hot Ham'N'Cheese	1	12	330	33%
Mushroom'N'Swiss Burger	1	27	490	50%
Quarter Pound Cheeseburger	1	29	500	52%
Regular Roast Beef	1	9	260	31%
The Lean 1	1	18	420	39%
Turkey Club	1	16	390	37%
SALADS & SPECIAL ITEMS				
Big Fry	1	23	500	41%
Chef Salad	1	15	240	56%
Chicken'N'Pasta Salad	1	3	230	12%
Chicken Stix	6 pieces	9	210	39%
	9 pieces	14	310	41%
Crispy Curls	1 Order	16	300	48%
Garden Salad	1	14	210	60%
Large French Fries	1	17	360	43%
Regular French Fries	1	11	230	43%
Side Salad	1	–	20	–

Food and Description	Amount	Fat Grams	Total Calories	% Fat Calories
SHAKES & DESSERTS				
Apple Turnover	1	12	270	40%
Big Cookie	1	13	250	47%
Cool Twist Cone				
chocolate	1	6	200	27%
vanilla	1	6	190	28%
vanilla/chocolate	1	6	190	28%
Cool Twist Sundae				
caramel	1	10	330	27%
hot fudge	1	12	320	34%
strawberry	1	8	260	28%
Shake				
chocolate	1	8	460	16%
strawberry	1	8	440	16%
vanilla	1	9	400	20%
JACK-IN-THE-BOX				
BEVERAGES				
Coca-Cola Classic	12 oz	–	144	–
Coffee	8 oz	–	2	–
Diet Coke	12 oz	–	1	–
Dr. Pepper	12 oz	–	144	–
Iced Tea	12 oz	–	1	–
Milk-lowfat	8.5 oz	5	122	37%
Orange Juice	1	–	80	–
Ramblin'Root Beer	12 oz	–	176	–
Shakes				
chocolate	11 oz	7	330	19%
strawberry	11.5 oz	7	320	20%
vanilla	11 oz	6	320	17%
Sprite	12 oz	–	144	–
BREAKFAST				
Breakfast Jack	1	13	307	38%
Canadian Crescent	1	31	452	62%
Grape Jelly	1 pkt	–	38	–
Hash Browns	1 Order	7	116	54%
Pancake Platter	1	22	612	32%
Pancake Syrup	1 pkt	–	121	–
Sausage Crescent	1	43	584	66%
Scrambled Egg Platter	1	40	662	54%
Supreme Crescent	1	40	547	66%
DESSERTS				
Cheesecake	1	17.5	309	51%
Hot Apple Turnover	1	24	410	53%
FINGER FOODS				
Chicken Strips	4 pieces	14	349	36%

Food and Description	Amount	Fat Grams	Total Calories	% Fat Calories
	6 pieces	20	523	34%
Egg Rolls	3 pieces	19	405	42%
	5 pieces	32	675	43%
Seafood Cocktail Sauce	1 pkt	–	32	–
Shrimp	10 pieces	16	270	53%
	15 pieces	24	404	54%
Sweet & Sour Sauce	1 pkt	–	44	–
Taquitos	5 pieces	16	363	40%
	7 pieces	22	508	39%
HAMBURGERS				
Bacon Cheeseburger	1	39	705	50%
Cheeseburger	1	14	315	40%
Double Cheeseburger	1	27	467	52%
Hamburger	1	11	267	37%
Jumbo Jack	1	34	584	52%
w/cheese	1	40	677	53%
Swiss & Bacon Burger	1	47	678	62%
Ultimate Cheeseburger	1	69	942	66%
MEXICAN FOOD				
Guacamole	1 pkt	5	55	82%
Salsa	1 pkt	–	8	–
Super Taco	1	17	288	53%
Taco	1	11	191	52%
SALADS				
Bleu Cheese Dressing	1 pkt	22	262	76%
Buttermilk House Dressing	1 pkt	36	362	90%
Chef Salad	1	18	295	57%
French-Reduced Calorie Dressing	1 pkt	8	176	41%
Mexican Chicken Salad	1	23	442	47%
Side Salad	1	3	51	53%
Taco Salad	1	31	503	56%
Thousand Island Dressing	1 pkt	30	312	87%
SANDWICHES				
Beef Fajita Pita	1	14	333	38%
Chicken Fajita Pita	1	8	292	25%
Chicken Supreme	1	36	575	56%
Fish Supreme	1	32	554	52%
Grilled Chicken Fillet	1	17	408	38%
Mayo-Onion Sauce	1 pkt	15	143	94%
Mayo-Mustard Sauce	1 pkt	13	124	94%
SIDE ORDERS				
French Fries	Small	12	221	49%
	Regular	19	353	48%
	Jumbo	24	442	50%
Onion Rings	1 Order	23	382	54%

Food and Description	Amount	Fat Grams	Total Calories	% Fat Calories
KENTUCKY FRIED CHICKEN				
EXTRA TASTY CRISPY CHICKEN				
Drumstick	1 piece	10.9	173	57%
Center Breast	1 piece	19.7	342	52%
Drumstick	1 piece	13.9	204	61%
Side Breast	1 piece	22	343	58%
Thigh	1 piece	29.8	406	66%
Wing	1 piece	18.6	254	66%
Hot Wings	6 pieces	24	376	57%
LITE N' CRISPY				
Center Breast	1 piece	11.9	220	49%
Drumstick	1 piece	7	121	52%
Side Breast	1 piece	12	204	53%
Thigh	1 piece	16.	246	61%
ORIGINAL RECIPE CHICKEN				
Drumstick	1 piece	8.5	146	52%
Center Breast	1 piece	15	283	48%
Thigh	1 piece	19.7	294	60%
Side Breast	1 piece	16.5	267	56%
Wing	1 piece	11.7	178	59%
KENTUCKY NUGGETS & SAUCES				
Nuggets	1	2.9	46	57%
Sauce				
Barbeque	1 oz	.57	35	15%
Honey	1 oz	–	49	–
Mustard	1 oz	.9	36	23%
Sweet & Sour	1 oz	.56	58	9%
OTHER KFC ITEMS				
Buttermilk Biscuits	1	11.9	232	46%
Chicken Littles Sandwich	1	10	169	53%
Cole Salw	1 order	6.57	119	50%
Colonel's Chicken Sandwich	1 sandwich	27	482	50%
Corn-on-the-Cob	1	3	176	15%
French Fries	Regular	11.9	244	44%
Mashed Potatoes & Gravy	1 order	1.6	71	20%
LONG JOHN SILVER'S				
A LA CARTE ITEMS				
Battered Fish	1 Order	8	150	48%
Battered Shrimp	1 Order	3	40	68%
Breaded Clams	1 Order	12	240	45%
Breaded Shrimp	1 Order	10	190	47%
Catfish Filet	1 Order	11	180	55%
Chicken Plank	1 Order	6	110	49%
Clam Chowder w/cod	1 Order	6	140	39%
Cole Slaw	1 Order	6	140	39%

Food and Description	Amount	Fat Grams	Total Calories	% Fat Calories
Corn on the Cob w/Whirl	1 Order	14	270	47%
Crispy Breaded Fish Sandwich	1	28	600	42%
Fries	1 Order	10	220	41%
Gumbo w/Cod & Shrimp Bobs	1 Order	8	120	60%
Homestyle Fish	1 Order	7	125	50%
Hushpuppies	1 Order	2	70	26%
Lemon Meringue Pie	1 Order	7	260	24%
Mixed Vegetables	1 Order	2	60	30%
Pecan Pie	1 Order	25	530	43%
Seafood Salad	1 Order	5	210	21%
Side Salad	1 Order	–	20	–
BAKED ENTREES				
Accompaniments				
Breadstick	1 serving	3	110	25%
Cole Slaw	1 serving	6	140	39%
Garden Vegetables	4 oz	6	120	45%
Green Beans	4 oz	< 1	30	15%
Rice Pilaf	5 oz	2	210	9%
Side Salad w/o dressing	1 serving	–	20	–
Vegetables	1 serving	6	120	45%
Seafood and chicken				
3-piece fish				
lemon crumb	5 oz	1	150	6%
light paprika	4.7 oz	< 1	120	4%
scampi sauce	5.2 oz	5	170	26%
2-piece fish w/rice & small salad				
lemon crumb	10 oz	4	320	11%
light paprika	10 oz	2	300	6%
chicken/light herb	4.1 oz	4	140	26%
cod	5.8 oz	< 1	150	3%
cod delight	6 oz	1	180	5%
cod supreme	6.2 oz	4	190	19%
shrimp scampi	5.7 oz	7	160	39%
CHILDREN'S MEALS				
1 Fish, Fries & 1 Hushpuppy	1 Order	20	440	41%
2 Planks, Fries & 2 Hushpuppies	1 Order	24	510	42%
1 Fish, 1 Plank, Fries & 1 Hushpuppy	1 Order	26	550	43%
CONDIMENTS				
Bleu Cheese Dressing	1 pkt	2	120	15%
Catsup	1 pkt	–	15	–
Club Crackers	1 pkt	2	35	–
Honey Mustard Sauce	1 pkt	–	60	–
Hot Honey Mustard Sauce	1 pkt	2	90	20%
Malt Vinegar	1 pkt	–	2	–
Ranch Dressing	1 pkt	3	140	19%

Food and Description	Amount	Fat Grams	Total Calories	% Fat Calories
Reduced Calorie Italian Dressing	1 pkt	1	18	50%
Sea Salad Dressing	1 pkt	7	140	45%
Seafood Sauce	1 pkt	1	45	20%
Sweet-n-Sour Sauce	1 pkt	–	60	–
Tartar Sauce	1 pkt	3	80	34%
ENTREES				
2-pc Fish & Fries/2 fish, fries	2 hush-puppies	30	660	41%
3-pc Fish & Fries/3 fish, fries	2 hush-puppies	38	10	42%
Fish & More/2 fish, fries, slaw	2 hush-puppies	37	800	42%
3-pc Fish Dinner/3 fish, fries, slaw	2 hush-puppies	44	60	41%
3-pc Chicken Plank Dinner 3 chicken planks, fries, slaw	2 hush-puppies	39	830	42%
4-pc Chicken Plank Dinner 4 chicken planks, fries, slaw	2 hush-puppies	44	40	42%
Shrimp, Fish & Chicken Dinner 2 battered shrimp, 1 fish, 1 chicken plank, fries, slaw	2 hush-puppies	40	840	43%
Fish & Chicken 1 fish, 2 chicken planks, fries, slaw	2 hush-puppies	40	870	41%
Seafood Platter 1 fish, 2 battered, shrimp clams, fries, slaw	2 hush-puppies	46	970	43%
Clam Dinner Clams, fries, slaw	2 hush-puppies	45	980	41%
6-pc Battered Shrimp Dinner 6 battered shrimp, fries, slaw	2 hush-puppies	37	740	45%
9-pc Battered Shrimp Dinner 9 battered shrimp, fries, slaw	2 hush-puppies	45	860	47%
13-pc Breaded Shrimp Feast Breaded shrimp, fries, slaw	2 hush-puppies	41	880	42%

Food and Description	Amount	Fat Grams	Total Calories	% Fat Calories
21-pc Breaded Shrimp Feast				
Breaded shrimp, fries, slaw	2 hush-puppies	51	1070	43%
Shrimp & Fish Dinner				
1 fish, 3 battered shrimp, fries, slaw	2 hush-puppies	37	770	43%
Catfish Fillet Dinner				
2 catfish fillets, fries, slaw	2 hush-puppies	42	860	44%
Homestyle Fish Sandwich Platter	1	38	870	39%
3-pc Homestyle Fish Dinner				
Homestyle fish, fries, slaw	2 hush-puppies	42	880	43%
4-pc Homestyle Fish Dinner				
Homestyle fish, fries, slaw	2 hush-puppies	50	1010	45%
6-pc Homestyle Fish Dinner				
Homestyle fish, fries, slaw	2 hush-puppies	64	260	46%
SALADS				
Garden Salad	1	8	140	51%
Ocean Chef Salad	1	9	250	32%
Seafood Salad	1	7	270	23%
MCDONALD'S				
BEVERAGES				
Coca-Cola Classic	12 oz	–	140	–
	16 oz	–	190	–
	22 oz	–	260	–
	32 oz	–	384	–
Diet Coke	12 oz	–	1	–
	16 oz	–	1	–
	22 oz	–	2	–
	32 oz	–	3	–
Grapefruit Juice	6 oz	–	80	–
Milk-2%	8 oz	4.7	120	35%
Orange Drink	12 oz	–	130	–
	16 oz	–	180	–
	22 oz	–	240	–
	32 oz	–	360	–
Orange Juice	6 oz	–	80	–
Shakes				
chocolate	~ 10.7 oz	10.6	390	24%
strawberry	~ 10.7 oz	10	380	24%
vanilla	~ 10.7 oz	10	350	26%

Food and Description	Amount	Fat Grams	Total Calories	% Fat Calories
Sprite	12 oz	–	140	–
	16 oz	–	190	–
	22 oz	–	260	–
	32 oz	–	380	–
BREAKFAST				
Biscuit				
w/bacon, egg, & cheese	1	26	440	53%
w/biscuit spread	1	12.7	260	44%
w/sausage	1	29	440	59%
w/sausage & egg	1	34.5	520	42%
Danish-apple	1	17.9	390	41%
cinnamon raisin	1	21	440	43%
iced cheese	1	21.8	390	50%
raspberry	1	15.9	410	35%
Egg McMuffin	1	11	290	34%
English Muffin w/butter	1	4.6	170	24%
Hashbrown Potatoes	1 Order	7	130	49%
Hotcakes w/butter & syrup	1 Order	9	410	20%
Pork Sausage	1 Order	16	180	80%
Sausage McMuffin	1	21.9	370	53%
Sausage McMuffin w/egg	1	26.8	440	55%
Scrambled Eggs	1 Order	9.8	140	63%
CHICKEN MCNUGGETS & SAUCES				
Chicken McNuggets	1 Order	16	290	50%
Sauces				
Barbeque Sauce	1 pkt	.5	50	9%
Honey Sauce	1 pkt	–	45	–
Hot Mustard Sauce	1 pkt	.5	70	6%
Sweet & Sour Sauce	1 pkt	–	60	–
DESSERTS				
Apple Pie	1	14.8	260	51%
Chocolate Chip Cookies	~ 2.3 oz	15.6	330	43%
HotCaramel Sundae	1	9	340	24%
Hot Fudge Sundae	1	9	310	26%
McDonaldland Cookies	~ 2.3 oz	9	290	28%
Soft Serve Ice-cream	1	4.5	140	29%
Strawberry Sundae	1	7	171	37%
SALADS				
Bacon Bits	1 Serving	1	16	56%
Chef	1	13	230	51%
Chicken Salad Oriental	1	3	140	19%
Chow Mein Noodles	1 Serving	2	45	40%
Croutons	1 Serving	2	50	36%
Dressings-Bleu Cheese	½ oz	6.9	70	89%
Caesar	⅓ oz	6	60	90%

Food and Description	Amount	Fat Grams	Total Calories	% Fat Calories
French	½ oz	5	58	78%
Lite Vinaigrette	½ oz	.5	15	30%
Oriental	½ oz	–	24	–
Peppercorn	½ oz	8.7	80	98%
Ranch	½ oz	8.6	83	93%
Red French low-cal	½ oz	1.9	40	43%
Thousand Island	½ oz	7.5	78	87%
Garden	1	6.6	110	54%
Side	1	3	115	24%
SANDWICHES				
Big Mac	1	32	560	51%
Cheeseburger	1	13.8	310	40%
Fillet-O-Fish	1	26	440	53%
Hamburger	1	9.5	260	33%
McLean	1	10	310	29%
McChicken	1	28.6	490	53%
McD.L.T.	1	36.8	580	57%
McRib	1	21.9	455	43%
Quarter Pounder	1	20.7	410	45%
w/cheese	1	29	520	50%
SIDE ORDERS				
French Fries	Small	5	220	21%
	Medium	17	320	48%
	Large	21	400	47%
PIZZA HUT				
HAND-TOSSED PIZZA				
Cheese	2 slices/			
	Medium	20	518	35%
Pepperoni	2 slices/			
	Medium	23	500	41%
Supreme	2 slices/			
	Medium	26	540	43%
Super Supreme	2 slices/			
	Medium	25	556	41%
PAN PIZZA				
Cheese	2 slices/			
	Medium	18	492	33%
Pepperoni	2 slices/			
	Medium	22	540	37%
Supreme	2 slices/			
	Medium	30	589	46%
Super Supreme	2 slices/			
	Medium	26	563	42%
PERSONAL PAN PIZZA				
Pepperoni	Whole Pizza	29	675	39%

Food and Description	Amount	Fat Grams	Total Calories	% Fat Calories
Supreme	Whole Pizza 28		647	39%
THIN'N CRISPY PIZZA				
Cheese	2 slices/ Medium	17	398	38%
Pepperoni	2 slices/ Medium	20	413	44%
Supreme	2 slices/ Medium	22	459	43%
Super Supreme	2 slices/ Medium	21	463	41%
ROY ROGERS				
BEVERAGES				
Coke	12 oz	–	145	–
Diet Coke	12 oz	–	1	–
Hot Chocolate	6 oz	2	123	15%
Milkshake				
chocolate	1	10	358	25%
strawberry	1	10	315	29%
vanilla	1	11	306	32%
BREAKFAST				
Crescent Roll	1	18	287	56%
Crescent Sandwich	1	27	401	61%
w/bacon	1	30	431	63%
w/ham	1	29	445	59%
w/sausage	1	29	449	58%
Egg & Biscuit Platter	1	27	394	62%
w/bacon	1	30	435	62%
w/ham	1	29	442	59%
w/sausage	1	29	460	57%
Pancake Platter				
w/syrup & butter	1	15	452	30%
w/bacon	1	18	493	33%
w/ham	1	17	506	30%
w/sausage	1	30	608	44%
SANDWICHES				
Bacon Cheeseburger	1	39	581	60%
Cheeseburger	1	37	563	59%
Hamburger	1	28	456	55%
Roast Beef	Regular	10	317	28%
w/cheese	Regular	19	424	40%
	Large	12	360	30%
w/cheese	Large	19	424	40%
RR Bar Burger	1	39	611	57%
CHICKEN				
Breast	1	24	412	52%

Food and Description	Amount	Fat Grams	Total Calories	% Fat Calories
Breast & wing combo	1	37	604	55%
Drumstick	1	8	140	51%
Nuggets	6	17	267	57%
Thigh	1	20	296	61%
Thigh & leg combo	1	28	436	58%
Wing	1	13	192	61%
DESSERTS				
Brownie	1	11	264	38%
Danish				
apple	1	12	249	43%
cheese	1	12	254	43%
cherry	1	14	271	47%
Strawberry Short Cake	1	19	447	38%
Sundaes				
caramel	1	9	293	28%
hot fudge	1	13	337	35%
strawberry	1	7	216	29%
SALAD BAR				
Bacon & Tomato Dressing	2 Tbs	12	136	79%
Bacon Bits	1 Tbs	1	33	27%
Beets-Sliced	¼ cup	–	15	–
Bleu Cheese Dressing	2 Tbs	16	150	96%
Broccoli	½ cup	–	20	–
Carrots-shredded	¼ cup	–	42	–
Cheddar Cheese	¼ cup	9	112	72%
Chinese Noodles	¼ cup	3	55	82%
Croutons	2 Tbs	1	70	13%
Cucumbers	6 slices	–	4	–
Eggs-chopped	2 Tbs	4	55	66%
Green Peas	¼ cup	–	7	–
Lettuce	1 cup	–	10	–
Low-Cal Italian Dressing	2 Tbs	6	70	77%
Macaroni Salad	2 Tbs	4	60	60%
Mushrooms	¼ cup	–	5	–
Potato Salad	2 Tbs	3	50	54%
Ranch Dressing	2 Tbs	14	155	81%
Sunflower Seeds	1 oz/ ~ 2 Tbs	14	160	79%
Thousand Island Dressing	2 Tbs	16	160	90%
Tomatoes	3 slices	–	20	–
SIDE ORDERS				
Biscuit	1	12	231	47%
Cole Slaw	1	7	110	57%
French Fries	Regular	14	268	47%
	Large	18	357	45%

Food and Description	Amount	Fat Grams	Total Calories	% Fat Calories
Hot Topped Potato	1	< 1	211	2%
w/bacon & cheese	1	22	397	50%
w/broccoli & cheeese	1	18	376	43%
w/margarine	1	7	274	23%
w/sour cream & chives	1	21	408	46%
w/taco beef & cheese	1	22	463	43%
Macaroni	1	11	186	53%
Potato Salad	1	6	107	51%
SHAKEY'S PIZZA				
Homestyle Cheese	1 slice	14	303	42%
Homestyle				
Mushroom & Sausage	1 slice	17	343	45%
Pepperoni	1 slice	15	343	39%
Sausage & Pepperoni	1 slice	20	374	48%
Homestyle Shakey's Special	1 slice	21	384	49%
Homestyle w/onion, green peppers, olives & mushrooms	1 slice	15	320	42%
Thick Crust				
cheese	1 slice	5	170	27%
green peppers, black olives, & mushrooms	1 slice	4	162	22%
pepperoni	1 slice	6	185	29%
sausage & mushroom	1 slice	6	179	30%
sausage & pepperoni	1 slice	8	177	41%
Shakey's Special	1 slice	8	208	35%
Thin Crust				
cheese	1 slice	5	133	34%
onion, green peppers, black olives, & mushrooms	1 slice	5	125	36%
pepperoni	1 slice	7	148	43%
sausage & mushroom	1 slice	6	141	38%
sausage & pepperoni	1 slice	8	166	43%
Shakey's Special	1 slice	9	171	47%
TACO BELL				
Bean Burrito/red sauce	1	14	447	28%
Bean Burrito/green sauce	1	14	447	26%
Beef Burito/red sauce	1	21	493	38%
Beef Burrito/green sauce	1	21	493	38%
Burrito Supreme/red sauce	1	22	503	39%
Burrito Supreme/green sauce	1	22	503	39%
Chicken Fajita	1	10	226	40%
Chicken Soft Taco	1	10	210	43%
Chilito	1	18	383	42%
Cinnamon Crispas	1 order	15	259	52%

Food and Description	Amount	Fat Grams	Total Calories	% Fat Calories
Cinnamon Twists	1 order	8	171	42%
Combination Burrito	1	16	407	35%
Double Beef Burrito Supreme/red	1	21.8	457	43%
Double Beef Burrito Supreme/green	1	21.8	451	44%
Enchirito/red sauce	1	19.7	382	46%
Enchirito/green sauce	1	19.7	371	48%
Guacamole	1 pkt	2	34	53%
Jalapeno Peppers	1 order	–	20	–
Mexican Pizza	1	36.8	575	58%
Meximelt	1	15	266	51%
Nachos	1 order	18	346	47%
Nachos Bellgrande	1 order	35	649	49%
Nachos Supreme	1 order	27	367	66%
Pico De Gallo	1	–	8	–
Pintos & Cheese/red sauce	1 order	8.7	190	41%
Pintos & Cheese/green sauce	1 order	8.7	184	43%
Ranch Dressing	1 pkt	24.8	236	95%
Salsa	1 pkt	–	18	–
Sour Cream	1 pkt	4	46	78%
Steak Fajita	1	10.8	234	42%
Steak Soft Taco	1	11	218	45%
Taco	1	10.8	183	53%
Taco Bellgrande	1	23	355	58%
Taco Light	1	28.8	410	41%
Taco Salad w/salsa	1 order	61	941	58%
Taco Salad w/salsa w/o shell	1 order	31	520	54%
Taco Salad w/o salsa or shell	1 order	31	502	56%
Taco Sauce	1 pkt	–	2	–
Taco Sauce-hot	1 pkt	–	2.5	–
Taco-soft	1	12	225	48%
Taco/Super Combo	1	15.9	286	50%
Taco Supreme-soft	1	15	230	59%
Tostada/red sauce	1	11	243	41%
Tostada/green sauce	1	11	237	42%

WENDY'S
BREAKFAST

Food and Description	Amount	Fat Grams	Total Calories	% Fat Calories
Bacon	2 strips	10	110	82%
Breakfast Sandwich	1	19	370	46%
Danish	1	18	360	45%
French Toast	2 slices	19	400	43%
Gravy-sausage	6 oz	36	440	74%
Home Fries	1 order	22	360	55%
Omelet #1-Ham & Cheese	1	17	250	61%

Food and Description	Amount	Fat Grams	Total Calories	% Fat Calories
Omelet #2-Ham, Cheese, Mushroom	1	21	290	65%
Omelet #3-Ham, Cheese, Onion, & Green Pepper	1	19	280	61%
Omelet #4-Mushroom, Onion & Green Pepper	1	15	210	64%
Sausage	1 patty	18	200	81%
Scrambled Eggs	1 order	12	190	57%
Toast w/margarine	1 order	9	250	32%
CHICKEN				
Chicken Fried Steak	1	41	580	64%
Crispy Nuggets, cooked in animal/veg oil	6 pieces	21	290	65%
Crispy Nuggets, cooked in vegetable oil	6 pieces	21	310	61%
Nuggets Sauce				
Barbecue	1 pkg	–	50	–
Honey	1 pkg	–	45	–
Sweet & Sour	1 pkg	–	45	–
Sweet Mustard	1 pkg	1	50	18%
DESSERTS				
Chocolate Chip Cookie	1	17	320	48%
Danish-Apple	1	14	360	35%
Cinnamon Raisin	1	18	410	40%
Frosty-Dairy	Small	14	400	32%
	Medium	18	520	31%
	Large	24	680	32%
Pudding				
Butterscotch	¼ cup	4	90	40%
Chocolate	¼ cup	4	90	40%
MISCELLANEOUS				
Special Sauce	1 Tbs	3	40	68%
Tartar Sauce	1 Tbs	9	90	90%
POTATOES				
Bacon & Cheese	1	30	570	47%
Broccoli & Cheese	1	25	500	45%
Cheese	1	34	590	52%
Chicken A la King	1	6	350	15%
Chili & Cheese	1	20	510	35%
Plain	1	2	250	7%
Sour Cream & Chives	1	24	460	47%
SALAD BAR				
Dressings				
Bleu Cheese	1 Tbs	9	81	100%
Celery Seed	1 Tbs	6	70	77%

Food and Description	Amount	Fat Grams	Total Calories	% Fat Calories
Creamy Peppercorn	1 Tbs	8	80	90%
French Dressing	1 Tbs	6	70	77%
Golden Italian	1 Tbs	4	50	72%
Oil	1 Tbs	15	135	100%
Ranch	1 Tbs	6	54	100%
Red French	1 Tbs	6	70	77%
Bacon & Tomato/low-cal	1 Tbs	4	45	80%
Italian Caesar	1 Tbs	8	72	100%
Italian/low-cal	1 Tbs	2	25	72%
Sour Topping-imitation	1 oz	4	45	80%
Thousand Island/low-cal	1 Tbs	4	45	80%
Thousand Island	1 Tbs	5	70	64%
Wine Vinegar	1 Tbs	–	2	–
Salad Ingredients				
Alfafa Sprouts	2 oz	–	20	–
American Cheese	1 oz	5	70	64%
Bacon Bits	⅛ oz	–	10	–
Bell Peppers	¼ cup	–	4	–
Blueberries	1 Tbs	–	8	–
Breadsticks	1	1	20	45%
Broccoli	½ cup	–	14	–
California Cole Slaw	2 oz	6	60	90%
Cantaloupe	2 pieces	–	4	–
Carrots	¼ cup	–	12	–
Cauliflower	½ cup	–	14	–
Cheddar Chips	½ cup	11	160	62%
Chow Mein Noodles	¼ cup	3	60	45%
Corn Relish-Old Fashion	¼ cup	–	35	–
Cottage Cheese	¼ cup	5	110	41%
Country Crock Spread	1 Tbs	7	70	90%
Croutons	18 pieces	1	30	30%
Crushed Red Peppers	1 oz	4	120	30%
Cucumbers	¼ cup	–	4	–
Eggs	1 Tbs	1	14	64%
Green Peas	½ cup	–	60	–
Jalapeno Peppers	1 Tbs	–	9	–
Lettuce-Iceberg	1 cup	–	8	–
Lettuce-Romaine	1 cup	–	10	–
Mozzarella Cheese	1 oz	7	90	70%
Mushrooms	¼ cup	–	6	–
Parmesan Cheese-imitation	1 oz	3	80	34%
Pasta Salad	¼ cup	–	35	–
Peaches	2 pieces	–	17	–
Pepperoni-sliced	1 oz	12	140	77%

Food and Description	Amount	Fat Grams	Total Calories	% Fat Calories
Potato Chili Cheese	1 oz	8	100	72%
Potato Salad-Red Bliss	¼ cup	9	110	74%
Pineapple Chunks	½ cup	–	80	–
Red Onions	1 Tbs	–	4	–
Salad Bar Imitation Cheese	1 oz	6	80	68%
Saltine Crackers	4 pieces	2	45	40%
Sunflower Seeds & Raisins	¼ cup	13	180	65%
Taco Chips	2 oz	10	260	35%
Taco Shells	1	2	50	36%
Three Bean Salad	¼ cup	–	60	–
Tomatoes	1 oz	–	8	–
Tortilla-flour	1	3	110	25%
Turkey Ham	¼ cup	2	46	39%
Watermelon	2 pieces	–	3	–
Sauces				
Alfredo	2 Tbs	2	50	36%
Cheese	2 Tbs	2	50	36%
Picante	2 oz	–	18	–
Spaghetti	2 Tbs	–	40	–
SANDWICHES				
(NOTE: All sandwiches are served "with everything" unless otherwise stated.)				
Bacon Cheeseburger				
¼ lb/white bun	1	28	460	55%
Bacon Cheeseburger Junior				
w/mayo	1	29	412	63%
w/o mayo	1	19	322	53%
Bacon Swiss Burger/Kaiser Bun	1	44	710	56%
Big Classic on Kaiser Bun	1	34	580	53%
Big Classic w/cheese-Kaiser Bun	1	40	640	56%
Bun-Multigrain wheat	1	3	200	14%
Bun-white	1	3	160	17%
Cheeseburger 2 oz/Kid's Meal	1	15	320	42%
Cheeseburger-small	1	15	320	42%
Cheeseburger ¼ lb/white bun	1	36	490	66%
Chicken Breast				
multigrain wheat bun	1	19	430	40%
Grilled Chicken	1	11	342	29%
Hamburger-small	1	9	260	31%
Hamburger ¼ lb Single				
multi-grain	1	17	340	45%
Hamburger ¼ lb Single				
white bun	1	22	430	46%
Hamburger ¼ lb Single-plain	1	16	350	41%
Hamburger ¼ lb Single w/cheese				
plain	1	22	410	48%

Food and Description	Amount	Fat Grams	Total Calories	% Fat Calories
Hamburger½ lb Double white bun	1	34	560	55%
Hamburger 2 oz/Kid's Meal	1	9	260	31%
Philly Swiss Burger/Kaiser Bun	1	24	510	42%
SIDE ORDERS				
Chef Salad (Take-out)	1	9	180	50%
Chili	8 oz	8	260	28%
	12 oz	12	360	30%
NEW Chili	9 oz	9	230	35%
French Fries	Small	14	280	45%
	Regular	15	310	44%
	Large	20	403	45%
Garden Salad (Take-out)	1	5	102	44%
Pick-up Window Salad	1 order	6	110	49%
Taco Salad (prepared)	1	37	660	51%
WHATABURGER				
BEVERAGES				
Orange Juice	6 oz	–	85	–
Vanilla Shake	Small	9	322	25%
BREAKFAST				
Breakfast on a bun	1	34	520	59%
Egg Omelette Sandwich	1	15	312	43%
Hash Browns	1 order	9	150	54%
Pancakes	1 order	2.9	199	13%
Pancakes w/sausage	1 order	21.9	407	48%
Pecan Danish	1	15.6	270	52%
Sausage	1 order	9	150	54%
SANDWICHES				
Whataburger	1	24	580	37%
Whataburger/cheese	1	32.6	669	44%
Whataburger, Jr.	1	13.5	304	40%
Whataburger, Jr./cheese	1	18	351	46%
Justaburger	1	11.5	265	39%
Justaburger/cheese	1	15.5	312	45%
Whatacatch	1	27	475	51%
Whatacatch/cheese	1	31	522	53%
Chatachick'n	1	31.7	671	43%
SIDE ORDERS				
Apple Pie	1	11.8	236	45%
Fajita Taco	1	11	301	33%
French Fries	Small	12	221	49%
	Regular	18	332	49%
Onion Rings	1 order	13	226	52%
TAQUITOS				
Plain	1	18.5	310	54%

Food and Description	Amount	Fat Grams	Total Calories	% Fat Calories
With Cheese	1	22.5	357	57%
Potato and Egg	1	14	311	41%
Potato and Egg w/cheese	1	18.8	358	47%
WHITE CASTLE				
White Bun Only	1	< 1	74	6%
Cheeseburger	1	11	200	50%
Chicken Sandwich	1	7.5	186	36%
Fish Sandwich-no tartar sauce	1	5	155	29%
French Fries	Regular	15	301	45%
Hamburger	1	8	161	45%
Onion Rings	Regular	13	245	48%
Sausage & Egg Sandwich	1	22	322	62%
Sausage Sandwich	1	12	196	55%
Tartar Sauce	1 Tbs	8	72	100%